# Emergency Management of the Trauma Patient

## CASES, ALGORITHMS, EVIDENCE

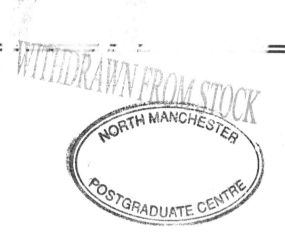

**Be prepared for any emergency with the Emergency Management series**

- Features clinical case scenarios of real-life emergency situations with questions that ask the reader to critically think through management decisions at every step
- Highlights literature and evidence that has molded EM clinical practice
- Includes pocket-sized card with algorithms for quick reference of protocols

*Emergency Management of the Coding Patient: Cases, Algorithms, Evidence*
A step-by-step guide of the clinical and leadership skills needed to run a hospital code with review of ACLS protocols

*Emergency Management of the Pediatric Patient: Cases, Algorithms, Evidence*
A must-have manual detailing effective strategies for initial stabilization and treatment of the critical pediatric patient including PALS review

*Emergency Management of the Trauma Patient: Cases, Algorithms, Evidence*
A practical resource covering emergency care of trauma patients with a complete review of ATLS protocols

# Emergency Management of the Trauma Patient

## CASES, ALGORITHMS, EVIDENCE

### Mark Bisanzo, MD

Emergency Medicine Resident
Brigham and Women's Hospital
Massachusetts General Hospital
Boston, Massachusetts

### Michael R. Filbin, MD

Attending Physician Department of Emergency Medicine
Massachusetts General Hospital
Clinical Instructor, Harvard Medical School
Boston, Massachusetts

### Kriti Bhatia, MD

Assistant Residency Director
Attending Physician Department of Emergency Medicine
Brigham and Women's Hospital
Massachusetts General Hospital
Boston, Massachusetts

Series Founder and Editor: **Michael R. Filbin, MD**

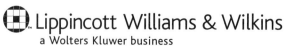
. Lippincott Williams & Wilkins
a Wolters Kluwer business
Philadelphia · Baltimore · New York · London
Buenos Aires · Hong Kong · Sydney · Tokyo

*Acquisitions Editor:* Donna M. Balado
*Managing Editor:* Selene Steneck
*Marketing Manager:* Jennifer Kuklinski
*Associate Production Manager:* Kevin P. Johnson
*Designer:* Holly Reid McLaughlin
*Compositor:* Schawk, Inc.
*Printer:* Victor Graphics

*Printed in the United States of America*

**Library of Congress Cataloging-in-Publication Data**
Bisanzo, Mark.
  Emergency management of the trauma patient : cases, algorithms, evidence / Mark Bisanzo, Kriti Bhatia, Michael R. Filbin.
    p. ; cm. — (Emergency management)
  Includes index.
  ISBN 1-4051-0487-2 (alk. paper)
  1. Emergency medicine—Case studies.  2. Emergency medical services—Case studies.  3. Wounds and injuries—Treatment—Case studies.  I. Bhatia, Kriti.  II. Filbin, Michael R.  III. Title.  IV. Series: Emergency management series (Baltimore, Md.)
  [DNLM: 1. Emergency Medical Services—methods—Case Reports.  2. Wounds and Injuries—therapy—Case Reports. WX 215 B621e 2007]
  RC86.7.B574 2007
  616.02'5—dc22

                                                    2006001607

To purchase additional copies of this book, call our customer service department at **(800) 638-3030** or fax orders to **(301) 223-2320.** International customers should call **(301) 223-2300.**

***Visit Lippincott Williams & Wilkins on the Internet: http://www.LWW.com.*** Lippincott Williams & Wilkins customer service representatives are available from 8:30 am to 6:00 pm, EST.

06 07 08 09 10
1 2 3 4 5 6 7 8 9 10

# About the Authors

**Mark Bisanzo** is a senior emergency medicine resident at the Harvard Affiliated Emergency Medicine Residency Program based at the Brigham and Women's and Massachusetts General Hospitals. He studied biochemistry at Middlebury College before attending Harvard Medical School in Boston. Mark loves backpacking as well as both telemark and alpine skiing, and he spends as much of his free time as possible in the mountains.

**Michael Filbin** is an attending physician in the Emergency Department at Massachusetts General Hospital. He received a bachelor's degree in aerospace engineering from the University of Washington in Seattle. He worked in manned space flight mission operations at the National Aeronautical and Space Agency (NASA) before attending medical school at Baylor College of Medicine in Houston. He completed residency at the Harvard Affiliated Emergency Medicine Residency Program in Boston where he now practices and teaches.

**Kriti Bhatia** is an attending physician in the Emergency Department at Brigham and Women's Hospital in Boston. She completed her bachelor's degree in psychology at Boston University. Prior to beginning medical school at Tufts University in Boston, she worked at the All India Institute of Medical Sciences in New Delhi in genetics research. She completed her residency at the Harvard Affiliated Emergency Medicine Residency Program in Boston where she is now Assistant Residency Director.

# Preface

*Emergency Management of the Trauma Patient: Cases, Algorithms, Evidence* is part of a new three-part series designed to address management of emergent medical situations. The other two books in this series, *Emergency Management of the Coding Patient* and *Emergency Management of the Pediatric Patient*, will provide a review of commonly encountered situations and emphasize the clinical skills needed to make important management decisions in these specialty areas.

*Emergency Management of the Trauma Patient: Cases, Algorithms, Evidence* provides a practical and realistic approach to managing a trauma code. Each chapter begins with the presentation of a trauma scenario in which the reader is asked to make decisions regarding management. Following the case, the chapter text covers main concepts encountered in real-life trauma management in the ED. Literature references are highlighted within the chapters and provide a discussion of important journal articles relevant to the topic at hand. Algorithms are integrated into the chapters to serve as a roadmap for management and to galvanize the information presented in the text.

The book begins with an introduction to trauma, including an overview of trauma center designation, the trauma team, and the essentials of running a trauma code. The following chapters address airway management and traumatic shock, including trauma arrest. The remaining chapters address specific injuries by system and by mechanism of injury. The two major mechanisms categories are blunt and penetrating trauma. The approach to management of these two mechanisms is significantly different for a given system. For example, the approach to blunt thoracic injury is different than that for penetrating thoracic injury. Several chapters at the end address special topics such as burn injury, trauma in pregnancy, and pediatric trauma.

Accompanying this text is a pocket card containing the most important algorithms presented in the book. These algorithms are what we believe the most essential information needed when managing a major trauma, including all major points to be considered depending on the clinical scenario. After reading the text and working through the practice code scenarios in the Appendix, we believe the pocket card will be all you need with you to be ready for any trauma code.

Although this text was designed with senior medical students and interns in mind, we believe it provides a depth of knowledge useful for senior surgery and emergency medicine residents. The responsibility of running trauma is great, given the time-sensitive nature of the disease. Being well versed in the major concepts of trauma management and current literature is essential. We feel the format of this text provides the most effective means of encapsulating this complex topic in order to help you provide excellent care to your trauma patients.

Mark Bisanzo, MD
Michael R. Filbin, MD
Kriti Bhatia, MD

# Reviewers

**Keli M. Kwok, MD**
Transitional Year Intern
LDS Hospital
Salt Lake City, Utah

**Melissa Bakar, MD**
Class of 2005
Albany Medical College
Albany, New York

**Gregory Tasian, MD, MSc**
PGY-1, Department of Surgery
University of California, San Francisco
San Francisco, California

# Acknowledgments

We would like to thank the staff at Blackwell Publishing, LWW, and Schawk for bringing this work to fruition. In particular we are grateful to Selene Steneck whose hard work left an indelible impression on the content of this book. We thank you for your guidance, expertise, and patience. We are also grateful to Bridget Nelson, Liz Clemmons, and Kristen Kriesant for pouring over the details and making the end-product look great on paper. We would especially like to express our appreciation for the attending physicians, residents, nurses, staff members, and patients at the Harvard teaching hospitals, without whom this book would not have been possible.

Mark Bisanzo
Michael Filbin
Kriti Bhatia

December 2005

# Contents

# ABBREVIATIONS

| | | | | |
|---|---|---|---|---|
| AC | Antecubital fossa | LOC | Loss of consciousness |
| ACL | Anterior cruciate ligament | LOS | Length of stay |
| ACS | American College of Surgeons | LR | Lactated Ringer's |
| AP | Anteroposterior | LWE | Local wound exploration |
| API | Aterial pressure index | MAP | Mean arterial pressure |
| ATLS | Advanced trauma life support | MCC | Motorcycle crash |
| BAI | Blunt aortic injury | MDCT | Multidetector CT |
| BCI | Blunt carotid injury | MRI | Magnetic resonance imaging |
| BP | Blood pressure | MVC | Motor vehicle crash |
| CK | Creatinine kinase | NRB | Nonrebreather oxygen mask |
| CK-MB | Creatinine kinase-MB fraction | NS | Normal saline |
| CNS | Central nervous system | OR | Operating room |
| CPP | Cerebral perfussion pressure | PCA | Patient controlled anagelesia |
| C-spine | Cervical spine | PCL | Posterior cruciate ligament |
| CT | Computed tomography | PRBCs | Packed red blood cells |
| CTA | CT angiogram | PT | Posterior tibial |
| CXR | Chest x-ray | RBC | Red blood cell |
| D5W | Sterile water with 5% dextrose | RCT | Randomized-controlled trial |
| DP | Dorsalis pedis | RR | Respiratory rate |
| DPL | Diagnostic peritoneal lavage | RSI | Rapid sequence intubation |
| ED | Emergency department | SBP | Systolic blood pressure |
| ETT | Endotracheal tube | SGW | Shotgun wound |
| Ex-lap | Exploratory laparotomy | SVC | Superior vena cava |
| FAST | Focused assessment with sonography in trauma | SW | Stab wound |
| GCS | Glasgow Coma Scale | TBI | Traumatic brain injury |
| GSW | Gun shot wound | TLS | Thoracic lumbar sacral spine |
| ICP | Intracranial pressure | TNI | Troponin-I |
| ISS | Injury severity score | TEE | Transesophageal echocardiogram |
| IV | Intravenous | US | Ultrasound |
| IVC | Inferior vena cava | WBC | White blood cell |

# CHAPTER 1

# Trauma Code

Over the past 30 years, the care of patients who suffer traumatic injuries has evolved significantly. During this time, civilian trauma management benefited from lessons learned for caring for the wounded in battle. The concept of creating a standardized approach to trauma began in Nebraska in the late 1970s, and the first version of the Advanced Trauma Life Support (ATLS) manual was released in 1980. The driving concept behind the manual was the idea that by improving trauma care, clinicians could save patients with salvageable injuries and prevent long-term disability and death; these are the patients in groups II and III in Table 1–1. By creating an organized approach to the trauma patient, doctors began treating the greatest life threats first. This method has evolved into an entire systematic approach to trauma that can be conceptualized on two levels: orchestration of trauma care (prehospital, hospital, and rehabilitation) and care of the individual patient.

## ORCHESTRATION OF TRAUMA CARE

### Prehospital Trauma Care

Prehospital trauma care is a subject of a great deal of debate in the trauma literature and in real world applications. It poses challenges to emergency medical technicians because they encounter patients in an uncontrolled environment, often outdoors with inadequate lighting or in areas with potential hazards (e.g., major highways, crime scenes). In general, prehospital care should focus largely on oxygenation, control of external bleeding, patient immobilization when appropriate, and rapid transport to the nearest suitable facility. In situations where multiple victims are present, the prehospital providers must triage the victims based on the availability of resources. When resources are limited, triage shifts to the principle of "do the most good for the most patients." This means that unsalvageable patients have lower priority in order to focus resources on those with a chance of survival.

### Trauma Centers

Individual hospitals can make a commitment to provide specific facilities, medical and nursing staff, and ancillary personnel in order to better care for trauma patients. The amount of resources a given institution has is designated by a level rating for that hospital in the trauma system. Prehospital personnel will preferentially transport patients to the appropriate center when one is accessible (Table 1-2).

### The Trauma Bay

Because the basis of trauma management is rapid diagnosis and treatment of life-threatening injuries, all the supplies needed to care for a critically-ill trauma patient should be readily available. Every trauma center has designated resuscitation rooms that contain standard supplies needed in trauma management (Box 1-1). Furthermore, these rooms should have adequate space for the resuscitation to be carried out.

### The Trauma Team

In most trauma centers, the trauma team is a combination of emergency physicians, trauma surgeons, and emergency department nurses. There is variability of roles and responsibilities from center to center; however, to provide the highest level of care, all members must work as a team. In many larger centers, there are various levels of activation of the trauma team. These are based on a variety of factors that loosely predict how critical the patient is or how likely it is the patient will need to go to the operating room (OR). Generally, this triage is based on mechanism of injury, prehospital vital signs, and nature of injuries detected by prehospital personnel. Ideally, the prehospital team communicates this information to the receiving facility prior to the patient's arrival. This advanced warning allows members of the trauma team to make preparations for the patient that may make the difference between life and death.

| TABLE 1-1 Distribution of deaths related to trauma | | |
|---|---|---|
| Peak | Time frame | Typical causes of death |
| I | Seconds to minutes | High spinal cord injury, cardiac lacerations, or aortic tears |
| II | Minutes to hours | Ruptured spleen, liver laceration, or epidural hematoma |
| III | Days to weeks | Sepsis or multisystem organ failure |

**BOX 1-1 Standard supply list for resuscitation rooms**

1. Standard airway equipment—endotracheal tubes (neonatal through large adult), stylets, $CO_2$ detector, 10 cc syringes, ambu bags, bag valve masks, suction, and oxygen
2. Difficult airway equipment—any combination of bougie, laryngeal mask airway, fiberoptic equipment, cricothyrotomy tray, and tracheostomy tube
3. Intravenous line equipment—large-bore IVs, intraosseous needles, IV tubing, central lines, normal saline, lactated Ringer's, warmed IV fluids, preferably a Level I Rapid Infuser, and blood warmer
4. Monitoring equipment for EKG, pulse oximetry, and blood pressure
5. Chest tube supplies—chest tubes, underwater-seal apparatus, and suture material
6. Thoracotomy tray
7. Diagnostic peritoneal lavage (DPL) kit/tray
8. Orthopedic splinting supplies
9. Foley catheters
10. Protective equipment for practitioners—gowns, gloves, sterile gloves, eye shields, and masks

In general, trauma teams are structured based on a standard scheme. In a Level I setting, typically a senior emergency medicine or surgical resident is designated a team leader. This physician controls the tempo of the resuscitation, often carrying out the primary and secondary surveys and calling out orders to other members of the team. Ideally, the team leader is not involved in procedures so that he or she is able to manage the flow of the code, including following trends in vital signs, paying attention to fluid and blood product administration, and monitoring activities of the entire team. Ideally, a trauma team has two additional physicians available to perform procedures (e.g., airway management and intubation, chest tube placement, central line placement). Two nurses should be present in the trauma bay initially, one to establish IV access and the other to place the patient on the monitor and obtain blood pressure and pulse oximetry readings.

The team leader should ensure that no unnecessary personnel are in the trauma bay. It is good practice for the team leader to identify team members and assign roles before the code begins. In a well run trauma code there is relative calm. All communication is through the team leader; therefore, the only voices heard should be the team leader giving instructions or a member talking to the leader. All orders should be issued by the team leader only, including those for procedures, fluid or blood product administration, medications, and laboratory or radiographic studies.

### Categorizing Severity: Trauma Scoring Systems

Trauma care uses multiple scoring systems that are generally based on physiologic or anatomic parameters. The purpose of a scoring system is to predict the severity of injury, level of resource utilization, and patient outcome. These scores are incorporated into triage algorithms, trauma research, and outcomes studies. No system is perfect, but it is important for those caring for trauma patients to have a basic understanding of these systems (Table 1-3).

| TABLE 1-2 Trauma center designation | | | | |
|---|---|---|---|---|
| Trauma center level | Typical location | Resources immediately available | Resources on call | Roles |
| I | Large city | Emergency physicians and surgeons | Surgical subspecialists | Research, teaching, community outreach, and trauma systems leadership |
| II | Regional | Emergency physicians | Trauma surgeon | Community outreach, definitive care to community trauma systems leadership role |
| III | Local community | Physicians | General surgeon | Provide initial stabilization and emergency surgery; transfer agreements with Level I or II |
| IV | Rural | Midlevel practitioner or physician | None required | Initial assessment and stabilization, prepare for transfer to Level I or II |

| TABLE 1-3 Trauma scoring systems | | | |
|---|---|---|---|
| **Scoring system** | **Score type** | **Brief description** | **Score interpretation** |
| Revised trauma score (RTS) | Physiologic | Combines GCS with SBP, RR, and capillary refill | Lower scores indicate more severe injury |
| Injury severity score (ISS) | Anatomic | Body divided into six regions, each assigned a severity value (1 = minor, 6 = major) | Sum of the square of three highest scoring regions |
| New injury severity score (NISS) | Anatomic | Each injury assigned a severity from 1 to 6, allowing multiple injuries in a body region to be considered | Sum of the square of three highest scoring injuries |
| Trauma and injury severity score (TRISS) | Combined | Attempts to predict mortality by combining anatomic and physiologic derangements | Calculates a probability of survival based on logistic regression of RTS, ISS, and age |

GCS, Glasgow Coma Scale; SBP, systolic blood pressure; RR, respiratory rate.

## CARE OF THE INDIVIDUAL PATIENT

The ABCs mnemonic has become the general algorithm for the approach to critically-ill patients, including trauma. Clinicians should initially evaluate all trauma patients in the order of the ABCs, return to A and start again whenever a significant change in the patient's condition occurs.

### Primary Survey

**A—Airway.** The airway refers to an open passageway for airflow to occur between the environment and the lungs. An intact airway refers to the absence of an obstruction between the mouth, oropharynx, larynx, and trachea. Blunt or penetrating trauma to the face or neck can distort anatomy, result in hematomas that cause compression, or fill these passageways with blood. An intact airway can be confirmed by inspection (i.e., looking for obvious distortion of face or neck anatomy), asking the patient to open his or her mouth or speak if conscious, or looking for signs of air movement. Airway disruption or obstruction must be addressed immediately before all else. This can usually be accomplished by orotracheal intubation. In some cases of severe airway distortion, a cricothyrotomy is necessary.

**B—Breathing.** Breathing refers to the movement of air to and from the lungs. This requires an intact airway and diaphragmatic contraction to create negative intrathoracic pressure. Breathing should be assessed by auscultating both lungs and looking for chest expansion with inspiration. A tension pneumothorax creates large positive intrathoracic pressures and prevents adequate ventilation. This can be detected by absent breath sounds on one side or tracheal deviation, in addition to low oxygen saturation.

This requires immediate chest tube placement to reestablish breathing.

**C—Circulation.** Circulation refers to cardiac output that provides oxygenated blood to vital organs. Circulation is assessed by checking a pulse (radial, femoral, or carotid) and blood pressure. In trauma, circulation can be compromised by loss of blood volume (i.e., hemorrhagic shock) or by decreased cardiac output (e.g., pericardial tamponade, cardiac contusion). The degree of circulatory shock is important to determine up front because it correlates with the severity of injury and subsequent mortality. Patients with signs of circulatory shock require aggressive resuscitation initially with blood products and operative management as soon as possible.

**D—Debilitation.** Debilitation refers to neurologic compromise, either global depression of consciousness or specific neurologic deficits (e.g., paraplegia, sensory level). Level of consciousness can be assessed with the Glasgow Coma Score (GCS) that is described in Chapter 4. GCS assesses alertness, ability to speak, and ability to follow commands. A follow-up to the primary survey of the ABCs should include a quick survey of peripheral motor and sensory function. Simply ask the patient to wiggle his or her toes or squeeze his or her hands, and ask him or her to identify which extremity is being touched. It is important to identify spinal cord injuries early to prevent further actions that may exacerbate the injury (i.e., moving or rolling the patient without proper precautions).

**E—Exposure.** Patients should be fully exposed so that no injuries are missed. Once a full inspection has been done, the patient should be covered again to prevent hypothermia. Trauma victims are often already hypothermic because of blood loss or environmental exposure. In these patients, passive and active rewarming techniques should be initiated early, including warmed fluids and blood products, warm blankets, or heat lamps.

**F—Foley.** Seriously injured trauma patients should have a Foley catheter placed to monitor urine output and check for hematuria. It is essential to do a rectal exam before the Foley catheter is placed in male patients to ensure normal prostatic position and thus urethral integrity. A retrograde urethrogram (RUG) to ensure intact urethral anatomy must be performed prior to Foley placement if the prostate is high-riding (i.e., displaced superiorly on exam) or if there is blood at the meatus.

**G—Gastric Tube.** An orogastric tube should be placed in all intubated patients to decompress the stomach, thereby reducing the risk of aspiration. While some argue that this tube will keep the lower esophageal sphincter open, thus making gastric reflux more likely, most agree that intubated trauma patients benefit from stomach decompression.

**H—History of Present Illness (HPI).** An HPI should be taken after the initial life threats are assessed and managed. The mechanism of injury is crucial and will often guide the secondary survey to look for suspected injuries. The mechanism is often provided by Emergency Medical Service (EMS) personnel after arrival and should be obtained while doing the primary survey. A patient's past medical history, medications, or allergies may influence management.

**I—Initiate Transfer.** During this initial survey and early resuscitation, the clinician should think if transfer to a higher-level trauma center is needed. If so, this process should be started early before the patient decompensates further. Also included at this point is consideration for whether the patient may need to go to the OR. If operative management is likely, a trauma surgeon and OR staff should be notified as soon as possible.

### The Secondary Survey

The secondary survey is a head-to-toe physical examination to identify all injuries sustained. While most of this may be self-evident, Box 1-2 highlights the crucial features of each part of the exam. If the patient deteriorates, the secondary survey should be abandoned to reasses the ABCs.

### Adjunctive Studies

In most centers there are standard tests obtained on every trauma patient, including basic blood work, a trauma series (plain films of the c-spine, chest, and pelvis), EKG, and now a FAST exams. While this remains dogma in ATLS textbooks, the utility of some of these interventions is debated in the trauma literature. Additional studies, including CT scan, echocardiograms, and diagnostic peritoneal lavage (DPL) will be discussed in the relevant chapters throughout the text.

---

**BOX 1-2  The secondary survey**

- *General:* Is the patient shivering, wet, nervous, or scared? Steps taken to make the patient more comfortable will make the resuscitation run more smoothly.
- *Head:* Palpate for step-offs or deformity (skull fracture). Inspect for lacerations. Note raccoon eyes or Battle's sign (basilar skull fracture).
- *Ears:* Check for hemotympanum (basilar skull fracture), blood in the ear canal (open temporal bone fracture), or CSF in the ear canal (skull fracture).
- *Eyes:* Look for bulging or proptosis (indicates retro-orbital hematoma and possible need for lateral canthotomy), pupil irregularity (globe rupture), "blown" pupil (uncal herniation), pinpoint pupils (narcotics use), unreactive pupils (diffuse axonal injury).
- *Nose:* Look for CSF rhinorrhea (skull fracture) and septal hematoma.
- *Mouth:* Assess midface stability (LaForte fracture). Check for loose teeth.
- *Neck:* Maintain c-spine precaution while opening the collar to assess the neck for penetrating injury or crepitus. Palpate the c-spine for midline tenderness.
- *Chest:* Reauscultate breath sounds; listen for distant heart sounds (pericardial tamponade); palpate the clavicles and chest wall, assessing for crepitus (pneumothorax) or tenderness (rib or sternal fractures); observe chest rise for asymmetry (flail chest).
- *Abdomen:* Look for evidence of trauma (e.g., ecchymosis, seatbelt sign); palpate the abdomen gently and then more deeply, assessing for peritoneal signs or localized tenderness.
- *Pelvis:* Apply pressure to both anterior superior iliac spines with one hand on each side. Feel for crepitus or shifting bone (unstable pelvic fracture).
- *GU:* In male patients check the urethral meatus for blood; in female patients check for vaginal bleeding. Check for ecchymosis along the perineum.
- *Rectal:* Assess rectal tone (spinal cord injury); check position of the prostate; check for presence of gross blood.
- *Extremities:* Palpate all extremities and range all joints (except in the case of obvious deformity).
- *Back:* The patient must be log rolled and the back assessed for the presence of puncture wounds, lacerations, or ecchymosis. The entire length of the spine should be palpated to assess for tenderness, step-offs, or deformity.
- *Neurologic:* Check strength and sensation in all extremities.

## The Trauma Series

In most centers, a standard trauma series is performed on each patient. This series of plain x-rays consists of a lateral c-spine, a supine anteroposterior (AP) chest x-ray, and an AP pelvis. In recent years, multiple studies have addressed this practice and sought to justify limiting its use to when it is absolutely necessary because ordering the full trauma series is time-consuming and not always useful. This is especially true in the age of the readily available CT scan for stable patients. The trauma series remains important in patients who are too unstable to go to CT scan. It should be remembered, however, that ATLS recommendations call for a complete trauma series on all patients. Thus, at many centers it will be standard to get these three films. However, those who practice in areas with limited resources or who are trying to conserve resources can safely limit the plain radiographs obtained as part of a trauma series.

The lateral c-spine has a sensitivity of approximately 85% for fracture, given an adequate film (i.e., visualization of the C7–T1 junction). This study is probably unnecessary in most cases where the patient is alert and with a normal neurologic exam. In this case, the patient can go to CT scan for c-spine imaging if necessary. The exceptions are those patients with severe neck pain or deformity. Similarly, patients with altered mental status or those with neurologic deficits should have a lateral c-spine x-ray immediately in the trauma bay. Patients who have gross misalignment on lateral c-spine x-ray may require c-spine traction to prevent further cord injury prior to transport or manipulation. However, in an alert trauma patient without severe cervical pain and a normal neurologic exam, this injury is rather unlikely.

The portable chest x-ray (CXR) is useful in patients with suspected hemothorax or pneumothorax based on exam or abnormal vital signs. This is especially true for patients who are either hypotensive or hypoxic. In hypotensive patients, a portable CXR is necessary to look for a source of bleeding, either a large hemothorax or aortic rupture, the latter implied by a widened mediastinum. In blunt trauma, the portable CXR is done with the patient supine because of the risk of cervical injury. This limits the sensitivity for detecting hemothorax because it layers posteriorly, thus resulting in haziness of the entire lung, rather than pooling in the costophrenic angle as it would in an upright CXR. The sensitivity for seeing a pneumothorax is similarly decreased. Secondary indications of pneumothorax such as subcutaneous air or a deep sulcus sign (a pointed costophrenic angle that appears to extend deeper into the abdomen than normal) should be sought. Overall, the portable CXR is more useful than the lateral c-spine x-ray, and it should be obtained in all patients with significant blunt trauma, penetrating tho-

racoabdominal trauma, those with altered mental status, chest pain, shortness of breath, or abnormal vital signs.

The portable AP pelvis x-ray is useful in patients with blunt trauma who have evidence of pelvic trauma (e.g., tender or unstable pelvis), dislocated hip (e.g., internal or external rotation of the leg), or those with hypotension. It is important to rapidly diagnose a pelvic fracture in the setting of hypotension as a potential source of significant bleeding. Pelvic fractures are associated with venous and arterial injury that can result in rapid blood loss, in which case the pelvis needs to be wrapped tightly with a sheet to tamponade internal bleeding. Similarly, a traumatic hip dislocation needs to be relocated immediately to prevent avascular necrosis of the head of the femur.

---

**CLINICAL PEARL** ● ● ● ● ● ● ● ● ● ● ● ● ● ● ● ● ● ● ● ●

## Laboratory studies in the trauma patient

Many centers send an extensive panel of lab studies on every trauma patient. In reality, few of these tests are clinically useful in most trauma patients. There has been extensive literature showing that liver function tests, amylase and lipase levels are neither sensitive nor specific for significant organ injury. This is especially true in light of CT scanning for patients with high mechanism trauma. In addition to expense and wasted resources, incidental small abnormalities often initiate extensive and even more expensive workups to no clinical benefit.

The basic trauma panel in significant trauma that may require surgery includes a hematocrit, basic electrolytes, blood bank sample, and urinalysis. Base deficit and lactate may have some value in the severely injured patient as will be presented later. Similarly, cardiac enzymes may have some utility in evaluating for cardiac contusion. Even the urinalysis is controversial given that only gross hematuria is clinically significant, and the presence of microscopic hematuria will precipitate an expensive search for clinically insignificant injuries. A coagulation panel (PT, PTT), although often obtained, is actually only useful in patients who are hemodynamically unstable or otherwise severely ill. In this minority of patients it is important to know whether a coagulopathy exists.

## LITERATURE REFERENCE

 **The trauma series**

The pelvic x-ray has been shown in several studies to have a limited utility in cooperative patients who have a stable pelvis on exam and have no pain to palpation. Most recently, Gross et al. conducted a prospective observational study of blunt trauma patients. In this study all patients ($n = 973$) received an AP pelvic film. Only two patients without pelvic pain or tenderness had occult fractures, neither being clinically significant, provided they had a GCS of 15, were not intoxicated, and did not have a significant distracting injury. Imaging based on these criteria would have eliminated almost half of AP pelvic x-rays **[Gross et al. *J Emerg Med* 2005;28(3):263–266].**

### The FAST Exam

The focused assessment with sonography in trauma (FAST) exam plays an important role in the management of trauma patients; however, the limitations of ultrasound must be understood. This exam should be done after the primary survey and initial resuscitation, and its purpose is to identify pericardial or intra-abdominal bleeding. The four basic views include Morrison's pouch (hepatorenal space), the splenorenal space, retrovesicular space, and a subxiphoid view of the heart. An intercostal oblique view can also be done to assess for hemothorax or pneumothorax. It is generally quoted that bedside ultrasound is able to detect accumulations of greater than 500 cc of intraperitoneal blood; however, a normal FAST exam should not exclude the possibility of intraperitoneal bleeding. The sensitivity of the FAST exam for detecting intraperitoneal injury is quoted as 70% to 90%, depending on the definition of the disease (any injury versus clinically significant injury versus injury requiring operative intervention). It must be understood that bedside ultrasound is only useful for detecting free intraperitoneal blood and is not useful for visualizing solid organ injury (splenic or liver lacerations).

## PUTTING IT ALL TOGETHER

Every trauma should be approached in a systematic fashion as is presented in this introductory chapter. Even though every situation is different and certain injuries may distract the caregiver, this systematic approach must be followed. With experience this comes

naturally, and as the patient is rolled into the trauma bay the first thought, before thoughts of placing a central line or obtaining a trauma series, is: Does this patient need to be intubated? The primary survey should always be the same, regardless of the injury. The same holds true for the secondary survey. Variation comes into play with imaging and workup of specific injuries. These variations will be covered in the following chapters, with emphasis placed on highlighted aspects of the primary and secondary surveys for specific injuries, imaging and workup, and rationale for these.

## KEY POINTS

- Trauma center designation made based on level of resources
  - Regional Level I centers with 24-hour in-house trauma surgeon and full OR capability
  - Emergency Department (ED) transfer to Level I or II center often necessary for critical patients after stabilization
- Advanced preparation is vital in trauma
  - Stocked trauma bay with readily-available airway equipment, chest tubes, and CV catheters
  - Advanced notification from prehospital providers essential
- Trauma team composed of emergency physicians, trauma surgeons, and nurses
  - Team leader orchestrates overall care and all communication goes through him or her
  - All orders should come directly from team leader
- Multiple trauma illness severity scores to predict resource utilization and outcomes
  - Important for research and triage but not useful in acute management
  - Methodical approach to evaluation is cornerstone to avoid missed injuries
- Primary survey includes ABCs, IV–$O_2$–monitor, life-saving procedures
  - Intubation, chest tubes, CV lines, crystalloid bolus, and blood transfusion
  - Primary survey revisited when patient's condition changes during workup
- Secondary survey is head-to-toe assessment once patient stabilized
- FAST exam has become an extension of the primary survey
- Trauma care evolving toward evidence-based practice in experienced centers
  - Limited laboratory workup to those that will change management
  - Importance of physical exam in limiting radiographic studies
  - Trend toward nonoperative management where previously exploration common

# OVERVIEW ALGORITHM

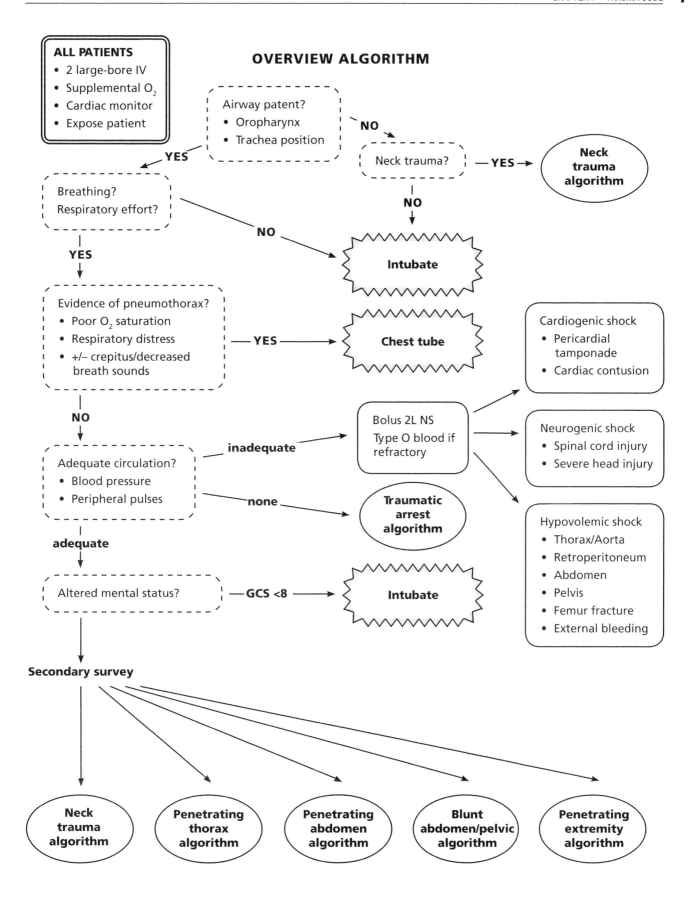

**ALL PATIENTS**
- 2 large-bore IV
- Supplemental O₂
- Cardiac monitor
- Expose patient

Airway patent?
- Oropharynx
- Trachea position

NO → Neck trauma? — YES → **Neck trauma algorithm**

YES

Breathing?
Respiratory effort?

NO → **Intubate**

NO

YES

Evidence of pneumothorax?
- Poor O₂ saturation
- Respiratory distress
- +/− crepitus/decreased breath sounds

— YES → **Chest tube**

Cardiogenic shock
- Pericardial tamponade
- Cardiac contusion

NO

Bolus 2L NS
Type O blood if refractory

Neurogenic shock
- Spinal cord injury
- Severe head injury

Adequate circulation?
- Blood pressure
- Peripheral pulses

inadequate

none → **Traumatic arrest algorithm**

adequate

Hypovolemic shock
- Thorax/Aorta
- Retroperitoneum
- Abdomen
- Pelvis
- Femur fracture
- External bleeding

Altered mental status? — GCS <8 → **Intubate**

**Secondary survey**

**Neck trauma algorithm**    **Penetrating thorax algorithm**    **Penetrating abdomen algorithm**    **Blunt abdomen/pelvic algorithm**    **Penetrating extremity algorithm**

# CHAPTER 2

# Trauma Airway

## CASE SCENARIO

A 23-year-old man is brought to the ED from the scene of a high-speed, rollover motor vehicle crash (MVC). At the scene, he was extricated from the car and was talking to EMS personnel. He was placed on a backboard and his c-spine immobilized. His vital signs during transport included a pulse of 108 and a blood pressure of 146/92. On arrival to the trauma bay, you note he has obvious facial trauma with swelling on the left side and blood from both nares. He is moaning but does not respond to your voice. On primary survey, he appears to be breathing, and you hear a gurgling sound in his upper airway. His teeth are clenched shut. His trachea is midline, and you feel a carotid pulse. During your primary survey, the nurse obtains vital signs that include a pulse of 112, blood pressure of 104/70, and oxygen saturation of 98%.

1. What is the next most appropriate step?
   a. Immediately intubate him using rapid sequence intubation
   b. Listen for breath sounds, and then prepare to intubate
   c. Place an oral or nasal airway, place on oxygen, and obtain a CXR
   d. Immediately obtain a head CT scan to evaluate for intracranial injury

This patient needs to be intubated immediately because there is evidence of airway obstruction and compromised ventilation (e.g., blood in the airway and likely aspiration, gurgling infers inability to protect his airway, decreased mental status). Given that the patient has a pulse, measurable blood pressure, and oxygen saturation, rapid sequence intubation (RSI) should be employed. If the patient were apneic or pulseless, then immediate intubation without medications would be attempted, defined as a "crash airway." In evaluating the ABCs, action is taken to correct life threats as they are discovered. For example, in assessing A if the patient is hypoventilating, has gurgling respirations from blood, or decreased mental status, then intubation is performed immediately before continuing the primary survey. If the airway is intact, then move to B and listen for breath sounds, and then move on to C and assess pulses and other signs of circulation.

2. What medications do you ask the nurse to draw up for intubation?
   a. Etomidate and succinylcholine
   b. Midazolam and vecuronium
   c. Lidocaine, etomidate, and succinylcholine
   d. Succinylcholine alone

Rapid sequence intubation (RSI) is a technique employed to render a patient rapidly unconscious and paralyzed, without having to provide bag-valve-mask (BVM) ventilations, to optimize conditions for direct laryngoscopy and orotracheal intubation. The two major pharmacologic components of RSI are an induction agent and a paralytic agent. Etomidate is the most common induction agent (to render patient unconscious) used today because it is fast acting, causes minimal cardiovascular depression (i.e., hypotension), and has a relatively short duration of action (about 10 to 15 minutes). Succinylcholine is the prototypical paralytic agent used for RSI. It has the effect of depolarizing the neuromuscular junction in skeletal muscle (i.e., depolarizing agent) and thus rendering the patient paralyzed within 45 seconds. Its duration of action is about 8 to 10 minutes, during which time the patient will be apneic.

In the setting of head trauma, some recommend pretreatment medications to blunt the reflex increase in intracerebral pressure (ICP) because of laryngeal stimulation of laryngoscopy. Lidocaine is the agent most widely used for this purpose (100 mg IV 2 minutes before paralysis); it is thought to decrease afferent nerve impulses from the larynx, thus decreasing the adrenergic response to laryngoscopy (i.e., increased heart rate and blood pressure) and to the resulting ICP elevation. Fentanyl and nondepolarizing neuromuscular blocking agents have also been recommended for this use as well, although the evidence for their effectiveness is only theoretical.

3. The patient is in a cervical collar, and you are worried about the potential for a c-spine fracture. How is this addressed during laryngoscopy?
   a. Clear the neck clinically before starting RSI
   b. Opt for fiber-optic intubation since laryngoscopy may worsen fracture
   c. Provide in-line stabilization with the collar undone to allow mandible mobility
   d. Perform laryngoscopy with the collar in place

C-spine injury should always be of utmost concern when intubating a trauma patient after blunt injury, especially in those with decreased mental status unable to provide a reliable history or exam. In-line stabilization is provided by a separate team member. Palms are placed bilaterally at the base of the skull with fingers running laterally the length of the neck. The purpose is to minimize anterior flexion of the c-spine during laryngoscopy while allowing anterior displacement of the mandible. This gives the operator a better view of the larynx, and a higher chance of success, while maintaining control of the c-spine.

The patient is intubated successfully and tube position confirmed with end-tidal $CO_2$ detection. You hear breath sounds bilaterally over the chest and visualize symmetric chest rise. A trauma series is ordered (i.e., portable x-rays of lateral neck, chest, and pelvis). You are continuing with the secondary survey when a repeat blood pressure of 84/46 is obtained.

4. What is the next step?
   a. Expedite the trauma series to look for tension pneumothorax
   b. Administer 1L normal saline bolus and recheck blood pressure
   c. Auscultate for breath sounds and perform needle decompression if absent
   d. Activate the operating room for likely exploratory laparotomy

Mechanical ventilation with positive pressure can convert a simple pneumothorax into a tension pneumothorax. Intrathoracic pressure is negative during normal respirations. Intubation and mechanical ventilation impart positive intrathoracic pressures during inspiration to force air into the alveoli. This also imparts pressure on the heart and decreases ventricular filling, thus decreasing cardiac output. Hypotension as a result of decreased cardiac output is also a common complication of intubation. A tension pneumothorax is an immediate life threat because the trapped air imparts a tremendous pressure on the heart and impedes cardiac output. Auscultation over the chest should reveal absent breath sounds over the affected side. Needle decompression should be performed immediately by placing a 14-gauge angiocatheter needle into the anterior chest between the second and third ribs. Answers: 1-a; 2-c; 3-c; 4-c

Airway management is the first priority of the primary survey in trauma. The primary survey should stop at A if the patient is not adequately ventilating and oxygenating (i.e., providing air to the alveoli for gas exchange to occur). Even if the patient is breathing and alert, the airway should be addressed by placing the patient on oxygen to increase blood oxygen concentration and tissue oxygenation. The first decision in managing the trauma patient is whether to establish a definitive airway (i.e., orotracheal intubation or cricothyrotomy). There are numerous indications for intubation that can be boiled down to the inability to ventilate and oxygenate. Additionally, situational control (e.g., aggressive head injury patient who needs a CT scan) and anticipated course (e.g., patient with gunshot wound to the abdomen who will need exploratory laparotomy in the OR) are also indications for intubation.

## RECOGNIZE THE NEED TO INTERVENE

Assessment of A and B of the ABCs seems straightforward, but in fact it is a subjective assessment that takes years of experience to master. It takes into account the overall gestalt of a patient, anticipated decompensation, or insidious signs of airway compromise. The first aspects to assess are mental status and obvious upper airway obstruction.

**CLINICAL PEARL** ● ● ● ● ● ● ● ● ● ● ● ● ● ● ● ● ● ● ●

## The challenge of c-spine immobilization

There has been a great deal of debate about the safety of oral intubation in c-spine injured patients. Concerns have been raised about causing spinal cord injury by manipulation of potentially unstable c-spine elements during direct laryngoscopy. As a result, blind nasotracheal intubation was once regarded as the intubation approach of choice in such patients. Although there has been no definitive study proving the safety of oral intubation in the setting of c-spine injuries, a number of studies have demonstrated no adverse outcomes using this approach. Oral intubation is now accepted as the intubation maneuver of choice as long as cervical immobilization is maintained throughout the procedure. This requires a second individual who kneels at the head of the bed, stabilizing the base of the skull and c-spine while the intubation is performed. Thus, during laryngoscopy, the mandible can be extracted upward, but the c-spine is not allowed to flex. This may make vocal cord visualization more challenging, and back-up equipment should be readily available (e.g., gum elastic bougie, laryngeal mask airway (LMA), lighted stylet).

Trauma patients who have a decreased level of consciousness (LOC) require immediate intubation (recommended for patients with GCS of 8 or less). These patients have decreased ventilatory drive and may unknowingly stop breathing if left to their own devices. They frequently vomit because of intoxication or head injury. When supine, the vomit has no place to go but down the trachea, and aspiration carries significant mortality. It is often tempting to forgo intubation in these patients because their vitals are stable, their oxygen saturation is above 95%, or they are breathing spontaneously. There are numerous excuses for not intubating these patients, but they are all wrong and place the patient at a higher risk of mortality.

Upper airway obstruction comes in several forms in the trauma patient, but the most common is blood. As with vomit, blood tends to go down the trachea in supine trauma patients. Copious bleeding into the oropharynx is a life threat, and a definitive airway (i.e., orotracheal tube) should be established. Another form of upper airway obstruction includes gross anatomic deformity from blunt trauma or a gunshot wound. In these cases, early definitive airway management is essential even though the patient may currently be breathing spontaneously. Over a short period of time, swelling or bleeding may result in total airway occlusion and intubation may be impossible. This is also the case with penetrating neck wounds with subcutaneous swelling. An injured carotid artery or internal jugular vein can cause an expanding hematoma. Initially the airway will appear normal, but it can rapidly become distorted making intubation impossible.

## PRIMARY SURVEY: AIRWAY AND BREATHING

As the patient is rolled into the trauma bay and transferred to the stretcher, a gestalt should be formulated (Table 2-1). The question should be: Does this patient need to be intubated? Sometimes this is obvious before the primary survey begins, and intubation should be performed immediately. Examples include circulatory collapse (e.g., decreased LOC, gray appearance, hypotensive in the field), obvious head injury with decreased LOC, or a gunshot wound associated with instability. As the patient is transferred to the stretcher, high-flow oxygen via a nonrebreather face mask should be placed.

The primary survey should begin with asking the patient his or her name. Ability to answer this question gives valuable information, such as degree of consciousness, control of laryngeal muscles (i.e., ability to protect against aspiration), and ability to ventilate. If a patient is unable to give his or her

**TABLE 2-1 Primary survey: Airway and breathing assessment**

| | |
|---|---|
| Obtain gestalt | Any obvious need for intubation? Comatose Circulatory shock Uncontrollably aggressive behavior |
| A—Ask patient his or her name | Establishes consciousness Ability to phonate (control of laryngeal muscles) Ability to ventilate |
| A—Inspect mouth | Look for blood, loose teeth, or swelling Assess difficulty of intubation |
| A—Inspect neck | Midline trachea Look for swelling or distortion |
| B—Auscultate lungs | Absent breath sounds suggest pneumothorax |
| B—Palpate chest | Crepitus suggests pneumothorax |

name, intubation is likely needed. Next, a quick inspection of the mouth should be done to look for blood, pooled secretions, and fractured or loose teeth. You can also get an idea of how difficult the intubation would be, if necessary, by looking at jaw and neck size, ability to open mouth, size of the tongue, and ability to visualize the oropharynx. The neck should be inspected quickly for tracheal deviation (i.e., implying tension pneumothorax or expanding hematoma), swelling, or hematomas that could compromise airway patency.

Breathing (ventilation) is assessed initially by level of consciousness (conscious patients are breathing). Breath sounds are auscultated to look for evidence of a pneumothorax, which would impair ventilation. Likewise, the chest wall is palpated to feel for crepitus, or subcutaneous air, which would also suggest pneumothorax. Vital signs are also part of the primary survey, and oxygen saturation should be obtained to help assess tissue perfusion. If there are clinical signs of a pneumothorax (e.g., absent breath sounds, crepitus, or low oxygen saturation), then a chest tube should be placed immediately before a CXR is obtained. If the diagnosis is in doubt, and the patient is hemodynamically stable and in no respiratory distress, then a CXR should be obtained first before placing the chest tube.

## RAPID SEQUENCE INTUBATION (RSI)

Airway management is a complex skill that requires formal training and years of experience to fully understand. The techniques involved in and knowledge required to manage the trauma airway could themselves fill a textbook. Here the focus will be on the medications commonly used and special considerations given to trauma patients.

RSI is a technique used to aid in the success of orotracheal intubation. Its purpose is to rapidly render a patient unconscious and paralyzed without having to give supplemental breaths, to facilitate laryngoscopy and orotracheal intubation. RSI has two main pharmacologic components: an induction agent (induction of rapid unconsiousness) and a paralytic agent (the ultimate muscle relaxant). Careful preparation must be undertaken before embarking on RSI with assembly of all necessary equipment completed (Box 2-1). This should be ready before the patient even arrives in the trauma bay if advance notice was given. Optimally, preoxygenation with high-flow oxygen via a nonrebreather facemask should be done. This allows for maximal blood and tissue oxygen saturations, and serum nitrogen wash-out, which is essential to prevent hypoxia during the period of paral-

**BOX 2-1  Equipment necessary for RSI**

- Suction device (Yankauer) with reservoir, tubing, and suction source
- Oxygen source with oxygen delivery device (facemask, nasal cannula)
- Airway adjuncts (nasopharyngeal airway, oropharyngeal airway)
- BVM apparatus connected to oxygen source
- Laryngoscope with operational light source
- Endotracheal tubes of various sizes
- Stylet to place into the endotracheal tube
- End-tidal $CO_2$ capnometer
- 10 mL syringe to inflate the ETT balloon
- Adjunct airway devices

ysis (and apnea) before successful tube placement. There are also a number of devices available to facilitate successful orotracheal intubation that can be useful in the setting of trauma (Box 2-2).

Etomidate is the most common induction agent used for RSI in trauma patients. Etomidate is an anesthetic that rapidly renders the patient unconscious (less than 30 seconds) and deeply sedated. The attractive feature of etomidate in trauma is that it results in little cardiovascular depression. This is important in patients with acute blood loss who may become hypotensive when induced for intubation. Midazolam (Versed) was previously used as an induction agent and is still used primarily in some EDs; however, being a benzodiazepine, it can cause significant hypotension in induction doses.

Succinylcholine is the predominant agent used for paralysis. It is a depolarizing agent, meaning that it causes depolarization of the motor end-plate in skeletal muscles. This accounts for the twitching, or fasciculations, seen after giving the medication. Once depolarization occurs, all skeletal muscle is paralyzed until succinylcholine metabolism takes place and repolarization can occur. This typically takes 8 to 10 minutes. Since irreversible brain damage occurs with about 6 minutes of hypoxia, orotracheal intubation must be achieved rapidly. If intubation is unsuccessful, it is important to provide BVM ventilation during this time of apnea.

Pretreatment agents are commonly used in the setting of head injury because of the premise that laryngoscopy results in adrenergic stimulation, which in turn results in increased ICP. The latter is hypothesized to have a deleterious effect in the setting of head injury. Of course the most important maneuver in minimizing increases in ICP is administering an induction and paralytic agent, which far outweigh the effects of any pretreatment agent. Lidocaine is most commonly given in the setting of head injury, optimally 2 minutes prior to induction and paralysis. It is hypothesized that

**BOX 2-2  Airway adjuncts used in trauma**

**Gum Elastic Bougie**: This device is a long plastic "wire" that can be used to locate the trachea if the vocal cords are not fully visualized. When placed in the trachea, the operator should be able to feel the "humps" of the tracheal rings (the esophageal walls are smooth). The endotracheal tube is then fed over the bougie.

**Fiber-optic Bronchoscope**: This technique requires both a skilled operator and a cooperative patient, although a low-dose sedative can be given (e.g., midazolam 2 mg IV) to facilitate the procedure. This is a good option for a patient with a known unstable c-spine fracture whose neck should not be hyperextended. This is an option only for patients who are somewhat stable and have no oral bleeding.

**Lighted Stylet**: This is a specially manufactured endotracheal tube with a light source at the tip that illuminates the anterior neck from within when the tip is correctly placed in the trachea. The light is not visible with esophageal intubation. The concept is to blindly place (without laryngoscopy) the tube into the trachea. This procedure takes some skill and practice; it should not be used in a critical airway situation. It is optimal for patients with c-spine fracture because it does not require laryngoscopy.

**Laryngeal mask airway (LMA)/Intubating LMA**: The LMA is a tube with a small rubber mask on the end that fits into the posterior pharynx. It is shaped such that it delivers air preferentially into the trachea, through the vocal cords, without inflating the stomach. It is typically placed blindly. This is a good rescue device in the case of a failed intubation where the patient is becoming hypoxic. The LMA is not a definitive airway device; it is a bridge until a definitive airway is provided. The intubating LMA is a variation of the original device that allows passage of an endotracheal tube through a hole in the device handle once the LMA is in place in the pharynx. Again this is good in the setting of suspected c-spine fracture because it does not require laryngoscopy.

**Combitube**: This is a rescue airway device used mostly in the pre-hospital setting. It has two tubes that bifurcate at the tip. When inserted, one tube goes into the trachea and one into the esophagus. Ventilation is then performed through the tracheal tube. The Combitube is also a good adjunct when other methods have failed and the patient is becoming hypoxic.

## LITERATURE REFERENCE

 ## Who should intubate the trauma patient?

There has been debate as to who should be responsible for trauma airway management. It is clear that only clinicians with extensive airway experience and adequate training, not only in trauma, should be responsible for the trauma airway, as the trauma airway in general can be the most challenging of airway scenarios. Prior to the 1970s, this role fell squarely on anesthesiologists for the most part. As emergency medicine evolved as a specialty, emergency physicians have become the most experienced in the management of trauma airways. There have been several studies comparing the success rate of physicians from various specialties. Omert et al. prospectively studied 11 months of trauma intubations at a Level I trauma center. All intubations were performed by emergency medicine physicians. A comparison was made with trauma intubation data from the previous year, where all trauma intubations were performed by anesthesiologists. There was no significant difference in success rate or number of attempts between the two groups **[Omert et al. *J Trauma* 2001; 51(6):1065–1068]**. Levitan et al. studied a total of 658 trauma intubations over a 3-year period, where the practice was to alternate between anesthesiologists and emergency medicine physicians on an even/odd day rotation. If the patient required immediate intubation prior to anesthesia arrival, the emergency medicine physician intubated the patient. There was no statistically significant difference in the success rate between the two specialties. The rate of crycothyrotomy compared favorably with other studies in which primary airway responsibility belonged to the anesthesiologist **[Levitan et al. *Ann of Em Med* 2004;43(1): 48–53]**.

| TABLE 2-2  Dosing of agents used in RSI | | |
|---|---|---|
| **Agent** | **Purpose** | **Dose** |
| Lidocaine | Pretreatment | 1.5 mg/kg |
| Etomidate | Induction | 0.3 mg/kg |
| Midazolam | Induction | 0.2 mg/kg |
| Succinylcholine | Paralysis | 1.5–2 mg/kg |

giving lidocaine at this time blunts afferent nerve impulses from the larynx and thus minimizes the reflex adrenergic response of laryngoscopy. Fentanyl and minidoses of nondefasciculating neuromuscular blocking agents are also thought to minimize ICP increases with laryngoscopy, but there has been no scientific proof to back this hypothesis (Table 2-2).

### The Difficult Trauma Airway

The trauma airway can pose challenges often not encountered in other patients. Distorted anatomy can result from blunt or penetrating trauma to the face or neck. It is important to assess for the ability to successfully intubate before administering a paralytic agent. This is sometimes difficult to predict with certainty based on external visualization and inspection of the oropharynx. A cricothyrotomy kit should be available and the neck prepped if orotracheal intubation is unlikely.

### When You Cannot Intubate or Ventilate, Perform a Cricothyrotomy

Cricothyrotomy is a critical procedure in the management of the trauma airway. It involves creating a direct opening to the trachea via the cricothyroid membrane through which a tracheostomy tube can be placed for ventilation (Box 2-3). This is required in the event of a failed airway by other methods or in the case of severe facial trauma that precludes orotracheal intubation. This procedure must therefore be performed rapidly and efficiently. As a note, children under the age of 10 are not candidates for cricothyrotomy because they have small, mobile larynxes and cricoid cartilages, making this procedure technically impossible. Percutaneous transtracheal ventilation is recommended in children.

---

**BOX 2-3  Cricothyrotomy: A lifesaving procedure**

Identify the cricothyroid membrane. Prepare the neck with antiseptic solution. If the patient is conscious, infiltrate lidocaine at the planned incision site. Immobilize the larynx by placing the thumb and middle finger on opposite sides of the laryngeal cartilage. A vertical, midline incision should be made through the skin approximately 2 cm in length. Next, incise the cricothyroid membrane with a horizontal incision. Insert the tracheal hook, and pull the upper portion of the trachea up and toward the head. Place dilator into incision to allow passage of the tracheostomy tube. Place tracheostomy tube between the blades of the dilator. Inflate the cuff and apply end-tidal $CO_2$ detector in line with the bag-valve apparatus to confirm placement and ventilate.

## KEY POINTS

- A and B of ABCs—primary survey
  - Assess airway patency and breathing
  - Immediate chest tube if symptomatic pneumothorax
- Does the patient need to be intubated?
  - Obstruction—blood, vomit, neck hematoma, or facial fractures
  - Hypoxia or shock
  - Hypoventilation—GCS <8
  - Anticipated deterioration—expanding neck hematoma, gunshot to chest
  - Aggressive behavior—concern for severe head injury
- Place on supplemental oxygen as part of ABCs: IV–$O_2$–monitor
- Rapid sequence intubation (RSI) is method of choice for intubation
  - Involves administration of induction agent and paralytic agent
  - Usually administer 20 mg of etomidate and 120 mg of succinylcholine
  - Allows deep sedation and paralysis for laryngoscopy
- C-spine immobilization important during laryngoscopy
- Back-up devices are important in trauma because of potential difficulty
- Be ready to perform cricothyrotomy quickly if all else fails

# CHAPTER 3

# Traumatic Shock and Arrest

## CASE SCENARIO

A 41-year-old male is brought to your ED after falling approximately 15 feet. He was found on the sidewalk below the window that he had been cleaning, holding his upper abdomen and moaning. His initial vital signs included a blood pressure of 110/70 and a heart rate of 108. He complained of abdominal pain. EMS personnel administered oxygen and placed a 16-gauge antecubital IV. On arrival to the ED, his vital signs include a heart rate of 126, blood pressure of 90/50 and an $O_2$ saturation of 99% on room air. As the trauma captain, you determine that his airway is patent and he does not require immediate airway management.

1. What is your next step?
   a. Auscultate for breath sounds, initiate aggressive fluid resuscitation, and proceed to secondary survey to determine the etiology of the hypotension
   b. Decompress his chest with a 14-gauge IV catheter to relieve a tension pneumothorax
   c. Consult surgery for exploratory laparotomy given his hypotension and abdominal pain
   d. Order uncrossmatched blood and transfuse after 1000 mL of normal saline

The patient is hypotensive and tachycardic. Given his mechanism, there are a number of possible etiologies for this. While surgery may be indicated, a systematic survey is warranted to determine the etiology of shock. Airway and breathing are first evaluated as two large-bore IVs are being placed and crystalloid administered. Uncrossmatched blood should be readily available and transfused if the blood pressure does not respond to a crystalloid bolus. The most immediate goal is to identify a source of bleeding, by both the secondary survey and ancillary imaging techniques available in the bay. This includes a CXR to look for evidence of hemothorax or aortic injury, a FAST exam to look for intraperitoneal blood, and pelvic x-ray.

The patient's blood pressure after 2 L of normal saline drops to 86/42, and his heart rate remains in the 120s. Red blood cells are transfused. On exam you note right chest wall tenderness with equal breath sounds, RUQ abdominal tenderness without rebound, a stable pelvis with tenderness over the pubic symphysis, and weak bilateral femoral pulses. His FAST exam is unremarkable.

2. What is the next most appropriate step?
   a. Operative ex-lap given the FAST is not 100% sensitive for intra-abdominal blood
   b. CT scan of his abdomen and chest
   c. Angiography for embolization given the tenderness over the pubis symphysis
   d. Obtain trauma series including lateral c-spine, chest, and pelvis

The primary and secondary surveys should always guide you to the appropriate interventions (e.g., intubation, chest tube placement, and administration of blood) and imaging studies (e.g., FAST exam, trauma series, and CT scan). The secondary survey includes a log roll to inspect for bleeding scalp lacerations, palpate the back, and perform a rectal exam. This patient is unstable and requires rapid stabilization and workup in the bay. This excludes CT scan and angiography for the moment. At this point, in addition to blood infusion, a trauma series (at least the chest and pelvic x-rays) should be done to look for a source of hypotension.

The supine CXR shows left-sided anterior ribs 6–10 fractured without obvious underying pneumothorax. The mediastinum is somewhat widened, and there is diffuse haziness of the left lung.

**3.** What is the most appropriate action?
   **a.** Intubate for pulmonary contusion
   **b.** Pericardiocentesis for pericardial tamponade
   **c.** Left-sided chest tube for hemothorax
   **d.** Operative thoracotomy for ruptured aorta

A hemothorax on a supine CXR will appear as diffuse haziness of the whole lung compared with the other side because of the pooling of blood posterior to the lung. This injury would be likely given the rib fractures and possible intercostal artery laceration. Anterior breath sounds are often unchanged in supine patients with a hemothorax given that the lung floats atop the blood. Pulmonary contusion might also be expected with rib fractures and will often result in hypoxia but not hypotension. A pericardial tamponade is characterized by Beck's triad of hypotension, distended neck veins, and distant heart sounds. Note most importantly, fluid would be seen in the pericardial sac on the FAST exam. A slightly widened mediastinum on supine CXR is common and does not always infer aortic injury, although this diagnosis is still a possibility.

A left-sided chest tube is placed with the drainage of 1,500 mL of blood. The patient suddenly becomes pale and loses consciousness. You do not feel a carotid pulse.

**4.** What do you do now?
   **a.** Intubate, CPR, internal jugular cordis, and autotransfuse blood from chest tube
   **b.** Intubate, CPR, and transport to OR for thoracotomy
   **c.** Intubate, CPR, epinephrine, and rapid blood transfusion
   **d.** Intubate, CPR, and ED thoracotomy

There are several indications for an ED thoracotomy, depending on whether the trauma is blunt or penetrating. The procedure is typically more successful in the setting of penetrating trauma given that the bleeding is often coming from a discrete lesion that can be repaired under direct visualization (e.g., laceration to left ventricle). The indication for ED thoracotomy for penetrating trauma is loss of vital signs in the field or in the ED. Cardiac arrest in patients with blunt trauma is typically less amenable to ED thoracotomy given the wider extent of injury. ED thoracotomy in blunt trauma is futile if the patient arrives to the ED without vital signs. It is indicated for blunt trauma patients who lose vital signs in the ED and have a suspected reversible cause for decompensation. Examples of this would be pericardial tamponade and massive hemothorax.          Answers: 1-a; 2-d; 3-c; 4-d

# DEFINITION

Shock is simply defined as inadequate end-organ perfusion as the result of increased oxygen demand in the setting of decreased supply. Inadequate tissue perfusion in trauma can result from any disruption of oxygen transport between the outside environment and peripheral tissue beds, including inability to ventilate (e.g., airway obstruction from facial or neck trauma), inability to oxygenate (e.g., pulmonary contusions, pneumothorax, or hemothorax), decreased cardiac output (e.g., decreased preload because of blood loss, cardiac tamponade, tension pneumothorax, or myocardial contusion), or decreased oxygen-carrying capacity (e.g., decreased red blood cells because of blood loss). Shock is typically characterized by hypotension; however, it is important to recognize shock in its early stages when only tachycardia or increased respiratory rate is present. Early aggressive treatment is essential and may require a procedure (e.g., intubation, chest tube, or exploratory laparotomy) or administration of PRBCs. Trauma victims tend to be a younger, healthier group of patients and will be able to compensate for large amounts of blood loss by increasing cardiac output and increasing peripheral vascular resistance. See Table 3-1 for the classification system used for traumatic shock based on clinical signs.

## Types of Shock

Hemorrhagic and cardiogenic shock are the two primary etiologies for shock in trauma victims. Neurogenic shock, a result of loss of peripheral vascular tone because of a high c-spine injury, is often talked about but rarely seen. Septic shock is not an issue for the acutely injured patient but may be a postoperative complication in severely injured trauma patients. Acute hemorrhage can result in shock by two mechanisms. First, loss of blood results in a lower red blood cell mass and thus a decreased capacity for transport of oxygen to tissues, which is a major component of tissue perfusion. The results are tissue hypoxia,

**TABLE 3-1 The classification of hypovolemic shock**

| For a 70 kg male | Class 1 | Class 2 | Class 3 | Class 4 |
|---|---|---|---|---|
| Blood loss (mL) | <750 | 750–1,500 | 1,500–2,000 | >2000 |
| Blood loss (%BV) | <15% | 15%–30% | 30%–40% | >40% |
| Heart rate (bpm) | <100 | >100 | >120 | >140 |
| Pulse pressure (mm Hg) | Normal | Normal | Decreased | Decreased |
| Respiratory rate (bpm) | 14–20 | 20–30 | 30–40 | >35 |
| Urine output (ml/hr) | >30 | 20–30 | 5–15 | Negligible |
| CNS/mental status | Slightly anxious | Mildly anxious | Anxious/confused | Confused/lethargic |
| Fluids transfused | Crystalloid | Crystalloid | Crystalloid/blood | Crystalloid/blood |

anaerobic metabolism, and metabolic acidosis. Second, decreased circulating fluid volume results in decreased blood return to the heart, decreased ventricular filling pressures, and a resultant decrease in cardiac output.

Cardiogenic shock is not typically associated with trauma but must be a consideration in the hypotensive trauma victim. This is especially true in elderly patients who may have underlying cardiac conditions. These patients may develop cardiac ischemia secondary to increased myocardial demand (e.g., response to pain, blood loss, or anxiety). Constrictive cardiogenic shock must also be considered as the result of increased intrathoracic pressure (e.g., tension pneumothorax, massive hemothorax, or increased pressure because of mechanical ventilation) or because of pressure exerted on the heart itself (e.g., pericardial tamponade from stab wound). Finally, blunt cardiac injury can also lead to a decreased ejection fraction and subsequent cardiogenic shock.

### Recognize Shock When It Is Present

Shock may be insidious and deadly, especially in young patients who are able to compensate for large losses of blood. The most underrated symptom of shock is altered mental status due to inadequate cerebral perfusion. Altered mental status commonly is mistaken for head injury, intoxication, or just baseline personality. A common symptom is agitation that may be interpreted as simple anxiety. Sleepiness and lethargy will also result from shock, which is often mistaken for intoxication. These signs may be hard to recognize since many trauma victims are intoxicated or have cantankerous personalities.

In addition to mental status changes, there are other symptoms of shock that are apparent on physical exam. Vitals are crucial in recognizing shock. Tachycardia and widened pulse pressure (i.e., difference between systolic and diastolic blood pressures) are also the hallmarks of early shock. Increased respiratory rate is another underrated sign of shock. It is because of the physiologic response to metabolic acidosis. Anaerobic metabolism produces lactic acid, causing acidosis, and production of serum carbonic acid (dissolved carbon dioxide). The physiologic response is increased ventilatory rate to eliminate carbonic acid and restore normal pH. Patients often are pale, cool, or sweaty. Hypoperfused extremities take on a grayish hue, often with mottling and decreased capillary refill.

Over a number of hours, urine output is a fair measure of cardiac output, with normal renal perfusion producing greater than 1.0 ml/kg/hour, or about 50 to 100 cc per hour for most adults. A much better measure of cardiac output and resulting tissue perfusion is central venous oxygen saturation. This is measured from blood gas analysis of venous blood returning to the heart via an internal jugular or subclavian catheter. Similarly, base deficit can be measured from a peripheral venous sample and is a good surrogate for tissue hypoperfusion. The base deficit is defined as the amount of strong base that would have to be added to a liter of blood to normalize the pH. It is calculated using the pH and the $PCO_2$.

## MANAGEMENT

The cornerstone of shock management is to begin treatment while determining the cause of shock. Once identified, it is important to treat the cause, not

**CLINICAL PEARL** • • • • • • • • • • • • • • • • • • • • •

## Utility of base deficit and lactate

The base deficit has been the subject of a great deal of attention and may be the most useful lab to send in the trauma patient. But remarkably it is not commonly utilized in most institutions. The base deficit is a calculated lab value that represents the amount of $H^+$ in mEq/L needed to titrate blood back to a normal pH after eliminating the metabolic derangements caused by altered $PCO_2$. There have been multiple studies showing that the initial base deficit is a predictor of mortality and that serial measurements can be used to assess adequacy of the resuscitation. This seems to be especially true in patients with blunt mechanisms and patients with GSWs. There are also multiple studies indicating that serum lactate, which is also another useful marker of tissue hypoxia, can predict mortality. While it is true that alcohol and drug use will falsely raise the base deficit and the lactate, several studies have shown that even in intoxicated patients, the lactate and base deficit are still predictive of mortality.

the numbers (e.g., low blood pressure). The empiric treatment of shock entails administration of IV fluids for presumed hypovolemia, which is the most common cause of shock in trauma patients. After an initial bolus of 1 to 2 L of crystalloid, unresponsive shock should be treated with rapid infusion of PRBCs. While this is occurring, the evaluation of the source of shock begins with the ABCs. Always consider inadequate oxygenation, inadequate ventilation, or alterations in intrathoracic pressure first. This is addressed as A and B of the ABCs. Practically, this entails ensuring an adequate airway by evaluating for obstruction (e.g., blood, facial trauma, or expanding neck hematomas leading to compression of the trachea), decreased ability to oxygenate (e.g., pneumothorax or hemothorax), or decreased ventilatory drive (e.g., altered mental status or comatose because of head injury or intoxication). Intubation should be performed immediately if any of these conditions are present. Listen for breath sounds to assess for a tension pneumothorax, and place chest tubes as indicated.

Next, assess circulation. Palpating peripheral pulses is only the first step in the assessment of circulation in traumatic shock. It is crucial to identify the source of blood loss, stop the bleeding, and administer blood products. The main internal sources of significant blood loss are the thoracic cavity, retroperitoneum, peritoneal cavity, pelvis, and thighs. These sources can be readily identified by using the FAST exam and trauma series early in the management of the trauma victim. A portable CXR may detect a large hemothorax that would require immediate tube thoracostomy (i.e., chest tube). Additionally, an enlarged heart may indicate the presence of a traumatic pericardial effusion. This can be further assessed using the subxiphoid view of the FAST exam. The FAST exam can also identify intra-abdominal bleeding, which in the setting of hypotension would warrant immediate ex-lap in the OR. The pelvis x-ray is performed to identify fractures. Pelvic fractures, midshaft femur fractures, and large bleeding lacerations (especially scalp lacerations) are common sources of large-volume blood loss and should be addressed during the initial phase of evaluation. In the setting of hypotension and shock, an unstable fractured pelvis should be wrapped with a sheet, a midshaft femur fracture placed in traction, and a bleeding scalp laceration quickly "whip stitched" or stapled. Note that x-rays of the pelvis and femur are not necessarily required to initiate these actions if the injury is obvious on physical exam.

Intravenous access is paramount in traumatic shock and should occur simultaneously with evaluating the ABCs as part of the IV–$O_2$–monitor routine. Two large-bore (14-gauge or 16-gauge) IV catheters should be attempted in the antecubital areas bilaterally. If there is any delay in peripheral IV access, then central venous access or, less commonly, a peripheral venous cutdown should be done. It is important to remember that for suspected abdominal vascular injury or in cases of severe shock, intravenous access must be obtained above the diaphragm as well.

Volume replacement should begin with crystalloid solution, although it should be switched over to PRBCs after 2 L of fluid have been given if hypotension still exists. To avoid hypothermia, warmed fluids are recommended. Two liters of fluid should be administered rapidly, and the hemodynamic response noted. If blood is needed urgently, O-negative or type-specific blood should be transfused immediately; typed and crossmatched blood should then be used once available. Though fresh frozen plasma (FFP) and platelets may be needed in the setting of massive transfusion to maintain coagulation system balance, their administration is not routinely advocated during the acute

## Is blood transfusion absolutely a good thing?

The standard ATLS recommendation is that any hypotensive trauma patient who has already received two liters of crystalloid solution be given a blood transfusion. However, there is mounting evidence that transfused blood may have detrimental immunomodulating and proinflammatory effects, especially if the blood has been stored for 2 weeks or more. This has been investigated in several recent studies. Malone et al. retrospectively showed that transfusion was an independent predictor of mortality, ICU admission, ICU length of stay, and hospital length of stay in a cohort of more than 15,000 trauma patients, even when ISS, GCS, age, race, and shock associated variables, e.g., base deficit, lactate, shock index were controlled for. **[Malone et al. *J Trauma* 2003;54(5):898–905; discussion 905–907].**

However, anemia was also an independent predictor of bad outcome, raising the question of what the transfusion threshold should be for trauma patients to balance these negative effects. Robinson et al. looked at this question specifically in patients with blunt hepatic and splenic injuries and also found that when injury severity and degree of shock were controlled for, blood transfusion was an independent predictor of adverse outcome **[Robinson et al. *J Trauma* 2005;58(3): 437–444; discussion 444–445].** Investigators are now attempting to determine whether transfusing leukocyte-reduced blood will mitigate this effect. Additionally, there are several polymerized hemoglobin molecules that are being tested in trauma patients to determine whether these will be able to replace traditional blood transfusions.

## Recombitant factor VIIa to control bleeding in trauma patients?

Current trauma management is lacking an effective hemostatic agent that is safe, noninvasive, easy to use, and able to stimulate local thrombotic processes without triggering widespread arterial or venous thrombosis. Recombinant factor VIIa (rfVIIa, Novoseven), which has been successfully used in the management of bleeding complications in hemophilia patients for years, may be the answer. It has come under investigation as an agent for trauma and operative patients without pre-existing coagulopathy. Several studies and reviews have addressed its feasibility in such patients. Posttraumatic coagulopathy is an established multifactorial entity. Martinowitz et al. reported its use in seven massively bleeding, multi-PRBC transfused trauma patients who were refractory to conventional hemostatic measures. Use of this agent resulted in a decreased transfusion requirement and shortening of both the PT and PTT. None of the seven patients died directly from bleeding **[Martinowitz et al. *J Trauma* 2001;51(3):431–438; discussion 438–439].** Geeraedts et al. conducted a retrospective review of eight patients who sustained life-threatening bleeding injuries after blunt trauma. Infusion of rfVIIa resulted in markedly decreased red blood cell, platelet, and fresh frozen plasma transfusion requirements. None of the eight patients died from blood loss. No adverse events were documented **[Geeraedts et al. *Injury* 2005;36(4):495–500].** Levi et al. performed a systematic review of clinical studies investigating rfVIIa between 1966 and 2004 to determine the efficacy and safety of its use. They analyzed 483 articles (28 clinical trials, 124 case series, 176 case reports). They concluded that more randomized controlled clinical trails are required to make a definitive statement on its use; however, existing evidence is promising. There was a reported 1% to 2% incidence of thrombotic complications **[Levi et al. *Injury* 2005; 36:495–500].**

phase of treatment. Recombinant factor VIIa, a blood product that works by restoring hemostasis at the injury site without systemic activation of the coagulation cascade, is being investigated as an adjunct for the bleeding trauma patient.

Vasopressors are not used in the management of hemorrhagic traumatic shock. The only effective treatment is to stop the bleeding and restore circulating blood volume. For severely hypotensive patients, this means massive blood transfusion and operative management. In a dire situation, vasopressors can be used while the patient is being transported to the operating room. For the rare case of neurogenic shock, with hypotension, a result of peripheral vasodilatation, phenylepherine or norepinephrine is generally the vasopressor of choice. The former is a pure α-receptor agonist and the latter has potent α-receptor as well as β-receptor agonist.

Penetrating trauma in the proximity of the heart or concern for overlying rib fractures and hemodynamic instability should always raise the consideration of pericardial tamponade. Beck's triad of hypotension, distended neck veins, and muffled heart sounds is rarely present. Measuring a pulsus paradoxus in the intensive resuscitative phase is a ridiculous notion. The FAST exam can be used to detect a large pericardial effusion, which would suggest cardiac injury and pericardial tamponade. Patients with penetrating chest wounds and hypotension should spend little time in the ED and should be managed in the OR. If the patient is dying and there is a delay to operative management, then an open thoracotomy must be performed in order to relieve pericardial tamponade and repair myocardial injuries.

### Traumatic Arrest

ED thoracotomy is performed as a lifesaving measure in moribund patients who are too unstable to survive to the operating room. In general, consideration is given to performing an ED thoracotomy only if the patient has no signs of life (i.e., unresponsive and pulseless) or persistent severe hypotension (systolic blood pressure <60 mmHg) and is too unstable for transport to the operating room. Despite several decades of literature on the procedure, there is no true consensus on the indications for ED thoracotomy. Most of the literature centers on case series, some of which are quite large (about 1,000 patients). The purported downside to the procedure includes risk of body fluid exposure for the operators, futile use of resources, and potential long-term survival of a patient with no neurologic function (vegetative state). On the other hand, the

procedure can clearly save lives, with some reports indicating that one third or more of patients arriving to the emergency department with minimal signs of life and an isolated stab wound to the chest survive neurologically intact when ED thoracotomy is performed. Additionally, there is some evidence that survival rates improve in centers where more thoracotomies are performed. This raises the ethical question of expanding the indications to include patients not typically thought to benefit significantly (e.g., blunt trauma patients who arrest en route to the ED).

---

**LITERATURE REFERENCE**

 ## When to perform an emergency department thoracotomy

Branney et al. have compiled perhaps the most authoritative data on the subject of ED thoracotomy, which is the basis for current practice. They reviewed 868 ED thoracotomies over the course of 23 years at a busy urban trauma center. The authors report that 34 patients survived and were discharged neurologically intact, while 7 more survived and were neurologically disabled. Only two patients who had blunt trauma and unobtainable vital signs in the field survived to hospital discharge, both of whom were neurologically devastated. Neurologically intact survival rate increased to 2.5% if the patient had vital signs on paramedic contact. Not surprisingly, this report found that patients with stab wounds who arrived with vital signs had the best survival rates. In contrast to blunt trauma, those with penetrating trauma and initially obtainable vital signs in the field accounted for 26.5% of survivors. Overall, the survival rates were highest for stab wounds to the chest (18%), followed by gunshot wounds to the abdomen (13%), with blunt mechanisms having a survival rate of 2%, half of whom were neurologically devastated. From this study the indication for ED thoracotomy has been derived: penetrating trauma with loss of vital signs in the field or in the ED and blunt trauma with loss of vital signs in the ED **[Branney et al. _J Trauma_ 1998;45(1):87–94; discussion 94–95].**

**LITERATURE REFERENCE**

## Should we keep the trauma arrest warm or cold?

Recent studies have demonstrated that mild hypothermia can be therapeutic and improve both neurologic and cardiac outcome from a host of ischemic and traumatic insults. This is in contrast to the classic teaching that hypothermia is detrimental to trauma patients. The most likely cause of this discrepancy is different physiologic effects between uncontrolled environmental hypothermia and controlled therapeutic hypothermia. Nozari et al. conducted a study to look at the effect of induced hypothermia on traumatized dogs. The investigators had previously demonstrated that dogs can survive neurologically intact after 120 minutes of induced atraumatic cardiac arrest with ice-cold saline (suspended animation). A follow-up study looked at the effects of major trauma. They exsanguinated 14 dogs over 5 minutes to induce cardiac arrest, as frigid saline was introduced into the femoral artery. Eight of the dogs underwent laparotomy and thoracotomy to simulate traumatic injury. Each dog underwent 60 minutes of no-flow cardiac arrest, reperfusion with cardiopulmonary bypass, followed by intensive care for up to 72 hours. All 14 dogs survived to 72 hours with histologically normal brains. Four of the eight trauma group dogs had neurologic deficits. This study suggests that cooling may be beneficial in patients with traumatic circulatory shock, although application to human patients requires more study [Nozari et al. *J Trauma* 2004;57(6):1266–1275].

Many studies have tried to assess survival by mechanism of injury, presenting cardiac activity, and presence or absence of vital signs in the field. Given the small number of patients in reported case series, it is difficult to derive statistically significant conclusions. However, several common themes from this literature can be derived and used in practice (Box 3-1).

**BOX 3-1  ED thoracotomy from multiple case series**

- Patients with SW who have vital signs on ED arrival and subsequently lose vital signs have the best survival rates.
- Patients with penetrating mechanisms who are without vital signs in the field can survive neurologically intact and should undergo ED thoracotomy.
- Patients with penetrating abdominal trauma may benefit from cross-clamping of the descending aorta and should undergo ED thoracotomy.
- Blunt trauma patients without signs of life or vital signs in the field should not undergo ED thoracotomy because the rate of neurologically intact survival is most likely because 0%.
- Blunt trauma patients who lose vital signs in the ED have a small chance of neurologic survival and should undergo ED thoracotomy.
- Presenting cardiac rhythm alone should not influence the decision to perform an ED thoracotomy.

## KEY POINTS

- Shock is inadequate end-organ perfusion
  - Increased oxygen demand in the setting of decreased supply
- Hemorrhagic shock is by far most common in trauma
  - Think of places where blood hides—thorax, abdomen, pelvis/retroperitoneum, or thigh
- Cardiogenic shock a consideration in chest trauma
  - Think pericardial tamponade and cardiac contusion
- Recognize signs of shock, do not fixate on blood pressure
  - Altered mental status (confusion, agitation) is a common harbinger
  - Early signs include tachycardia and increased respiratory rate
  - Cool or mottled extremities and difficult-to-find pulses should alert to shock
- Cornerstone to treatment is aggressive volume resuscitation and finding underlying cause
  - Initial IV crystalloid bolus should be followed by rapid blood transfusion (type O)
  - Physical exam, FAST exam, and trauma series helpful in identifying internal bleeding
  - Rapid intervention is crucial before it is too late
- ED thoracotomy if patient loses vital signs
  - Most effective in penetrating chest trauma to relieve pericardial tamponade
  - Aortic cross-clamp can be temporizing in massive abdominal or pelvic bleeding

# TRAUMATIC ARREST

Arrest: Loss of vitals or SBP <60 mmHg despite resuscitation

Primary medical etiology likely?
(suspected MI, PE, stroke prior to trauma)

**YES** → **ACLS algorithms**

**NO**

Mechanism of trauma?

**Blunt**

**Penetrating**

Signs of circulation prior to ED arrival?

**YES** → **ED thoracotomy**

**NO**

**Stop resuscitation**

Blood in pericardial sac?

**YES**

**NO**

- Pericardiotomy
- Isolate and control bleeding
- Aggressive resuscitation
- Consider cross clamp aorta
- Consider open cardiac massage

- Cross clamp aorta
- Aggressive resuscitation
- Consider open cardiac massage

**Vital signs restored?**

**YES**

**OR**

# CHAPTER 4

# Head Injury

## CASE SCENARIO

A 23-year-old male is brought in by EMS with a collar but no backboard, after being found on the street outside of an expensive local restaurant. His initial vital signs include a pulse of 110, blood pressure 135/84, respiratory rate of 18, and oxygen saturation 100% on room air. He is well dressed but somewhat uncooperative. He is repeatedly asking for lip balm. He is oriented to person and place. He does not recall who the president is but does recall that he ate dinner at the restaurant and that he had "a ton of beers." He does not smell of alcohol. He has some abrasions on his forehead and swelling along with a laceration over his right temple. The remainder of his exam is significant only for left ankle swelling.

1. What is the best initial plan for this patient?
   a. Immediate head CT scan
   b. CT scan if ethanol level and tox screen are normal
   c. Treat potential alcohol withdrawal with benzodiazepines and observe clinically
   d. Serial neurologic exams and head CT if his condition deteriorates

This patient is talking to you therefore his airway and breathing are intact. He also has adequate circulation given his blood pressure. It is unclear whether he is intoxicated, and there is a good possibility he has sustained a head injury although he only has abrasions. He should receive an immediate head CT given his altered mental status, possibility of head trauma, and lack of obvious intoxication.

You complete a secondary survey that reveals no significant injury. The patient's sister and girlfriend arrive and supply more information. He is a student at a local graduate school and is studying politics. He had been out to dinner with his girlfriend and had not been drinking to her knowledge. He left the restaurant to get the car, but when she came out to meet him, she found him on the ground unconscious and called 911.

2. Based on the history, age, and physical exam, what is the most likely potential head injury?
   a. Epidural hematoma
   b. Subdural hematoma
   c. Traumatic subarachnoid hemorrhage
   d. Diffuse axonal injury

An epidural hematoma would be expected given the laceration over the right temple. The middle meningeal artery runs just under the temporal bone, which is the thinnest bone of the skull and susceptible to injury. An epidural hematoma is by definition an arterial bleed, as the arteries run in the epidural space, and therefore are prone to rapid expansion. After the initial injury, there may be a time of relative well-being before the patient's condition deteriorates. This is referred to as the lucid interval. An epidural hematoma mandates immediate surgery and evacuation.

You order a CT scan and return to re-examine the patient, who is becoming more somnolent and now has a GCS score of 8.

3. What is your first priority in managing this patient?
   a. Take the patient to CT scan immediately
   b. Intubate the patient for airway protection
   c. Call the lab to check on the results of the tox screen and blood alcohol level
   d. Administer a "coma cocktail" of IV glucose and naloxone

In the course of a trauma resuscitation and workup when the patient's condition changes, go back to the ABCs. It is becoming evident that he is deteriorating and cannot go to CT without securing the airway. You intubate him using RSI with lidocaine 100 mg, etomidate 20 mg, and succinylcholine 120 mg. You confirm tube placement with $CO_2$ capnometry. As you are preparing him to travel to the CT scanner, you notice his right pupil is dilated and no longer reactive to light. His pulse has slowed to 48.

4. What should you do?
   a. Continue to CT as this is likely a consequence of medications used for intubation
   b. Administer mannitol 1.4 g/kg and place an arterial line to monitor his blood pressure
   c. Take patient directly to the OR for a burr hole and craniotomy without the CT scan
   d. Manually hyperventilate the patient on the way to CT scan

A blown pupil is evidence of brain herniation and is a terminal event. At this point the patient should go directly to the OR for a burr hole followed by craniotomy. Given his precipitous decline and evidence of the Cushing's response (i.e., bradycardia), time cannot be spared to first get a CT scan.

Answers: 1-a; 2-a; 3-b; 4-c

## BACKGROUND

Head injury, along with accompanying traumatic brain injury (TBI), is exceedingly common in polytrauma victims. Head injury can occur without any associated neurologic deficits. TBI, however, is defined as brain injury from external mechanical force that causes temporary or permanent impairment of some aspect of cerebral functioning (e.g., cognition, psychosocial, or physical). TBI is more common in men than women overall; but in the older population, where falls account for a significant number of cases, the ratio evens out. The incidence of TBI peaks between the ages of 15 and 30 years. Mechanisms are somewhat predictable, with motor vehicle crashes, falls, and firearm injuries topping the list. Alcohol usually plays a role in these injuries.

The severity of TBI is defined based on the Glasgow Coma Scale (GCS) score (Table 4-1). It is important to remember that the patient's condition may fluctuate, along with his or her GCS score. Therefore, frequent reassessment is critical. Furthermore, it is important to consider that drugs and alcohol can influence the score. In general though, patients with a GCS of 14 to 15, which account for 80% of the head injuries seen in the ED, are said to have minor head injury. Moderate head injury (GCS of 9 to 13) is present in 10%. The remaining 10% have a GCS of less than 8 and are said to have severe head injury. Obviously, the severity of TBI will determine management and workup.

The pathophysiology of head injury can be divided into two phases, primary injury and secondary injury. Primary injury encompasses the injury caused directly by the external forces acting on the cranium, which include injury evident on physical examination and on CT scan. Secondary injury occurs in the hours to days following the primary injury, where further cellular damage occurs related to two main factors: a) lack of oxygen delivery and b) increased intracranial pressure (ICP).

Neuronal viability is dependent on oxygen delivery, which in turn is a function of blood oxygen content and cerebral blood flow. The first is maintained with oxygenation, ventilation, and hematocrit. Cerebral perfusion pressure (CPP) is an important measure of cerebral blood flow, and it is related to the mean arterial pressure (MAP) and intracranial

**TABLE 4-1  Glasgow Coma Scale**

| Category | Response | Score |
|---|---|---|
| Eye opening | Spontaeous | 4 |
| | To voice | 3 |
| | To Pain | 2 |
| | None | 1 |
| Verbal response | Oriented | 5 |
| | Confused conversation | 4 |
| | Inappropriate words | 3 |
| | Incomprehensible speech | 2 |
| | None | 1 |
| Motor response | Normal movements | 6 |
| | Withdraws to touch | 5 |
| | Withdraws to pain | 4 |
| | Flexion posturing | 3 |
| | Extension posturing | 2 |
| | Flaccid | 1 |

pressure (ICP), that is (CPP = MAP − ICP). Therefore, low MAP or increased ICP will adversely affect CPP. Unfortunately, trauma victims may have low MAPs because of hemorrhagic shock. Increased ICP is primarily the result of extra-axial blood collections (traumatic blood between the arachnoid layer of the brain and the skull) and cerebral edema. Cerebral edema is the result of contused neurons and resulting exudate of cell contents. Furthermore, autoregulation is impaired by a disrupted blood-brain barrier, which results in further edema.

# MANAGEMENT

The basic principles of management for head injured patients follow the ABCs. Generally, patients with a GCS *less than* 8 require intubation. In the event that a patient needs to be intubated, a cursory neurologic exam should be performed to obtain a baseline as summarized by the GCS score. This includes level of consciousness, verbal responsiveness, and motor function. The latter is as simple as asking a patient to make a fist or wiggle his or her toes. Withdrawal to pain should be assessed in unresponsive patients. This exam should take no longer than 10 to 15 seconds.

## Oxygen Delivery

As discussed above, oxygen delivery is the most important ingredient to neuronal survival. Therefore, hypoxia and hypotension should be treated aggressively. Intubation and mechanical ventilation with 100% oxygen dramatically increases pulmonary oxygen delivery and should be considered early if there is evidence of significant head injury. However, the effectiveness of prehospital intubation for TBI is still in question. Treatment of hypotension can start with crystalloid fluid such as normal saline but should include PRBCs early if hypotension persists. PRBCs provide hemoglobin to increase blood oxygen content and oxygen delivery to the brain. Some postulate that crystalloid may result in increased cerebral edema by decreasing serum osmolarity; therefore, administration of large volumes of crystalloid should probably be avoided in patients with suspected head injury.

## Hyperventilation

Much has been made of hyperventilation for patients with TBI, and until the mid-1990s, most experts recommended its routine use despite the lack of evidence supporting its value or safety. The theoretical benefit of hyperventilation is the reduction of $PaCO_2$ leading to reflex cerebral vasoconstriction and decreased cerebral blood volume and, in turn, decreased ICP. However, it must be recognized that this comes at the cost of decreased cerebral perfusion pressure and potential decreased oxygen delivery. Some evidence indicates that the change in blood volume is much smaller than the change in blood flow, and that hypocarbia may actually induce a reflexive increase in ICP. Therefore, current recommendations call for a target $PaCO_2$ of 35 mm Hg, with the role of hyperventilation limited to patients who are showing acute signs of herniation.

## Mannitol

Mannitol is an osmotic diuretic that increases serum osmolarity without crossing the blood-brain barrier, thus theoretically having the effect of drawing fluid out of the brain and decreasing ICP. Another proposed mechanism is through decreased blood viscosity and thus increased cerebral perfusion. It does have a diuretic effect, and it should be kept in mind that urinary losses need to be replenished by maintenance fluids. Mannitol has been used by neurosurgeons since the 1950s despite the absence of randomized controlled trials to support its efficacy. Common practice is to administer mannitol 0.5 to 1.0 g/kg (typically 50 g) over 30 to 60 minutes to head injury patients amenable to surgery while the operating room is being mobilized, provided the patient is not hypotensive. There is some evidence that a second dose of mannitol 0.5 to 1.5 g/kg significantly reduces ICP in patients with acute subdural hematoma. There is also some experimental evidence that high-dose mannitol is beneficial in cases of severe diffuse cerebral edema (GCS = 3), although its use in this setting is not well established.

## Seizure Prophylaxis

Approximately 2% of all patients who seek treatment for head injury develop posttraumatic seizure. While posttraumatic seizures have multiple physical and psychological effects and complicate recovery, antiepileptic drugs may also have adverse side effects, some of which are significant. According to the latest guidelines from the American Academy of Neurosurgeons (AAN) published in 2003, the weight of the evidence favors giving patients with severe TBI prophylaxis against early posttraumatic seizures. Phenytoin has been the most rigorously studied drug for this purpose and is recommended by the AAN. The patient should then be continued on therapeutic doses of oral phenytoin 7 days postinjury. The medication can be stopped if the patient remains seizure-free.

**Prehospital intubation of the head injury patient**

Intubation in the prehospital setting is a topic of great controversy and debate, especially in head trauma patients. The debate began with the publication of a retrospective study that showed improvement in mortality in patients with a GCS ≤8 and blunt head injury, who were intubated in the field **[Winchell et al. *Arch Surg* 1997;132(6):592–597]**. This study was done at a time when the ground paramedics could only intubate patients who could be intubated without neuromuscular blocking agents and who were having agonal or ineffective respirations. The recommendation by the authors was to expand the prehospital indications for intubation in head trauma patients. In the same EMS system, a prospective study, with historical controls, was conducted in which patients with a GCS of ≤8 were intubated with the use of neuromuscular blockade if intubation was unsuccessful without pharmacological treatment. This study demonstrated that paramedics could intubate a greater percentage of TBI patients successfully if given the ability to perform rapid sequence intubation (RSI), but no data was collected to determine whether or not this improved outcome **[Davis et al. *J Trauma* 2003;55(4):713–719]**.

The same investigators later showed that, matched to nonintubated historical controls, RSI in the field actually worsened outcomes of patients with severe TBI. It is important to note that the controls were not matched for GCS because this was not typically reported prior to institution of the RSI protocol. The authors proposed that this negative outcome may have been because of longer scene times needed to perform RSI, transient hypoxia after paralysis, or excessive hyperventilation **[Davis et al. *J Trauma* 2003;54(3):444–453]**. A later study by the same investigators documents significant hypoxia in patients who underwent RSI, even though their oxygenation status was adequate prior to airway manipulation **[Dunford et al. *Ann Emerg Med* 2003;42(6):721–728]**. While the study did not specifically look at the effect on mortality, given that hypoxia is known to worsen outcome in TBI, RSI would seem to be harmful to these patients. In a subgroup analysis done as part of a follow-up to the study showing worse outcomes with RSI, the authors determined that over-aggressive hyperventilation ($PaCO_2$ <25 mm Hg) adversely affected outcome **[Davis et al. *J Trauma* 2004;56(4):808–814]**. Given that this was only a subgroup analysis, further study was done with patients who had electronically recorded $ETCO_2$ and $SPO_2$ data available. The conclusion was that both hyperventilation and oxygen desaturation (less than 70%) led to worse outcomes. The effect of these two variables did not fully explain the difference in mortality, so the question of why RSI is deleterious for TBI patients was not fully answered **[Davis et al. *J Trauma* 2004;57(1):1–8; discussion 8–10]**.

## SPECIFIC INJURIES

### Epidural Hematoma

An epidural hematoma (EDH) is a collection of blood between the inner table of the skull and the dura. EDH occurs in only 0.5% of severely head-injured patients and typically results from injury to the middle menigeal artery, which is associated with temporal bone fractures. EDH can also result from a dural sinus tear. Although it occurs in only 15% to 30% of EDH, the lucid interval is described as a period of mental clarity after an initial period of unconsciousness. As the hematoma expands and herniation ensues, the mental status deteriorates again. EDH is rare in elderly patients and in children younger than 2, because the dura and the periostium tend to be closely opposed in these two age groups. If EDH is diagnosed prior to deterioration of mental status and the patient is promptly taken to the OR, the prognosis is excellent. On CT scan, EDH appears biconvex (ovoid in shape) and hyperdense. Because of dural attachements at suture lines, epidurals generally "respect" the suture lines and do not extend across them. If the density of the lesion appears mixed, there may still be active bleeding.

### Subdural Hematoma

Subdural Hematoma (SDH) is the most common traumatic mass lesion and is present in 20% to 40% of patients with severe head injury. The bleed occurs in the potential space between the dura and arachnoid layers, and the source is predominantly from the bridging veins between the cortex and the venous sinuses. The mechanism usually entails the brain moving relative to the skull. Thus, SDH is common in patients with brain atrophy (e.g., alcoholics, the elderly). SDHs are classified as acute, subacute, or chronic based on the time since the injury (less than 24 hours, 24 hours to 2 weeks, and greater than 2 weeks, respectively). This is based on the history and confirmed by CT findings.

An SDH appears as a crescent shape on CT scan and can run anywhere along the plane between the dura and the arachnoid, including areas adjacent to the falx or tentorium away from the skull. While these bleed tends to be relatively slow, SDH can still exert mass effect and precipitate herniation. If the bleed is acute, it will be hyperdense (bright white on CT scan), while the subacute and chronic bleeds appear hypodense or isodense (blending in with adjacent cerebral tissue on CT scan). Because chronic and subacute SDH may be more difficult to identify, it is important to look for secondary signs, including effacement of the adjacent sulci, midline shift, or ventricular compression.

### Subdural Hygroma

Subdural hygromas (SDHG) occur in up to 10% of patients with severe head injury, and their pathogenesis is still unclear. They are likely the result of small tears in the arachnoid, which allows CSF to leak out, forming a xanthochromic fluid collection in the subdural space. Both immediate and delayed accumulation of SDHG have been described. The presentation is similar to that for other extra-axial fluid collections. On CT, they appear crescent shaped (similar to SDH) but are generally similar in density to CSF. SDHG are often bilateral. If the patient is asymptomatic, these collections may be managed nonoperatively; otherwise surgical evacuation should be carried out as it would for other extra-axial collections.

### Subarachnoid Hemorrhage

Subarachnoid hemorrhage (SAH) is characterized by free blood in the space between the arachnoid layer and the pia. In the setting of atraumatic intracranial hemorrhage, SAH is usually caused by a ruptured cerebral arterial aneurysm. In this case, the SAH tends to be widespread, often filling the ventricles, and neurologically devastating. In the setting of trauma, focal collections of subarachnoid blood can be present via torn subarachnoid vessels. SAH is present in up to one third of all patients with severe head injury and, when present, is associated with a poorer prognosis. This is likely the result of cerebral vasospasm, which induces secondary ischemia. Nimodipine, a calcium channel

blocker, is used to mitigate vasospasm. In cases of isolated, focal SAH the prognosis is good, and no specific treatment is indicated other than nimodipine and observation.

### Parenchymal Contusion and Hematoma

Parenchymal contusions are essentially bruised brain tissue, generally caused by impact injury leading to rupture of parenchymal blood vessels. The lesion located on the side of the impact is referred to as a coup injury, while that occurring on the opposite side of the brain is a contracoup injury. The contusion is formed by the coalescence of multiple petechial hemorrhages and is typically focused in the gray matter. But it can extend into the white matter and may generate significant surrounding edema, creating mass effect and local tissue ischemia. Subarachnoid blood is also commonly present in the area surrounding a contusion. Parenchymal hematomas occur deep within the brain parenchyma and can also occur in the cerebellum, although they are more common in the cerebral cortex. They result from the coalescence of small petechial hemorrhages from disrupted deep arterioles as the brain is forcibly propelled against the irregular surfaces of the inner skull. These are typically present on initial CT scan as well-demarcated and hyperdense lesions but can present in a delayed fashion up to several days later. These lesions can cause surrounding edema and may raise ICP, necessitating emergent evacuation.

### Diffuse Axonal Injury

Diffuse axonal injury (DAI) is the most common CT finding in severely head-injured patients, resulting from shear forces which disrupt the neuronal axons in the brain. The distal portion of the disrupted axons will subsequently undergo Wallerian degeneration. The more axons disrupted, the greater the resulting deficits, explaining the variable prognosis of patients with DAI. The findings on CT may be quite subtle in the immediate period after the injury, but small petechial hemorrhages in the white matter and surrounding the third ventricle may be present. Profound coma can result despite the apparent lack of CT pathology. There is no way to predict the severity of DAI clinically or radiographically. Patients who do not show neurologic improvement within 24 hours ultimately do poorly.

### Skull Fractures

A significant amount of force is required to fracture the skull. While many patients have skull fractures in the absence of intracranial injury, the presence of a skull fracture increases the likelihood that the patient has an associated TBI. Isolated skull fractures, significant only if they extend into a sinus or introduce intracranial air, are open (have an overlying laceration) or are depressed below the inner table of the skull. *Linear skull fractures* are fractures that extend through the entire thickness of the skull but are not comminuted or depressed. There is no specific treatment for these injuries. However, if they cross one of the major venous sinuses or the course of the middle meningeal artery, they are associated with extra-axial bleeding, and an overnight observation is warranted. *Comminuted skull fractures* are multiple linear fractures radiating out from the impact site and imply a higher mechanism. *Depressed skull fractures* are much more likely to be associated with TBI because a portion of bone is forced below the plane of the skull, often lacerating the dura or puncturing underlying brain tissue. These fractures generally require operative elevation when the depressed bone lies below the inner table of the skull. Any patient with an identified depressed skull fracture, even in the absence of underlying TBI, requires admission for observation. *Basilar skull fractures* are simply linear fractures occurring at the base of the skull. These fractures generally occur in the temporal bone and can result in hemotympanum or Battle's sign (Box 4-1). Given the myriad of important structures that are found in close proximity to these fractures, several complications are possible, including cranial nerve entrapment, disruption of the auricular apparatus (with subsequent hearing loss or vertigo), extension into the cavernous sinuses, or injury to the carotid artery (pseudoaneurysm or AV fistula formation). *Open skull fractures* occur when a laceration overlies or is in close proximity to an underlying skull fracture or when the fracture extends into the paranasal sinuses or middle ear. These fractures can be irrigated thoroughly in the ED, and the laceration closed primarily. It is standard to give antibiotics for open fractures, although the data to support this practice is lacking.

### BOX 4-1  Classic physical exam findings in patients with basilar skull fracture

Battle's sign (retroauricular ecchymosis)
Raccoon eyes (circumferential periorbital ecchymosis)
Blood in the ear canal
Hemotympanum
CSF rhinorrhea or otorrhea
- Blood mixed with CSF produces double ring when dropped on paper
Evidence of cranial nerve deficit
- Vertigo, tinnitus, hearing loss, facial paralysis, or extraocular motion deficit

### LITERATURE REFERENCE

 **Repair of scalp lacerations**

In general, scalp lacerations heal well and have a low infection rate because the scalp receives an excellent blood supply. The principles that govern the closing of these wounds are similar to wounds elsewhere, but there are certain complexities worth mentioning. First, there is no data to suggest that trimming or shaving the hair around the wound reduces the infection rate or is necessary or useful. Second, lidocaine with epinephrine should be used to anesthetize the wound so that vasoconstriction provided by the epinephrine will decrease bleeding. Third, sutures or staples are both acceptable methods to close scalp wounds as long as the wound does not extend onto the face or through the hairline. Lastly, in cases where the galea is clearly disrupted, it is necessary to close the galea first with absorbable suture and then close the more superficial layer of skin.

Of interest, Hock et al. suggest that in patients with linear scalp wounds less than 10 cm long and hair greater than 3 cm in length, scalp wounds can be closed by apposing hair on either side of the wound with a single twist and then applying tissue glue to the hair. This was shown to produce less pain and equal or better cosmetic results, as well as fewer complications than standard repair **[Hock et al. *Ann Emerg Med* 2002;40(1):19–26].**

### Concussion

Concussion is a form of mild traumatic brain injury that induces some alteration in consciousness. The classic signs and symptoms are amnesia and confusion, both of which may occur immediately after the injury or several minutes later. Patients may complain of headache, vertigo, nausea or vomiting, and concentration difficulties. Patients may experience emotional lability, memory dysfunction, and fatigue for weeks after the injury. Concussion is, in effect, "stunning" of the brain parynchema without actual identifiable injury. One concern with concussion is second impact syndrome, occurring in those who sustain a concussion and then sustain a second head injury. It is thought that the brain is more susceptible after concussion to reinjury, including cerebral edema with subsequent long-term sequelae or even death. For this reason, the AAN has classified concussion into three types: a) mild

## The need for head CT in patients with minor head trauma

There has been a good deal of study regarding which patients with minor head injury require a head CT, and at least two well-circulated rules have been developed based on prospective studies of a large number of patients with minor head injury. These include the New Orleans criteria and the Canadian Head CT rules. The New Orleans rules are based on a study whose inclusion criteria were all patients must be over 3 years old with GCS of 15 in the ED and a history of head injury within the preceding 24 hours that involved LOC. The seven predictors in the New Orleans rule were validated by the investigators in a series of 909 patients and found to have sensitivity of 100% for any intracranial injury, regardless of whether an intervention other than observation was needed. Implementation of this rule would have only eliminated the need for CT scan in 22% of the patients **[Haydel et al. *N Eng J Med* 2000;Jul 13;343(2):100–105]**.

Stiell et al. studied 3,121 patients to generate the Canadian Head CT rules. The cohort was made up of adults (older than 16 years old) with LOC after head injury and a GCS of 13 to 15 in the ED, 80% of whom had a GCS of 15. Patients taking anticoagulants or who had a seizure were excluded. The goal of this study was to identify patients who need neurologic intervention. The high-risk criteria were 100% sensitive for this and required that only 32% undergo CT scan. It is important to note that in the Canadian study not all patients underwent head CT, but those who did not were interviewed over the phone 2 weeks after the injury to determine presence of symptoms and to assess level of impairment. The investigators found that their high-risk criteria identified all patients who would need neurologic intervention, but only 92% of patients who had any head injury on CT. In this study, none of the patients who would have been missed by the rule required intervention. As a result, Stiell et al. recommends a period of observation for patients having any of the medium risk criteria if CT is not performed **[Stiell et al. *Lancet* 2001;357(9266):1391–1396]**.

Additionally, there are certain groups that have been shown to be at higher risk and require CT scan even when they present with minor head injury. These include intoxicated patients (intracranial injury rate of 2.4% to 8.4% with minor head injury), patients with a coagulopathy or who were medically anticoagulated, and patients with ventricular shunts.

| Which patients with minor head injury need a CT scan? | |
| --- | --- |
| **New Orleans criteria** | **Canadian Head CT rules** |
| Headache | *High risk (for neurosurgical intervention):* |
| Vomiting | GCS <15 two hours after injury |
| Age greater than 60 years | Suspected open/depressed skull fracture |
| Drug or alcohol intoxication | More than two episodes of vomiting |
| Deficits in short-term memory | Physical evidence of basilar skull fracture |
| Seizure | Age greater than 65 years |
| Evidence of trauma above the clavicles | *Medium risk (for brain injury on CT):* |
| | Amnesia for events >30 minutes prior to injury |
| | High mechanism |

(symptoms less than 15 minutes), b) moderate (symptoms greater than 15 minutes), and c) severe (associated LOC). In general, it is recommended that contact sports be avoided for 1 week following a concussion. Two weeks is recommended if LOC was prolonged.

A concussion, by definition, is associated with a normal head CT. This begs the question of which patients need a head CT at all. It is generally accepted that patients do not need a head CT if the injury was low mechanism and there are no other serious associated injuries. Symptoms and signs that are concerning for intracranial hemorrhage include severe headache, vomiting, altered mental status, or abnormal neurologic exam. Intoxicated patients are difficult because their altered mental status may be a result of alcohol or intracranial injury; there should be a low threshold for obtaining a CT scan in these patients. Of note, LOC at the scene has never been associated with intracranial injury when the patient has a normal mental status in the ED.

## KEY POINTS

- Traumatic brain injury (TBI) is defined as an injury that causes either permanent or temporary impairment of cerebral function
- Glascow Coma Scale (GCS) is used to assess consciousness and neurologic function
    - Components include eye opening (4 points), verbal ability (5 points), and motor ability (6 points)
- Primary injury refers to initial injury because of traumatic force
    - Evidence on CT scan—skull fracture, cerebral contusion, or intracranial blood
- Secondary injury refers to delayed neuronal injury
    - Because of tissue hypoxia and increased intracranial pressure (ICP)
    - Cerebral perfusion pressure (CPP) = MAP − ICP
    - Systemic hypotension, hypoxia, and high ICP result in increased secondary injury
- ABCs are crucial to maintain tissue oxygenation and CPP
    - Intubate for respiratory difficulty, hypoxia, or GCS <8
    - Aggressive crystalloid and blood resuscitation for hypotension
- Hyperventilation reserved for those with evidence of herniation
- Mannitol used for patients with TBI awaiting surgery
- Phenytoin recommended in TBI to prevent seizure

# CHAPTER 5

# Penetrating Neck Injury

## CASE SCENARIO

A 48-year-old female is brought into the ED after being shot with a pellet gun in the anterior neck at the level of the cricothryoid membrane. She is alert and oriented but is beginning to complain of hoarseness. Her vitals signs include a pulse of 120, blood pressure 110/54, respiratory rate of 18, and oxygen saturation 99% on a nonrebreather mask. EMS placed a 14-gauge IV in her right antecubital fossa. Her c-spine is immobilized. She has no medical history and takes no medication.

1. What is the first priority in managing this patient?
   a. Obtain a STAT portable lateral neck x-ray to determine location of bullet
   b. Airway assessment
   c. Rapid exam to assess baseline neurologic function
   d. Establish a second large-bore IV

Trauma evaluation begins with airway assessment. She has normal mouth opening, and her oropharynx looks clear. You see a small wound just below the cricothyroid membrane with surrounding ecchymosis and swelling. She has bilateral breath sounds. You recall that a projectile must have a speed 350 ft/sec to pierce bone and that pellet guns are unlikely to generate muzzle speeds of greater than 300 ft/sec; but you agree with the prehospital providers that her c-spine needs to be immobilized until it is fully evaluated.

2. Which of the following is your best option for intubation?
   a. Cricothyrotomy
   b. Rapid sequence intubation
   c. Fiber-optic nasotracheal with topical anesthesia and mild sedation (1 to 2 mg of Versed)
   d. Simple nasotracheal intubation

There are several methods of establishing a definitive airway. The method chosen depends on the situation at hand and the experience of the operator. Rapid sequence intubation (RSI) should be the bread-and-butter of your repertoire when managing the trauma airway. Again, it consists of rendering the patient unconscious and paralyzed rapidly so as to optimize the conditions for laryngoscopy. Other methods can be employed when certain difficulties are anticipated, as might be the case here. The concern is that the trachea is being compressed by hematoma and that total airway closure is impending. Laryngeal view with laryngoscopy should not be impaired because of the injury; however, passing the tube may be difficult if tracheal narrowing exists. You will want to have several smaller sized tubes available just in case.

Despite the possible difficulties, the intubation goes smoothly. She had blood in her oropharynx but no obvious injury to her larynx or trachea. The remainder of her exam is significant for a small midline wound just below the level of the cricoid membrane that is oozing blood. There is no air bubbling in the wound, but she does have extensive subcutaneous air. Prior to intubation you observed that she was moving all four extremities.

3. What is the next step in her management?
   a. Call interventional radiology to obtain bilateral carotid angiograms
   b. Call GI to perform an emergent esophagoscopy to be followed by a barium swallow
   c. Prophylactic antibiotics, ICU admission, and careful observation for developing hematoma
   d. Portable chest and lateral neck x-rays to determine location of the bullet and then open exploration

This is an injury on the border between zones I and II of the neck. Zone II injuries, given the exposure of anatomic structures and the density of vital structures, are often taken to the OR for exploration if there are hard signs of injury (e.g., obvious laryngeal or tracheal injury or expanding hematoma). There is little doubt in this case that the trachea has been injured; therefore, open exploration in the OR is indicated.

Before you can carry out your management plan, the respiratory therapist reports that her peak airway pressures have risen sharply. She has taken the patient off the ventilator and notes she is becoming hard to bag. Her oxygen saturation tracing reads 85% with a good waveform, and her blood pressure has dropped to 70/30 with an accompanying tachycardia to 140. Repeat capnography confirms good end-tidal $CO_2$. Her breath sounds may be slightly greater on the left, but they seem relatively equal.

4. What immediate action is required to save this patient?
   a. Go straight to OR for probable carotid artery injury
   b. Place bilateral chest tubes
   c. Call the blood bank for a STAT transfusion of 2 units of PRBC
   d. Obtain STAT CTA since she is too unstable for angiography

Given that upper lobes of the lungs are in zone I of the neck, pneumothorax must be considered with penetrating neck injures to this area. This patient is deteriorating quickly, indicating a likely tension pneumothorax. A needle decompression should be performed by placing a 16-gauge angiocatheter in the anterior chest between the first and second ribs. When there is doubt as to which side is affected and the patient is deteriorating rapidly, it should be done on both sides.

A rush of air is obtained from the catheter as you place it in the right side. You then place a chest tube, and her blood pressure and oxygenation improve. She is then taken to the OR for exploration of the neck.                    Answers: 1-b; 2-b; 3-d; 4-b

## BACKGROUND

The neck is a unique part of the body because it is a small unprotected area that contains multiple critical structures, some of which are relatively superficial and highly susceptible to injury. The major body systems of concern in neck trauma are: a) vascular, b) airway/pulmonary, c) digestive, and d) neurologic. The latter, for the most part, is dealt with separately in a chapter on spinal cord injuries. Given the proximity of these structures to each other, it is not - uncommon for multiple systems to be involved in a given trauma patient. Because injuries are not always immediately obvious and the surgical approach varies greatly depending on the exact location of the injury, a rapid and thorough assessment of all possible injuries is critical.

Surgical management of neck trauma has evolved over the past 75 years from a policy of nonoperative management before World War I (with an accompanying high mortality rate) to mandatory exploration for all deep wounds (beginning in the 1950s) to a more selective management style that is still being developed today. Given the emphasis on selectively operating on patients, it is incumbent on clinicians to have highly sensitive methods for diagnosing occult injuries in a timely fashion. Additionally, these methods must be readily available at all times of the day and

night. The ideal approach to patients with these injuries is still being developed.

## CLINICAL ANATOMY

Having a firm grasp on the anatomy of the neck is of tantamount importance for all clinicians managing neck trauma because much of the clinical decision making is based on the depth and location of the wound. The depth, which is specific to penetrating trauma, will be discussed below; but suffice it to say that the decision point centers on whether or not the wound violates the platysma, a superficial muscle that completely envelops the anterior neck.

There are multiple ways to conceptualize the location of neck wounds and their relation to the anatomy of the neck. For the purposes of trauma management, the system of zones is usually favored. This system divides the neck into three zones that have identifiable landmarks (Figure 5-1 and Table 5-1). Zone I runs from the clavicles to the cricothyroid membrane, which lies just above the level of the sixth cervical vertebra. Of note, this zone is contiguous with the thorax and the vital structures contained within. Zone II extends from the cricothyroid membrane to the angle of the mandible. Finally, Zone III is superior to the angle of the mandible. The landmarks were

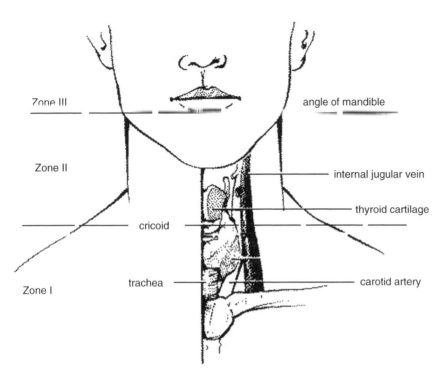

**FIGURE 5-1** Zones of the neck

| TABLE 5-1 Clinically relevant structures of the zones of the neck | | |
|---|---|---|
| **Zone I**<br>**Clavicles to cricothyroid membrane** | **Zone II**<br>**Cricothyroid membrane to angle of mandible** | **Zone III**<br>**Above angle of mandible** |
| *Vascular structures*<br>  Carotid artery<br>  Vertebral artery<br>  Subclavian artery<br>  Subclavian vein<br>  Internal jugular vein<br>  External jugular vein<br>  Anterior jugular vein<br>  Subclavian vein | *Vascular structures*<br>  Common carotid artery<br>  Internal carotid artery<br>  External carotid artery<br>  Vertebral artery<br>  Internal jugular vein<br>  External jugular vein<br>  Anterior jugular vein | *Vascular structures*<br>  Internal carotid artery<br>  Internal jugular vein<br>  External jugular vein |
| *Airway structures*<br>  Trachea<br>  Dome of the lungs | *Airway structures*<br>  Pharynx | *Airway structures*<br>  Oropharynx |
| *Digestive system structures*<br>  Esophagus | | |
| *Nervous system*<br>  Major cervical trunks<br>  Brachial plexus | *Nervous system*<br>  Spinal cord<br>  Recurrent laryngeal nerve | *Nervous system*<br>  Spinal cord |
| *Other*<br>  Thyroid gland<br>  Thoracic duct | | *Other*<br>  Submandibular gland |
| **Angiography first unless<br>hemodynamically unstable** | **Direct to OR if any hard signs** | **Angiography first unless<br>hemodynamically unstable** |

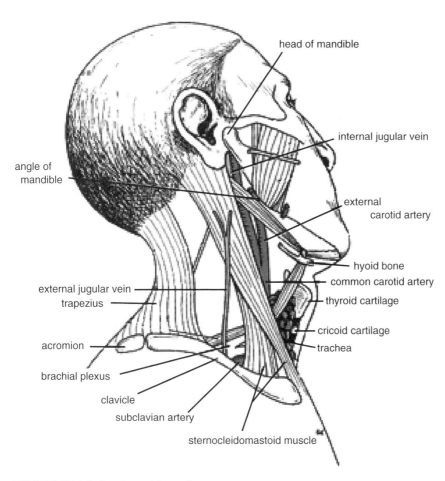

head of mandible

internal jugular vein

angle of mandible

external carotid artery

hyoid bone

common carotid artery

external jugular vein

thyroid cartilage

trapezius

cricoid cartilage

acromion

trachea

brachial plexus

clavicle

subclavian artery

sternocleidomastoid muscle

**FIGURE 5-2** Detailed anatomy of the neck

chosen because they delineate the cut-off for the different surgical approaches to neck trauma. It is important to keep in mind that in cases of penetrating trauma, missiles may enter the neck in one zone but affect structures in another zone.

Given the plethora of visible, or at least palpable, landmarks in most patients, it is quite useful to be able to identify the course of structures that traverse the neck, as well as the location of structures that are wholly contained within the neck. These in turn can be used as guides for location of the deeper, less palpable structures (Figure 5-2 and Table 5-2). The palpable structures also allow us to divide the neck into a group of triangles (anterior and posterior, bilaterally), as is taught in most anatomy classes. The anterior triangle is bordered by the medial aspect of the sternal belly of the sternocleidomastoid (SCM) muscle, the midline neck, and the lower edge of the mandible. This triangle contains the majority of vital structures in the neck, thus penetrating wounds to this area are more likely to cause damage requiring intervention. The posterior triangle is bordered anteriorly by the lateral aspect of the clavicular belly of

the SCM, inferiorly by the clavicle, and posteriorly by the trapezius muscle. Although the vertebral artery is found in the posterior triangle, the main concern with penetrating injuries in this area is damage to the spinal cord. Note that there is a small area between the medial aspect of the clavicular belly of the SCM and the lateral aspect of the sternal belly that is in

**TABLE 5-2  Palpable midline anatomy of the neck**

| Palpable structure | Cervical level | Relevant deep structures |
|---|---|---|
| Hyoid bone | C3 | Oropharynx |
| Notch of thyroid cartilage | C4 | Pharynx |
| Cricoid cartilage | C6 | Junction of pharynx and esophagus |
| Thyroid isthmus | C7 | Tracheal rings 2–4, esophagus |
| Suprasternal notch | T2 | Trachea, esophagus |

---

**BOX 5-1 The deep fascial layers of the neck**

Superficial → Deep

*Investing layer*—surrounds the neck and splits to encase the trapezius and SCM

*Pretracheal layer*—adheres to anterior surface of the cricoid and thyroid cartilages, tracts behind the sternum, and inserts on the pericardium anteriorly

*Prevertebral layer*—surrounds the prevertebral muscles and extends to form the axillary sheath, which surrounds the subclavian vessels

---

neither triangle, through which the carotid artery and the internal jugular vein run.

Finally, it is worth considering the fascial layers of the neck, which can be thought of as being either superficial or deep. The superficial layer, which has no clinical relevance in neck trauma, is just deep to the skin and covers the platysma muscle. The deep fascia, however, is quite important. It has three parts (Box 5-1). One of these, the pretracheal fascia, communicates directly with mediastinal structures, allowing bacteria and oral secretions from missed aerodigestive injuries to track inferiorly leading to mediastinitis. Having a firm grasp on this anatomy allows the clinician to manage a patient with a neck injury in a clear and organized manner.

## MANAGEMENT

There are three principle mechanisms of injury in neck trauma: a) penetrating, b) blunt, and c) strangulation (near hanging). Each mechanism has its own injury patterns, which will be discussed separately, followed by a discussion of specific pathology that can be found in patients with one or more of the mechanisms. However, as always, assessing the ABCs is the first priority. Given the density of vital structures, any injury causing edema or bleeding has high potential to complicate airway management. Thus, intubation in these patients is best done in a well-planned manner, possibly with the use of fiber-optic equipment. Any report of change in the pa-

tient's voice, findings of neck swelling or crepitence, should be acted on immediately. Careful consideration should be given to intubation in all patients being transferred to another facility. If positive-pressure ventilation is initiated for airway protection, the patient should be monitored closely for signs of tension pneumothorax, given that the lung apices extend into Zone I.

### Penetrating Neck Trauma

Once the airway of a patient with a penetrating neck wound is secured, circulation is assessed. If the patient is in refractory shock, he or she should go immediately to the OR without further workup, regardless of the location of the wound. Zone II wounds are relatively easy to explore, and gaining proximal and distal control of bleeding vessels is generally not a problem. However, zone I and III injuries are more complicated to deal with, especially when the patient is not stable enough for further workup (Table 5-3).

After the ABCs are assessed and deemed stable, the first question that needs to be answered is whether or not the wound violated the platysma muscle. This superficial muscle arises from the fascia of the pectoralis major and deltoid muscles bilaterally. It extends in a broad swath diagonally on either side of the neck to the inferior border of the mandible, covering all but the superior and posterior aspects of the posterior triangle and the inferomedial portion of the anterior triangle. To determine whether or not the platysma has been penetrated, careful exam under direct visualization is required. Blind probing of the wound tract with a finger or other instruments is *not* acceptable, as further injury can be induced or a clot dislodged, leading to bleeding and airway compression. If the weapon did not penetrate the platysma and the remainder of the patient's exam is reassuring, the wound can be irrigated and sewn closed.

In cases where the platysma is violated, the next questions should assess in what zone the injury is located and whether or not the physical exam indicates there is an immediate indication for surgery. Some authors refer to these as the hard signs of

---

**TABLE 5-3 The hard signs of penetrating neck trauma**

| Airway compromise | Circulatory compromise | Active bleeding |
|---|---|---|
| Tracheal deviation/stridor | Refractory shock | Expanding hematoma |
| Need for intubation | Evidence of cerebral stroke | Pulsative hematoma |
| Subcutaneous emphysema | Vascular bruit | Large hemothorax |
| Air bubbling in wound | Upper extremity ischemia | |

| **TABLE 5-4  Surgical exposure of the zones of the neck** | |
|---|---|
| **Zone** | **Surgical approach** |
| I | 1. Supraclavicular incision +/− removal of the head of the clavicle or<br>2. "Trap door" approach—supraclavicular incision, median sternotomy, and anterolateral thoracotomy |
| II | 1. Standard vertical neck incision along anterior border of SCM or<br>2. Transverse collar incision |
| III | 1. Cephalad extension of incision along anterior border of SCM +/− disarticulation or partial resection of the mandible +/− limited craniotomy |

penetrating neck trauma (see Table 5-4). While the number of indications varies from author to author, the hard signs can be grouped into three categories: a) evidence of airway compromise or injury b) evidence of circulatory compromise, and c) evidence of active bleeding. If any of these signs is present and the wound is in Zone II, the patient generally goes to the OR. If hard signs are present and the wound is in Zone I or III, an attempt to further characterize the injuries with ancillary testing prior to going to the OR is usually made to optimize operative planning. If none of these signs are present, the workup becomes more controversial and somewhat institution- and surgeon-dependent, as the sensitivity of the physical exam is variable. The options include laryngoscopy, bronchoscopy, esophagoscopy, esophagram, arteriography, noninvasive Doppler studies, CT scan, and in cases of asymptomatic Zone II injuries, observation alone. The general trend is toward less invasive techniques, and several high-volume centers are studying new algorithms to validate this.

### Blunt Neck Trauma

Motor vehicle crashes are the most common mechanism for blunt neck injury; however, patients can suffer "clothesline" or other direct injuries while riding snowmobiles, all-terrain vehicles, personalized watercrafts, motorcycles, and bicycles. While the general management principles for these injuries are relatively similar to that for penetrating trauma, there are different patterns of injuries, and the clinician does not have the benefit of a wound tract to assist in diagnosis. Thus, a full range of injuries, including c-spine fractures, should be considered. The workup of these injuries is still somewhat in flux; however, the preceding discussion regarding the workup of penetrating trauma can be broadly applied to blunt

trauma as well. Patients who have isolated neurologic deficits generally should undergo imaging since dissection of both the carotid and vertebral arteries is possible.

### Strangulation Injuries

The pattern of injury in strangulation and suicidal hanging, or near hanging, injuries is quite similar. It is important, however, to understand the difference between these injuries and complete hanging, or judicial hanging, in which the victim has a ligature around his or her neck and typically falls from a height that is equal to or greater than the body height. These patients typically suffer high cervical fractures, transecting the spinal cord, and leading to respiratory arrest. Patients who suffer near hanging injuries often fall from a lower distance, and cervical fractures are uncommon. In strangulation and near hanging the lethal injuries are carotid and internal jugular obstruction, in addition to airway occlusion. The patient experiences pain, then becomes unconscious and suffers brain damage secondary to anoxia.

It has been well documented in the literature that the majority of patients who survive attempted strangulation may not have any physical findings on neck exam, with a significant minority having only minor findings. Thus, the clinician should rely heavily on the history and seek out secondary signs of injury, such as presence of subconjunctival hemorrhages, facial petechiae, hoarseness, evidence of aspiration pneumonitis, or pulmonary edema secondary to forced inspiration against a closed glottis. There is also a risk of delayed encephalopathy from strangulation injuries that may progress to death. The workup is not well defined, but it is reasonable to start with a thorough physical exam, pulse oximetry, CXR, and then supplement that with fiber-optic examination of the larynx in patients who have complaints of voice changes or laryngeal pain. Neck CT angiography may be needed in some cases as well, although there is probably a low incidence of carotid injury from strangulation. Given the complex social situation of these patients, most will likely need to be admitted for neurologic checks, observation, and social services or psychiatry consultation.

## SPECIFIC INJURIES

### Pharyngoesophageal Injuries

While relatively rare in penetrating and blunt trauma, these injuries carry a significant mortality, which increases if the diagnosis is delayed more than 12 hours. There are no pathognomonic signs, but several symptoms and physical findings are suggestive (Table 5-5). Additionally, there have been strong suggestions in the

## LITERATURE REFERENCE

# Physical exam and CT in penetrating neck trauma

There have been a significant number of studies in the literature that have attempted to determine the sensitivity of the physical exam, especially for vascular injury, in penetrating neck trauma. Some of the studies report excellent sensitivity and negative predictive value for clinically significant injuries, while others call this into doubt. Many of these studies are plagued by the lack of objective criteria for a positive physical exam (e.g., extensive subcutaneous air versus subcutaneous air) and failure to define what constitutes a positive angiogram (e.g., an injury that alters management versus any abnormal finding). Finally, there is also some doubt as to whether or not patients with small injuries (e.g., intimal flap or psuedoaneurysm) should be anticoagulated, undergo endovascular repair, or just be observed. There does seem to be general consensus in the literature that the physical exam is severely limited in the detection of esophageal injury.

Given this debate and the fact that many trauma centers are attempting to make more efficient use of limited resources, there is much interest in seeing whether or not CTA of the neck can answer all of these questions. There are reports **[Gonzalez, et al. *J Trauma* 2003;54(1):61–64; discussion 64–65]** that CT offers no advantage over physical exam alone although these studies did not include more advanced CTA technology. Other reports **[Munera, et al. *Radiology* 2002;224(2):366–372]** have indicated the sensitivity and specificity of CTA of the neck is excellent and approaches that of angiography. As we gain more experience with mutltidetector scanners and approximating the track of wounds based on finding in the soft tissues on CT, we will likely be able to rely on this technology more and more. For now, however, even in institutions where CTA is the first-line study and the need for other studies such as esophagoscopy are based on the results of the CTA, patients are observed clinically for delayed complications or presentation of injury, despite a normal CTA.

literature that not all these patients are symptomatic. It should be noted that in penetrating trauma, there is a high coincidence of tracheal and esophageal injuries, implying that if one is suspected or found the other should also be sought.

The workup of these injuries remains in flux because there has not been an adequately large case series to evaluate the use of CT as compared to the traditional techniques of flexible esophagoscopy,

esophagram, and rigid esophagoscopy. The traditional techniques, when used in combination, are thought to have sensitivities approaching 100% but obviously are labor intensive and require that the patient undergo at least conscious sedation and, ideally, intubation. Therefore, in blunt trauma if the patient is awake and alert, exhaustive evaluation is done only if the patient is symptomatic or has secondary signs of esophageal injury, excluding isolated pneumomediastinum that is much more likely secondary to bronchial injury.

In penetrating trauma, a workup, either exploration or esophagram and esophagoscopy, is required if the wound is in close proximity to the esophagus. It is likely that as CT technology continues to improve, it will play a role in the diagnosis of both penetrating and blunt neck trauma: in penetrating trauma to determine the course of the wound and in blunt trauma to assess for secondary signs of esophageal injury (e.g., wall thickening, pleural effusion, periesophageal fluid). In any event, once esophageal injury is suspected, broad spectrum antibiotics including anaerobic coverage should be instituted while the workup is in progress.

| TABLE 5-5 Signs and symptoms of pharyngoesophageal injury | |
|---|---|
| **Signs** | **Symptoms** |
| Hematemesis | Dyspnea |
| Subcutaneous emphysema | Hoarseness |
| Blood in saliva | Odynophagia |
| Neck pain or tenderness | Cough |
| Reistance to passive neck motion | |
| Stridor | |
| Pneumomediastinum | |

## Laryngotracheal Trauma

Injuries to the larynx and the trachea can occur by both penetrating and blunt mechanisms. The main concern with these injuries is airway obstruction, which may be difficult to remedy because it is generally difficult for even experienced trauma surgeons to access the distal trachea rapidly enough to prevent cerebral hypoxia. Airway obstruction in blunt laryngotracheal trauma is of even greater concern in children, given the lack of cartilaginous calcification to help maintain a patent trachea.

The workup of these injuries is straightforward compared to that for pharyngoesophageal injuries. Injury can usually be determined by direct laryngoscopy or nasopharyngoscopy, with bronchoscopy being performed when more distal tracheal injuries are suspected (Table 5-6). Again, as technology evolves, CT will likely play a greater role in diagnosis of these injuries in both penetrating and blunt trauma, although currently its sensitivity is not adequate to obviate the need for bronchoscopy in most patients. Even in patients going for operative exploration, laryngoscopy should be done to assess the function of the vocal cords and thus potential injury to the recurrent laryngeal nerve, which lies adjacent to the trachea and

esophagus. Finally, laryngotracheal injuries are generally repaired operatively although luminal injuries involving less than one-third the circumference of the airway can be managed with close observation, voice rest, humidified air, prophylactic antibiotics, and follow-up bronchoscopy.

### Venous Injuries

The management of venous injuries is somewhat determined by the patient's stability. Given the proximal location of the vascular structures of the neck to the airway, bleeding from the jugular veins can significantly distort airway anatomy. Generally, operative intervention is dictated by the presence of hard findings on physical exam or CT scan findings as discussed previously. Prompt ligation is the rule for venous injuries in hemodynamically unstable patients.

### Arterial Injuries

Carotid artery injuries are more common in penetrating than in blunt trauma. Patients often present asymptomatically and then deteriorate later in the course. Also of importance, a significant percentage, 20% by some estimates, of blunt trauma patients will have no other significant injury. Although, the classic blunt mechanism is a direct blow to the neck, some series have shown that hyperextension injuries with rotation of the neck may be the most common cause. While angiography is technically still the gold standard, CT angiography is quickly gaining acceptance because it is less invasive, easier to perform, and more readily available around the clock. In patients with carotid artery injury, the best course of treatment is often determined by clinical status. A more aggressive approach to repair is indicated in patients who are still neurologically intact, while those who are comatose are managed expectantly. Most authors recommend anticoagulation, especially for cases of dissection, although there are no large studies to prove this is beneficial.

| TABLE 5-6  Signs and symptoms of laryngotracheal injury | |
| --- | --- |
| **Signs** | **Symptoms** |
| Bubbling in wound | Dyspnea |
| Dysphonia/aphonia | Neck tenderness |
| Stridor | Laryngeal/tracheal tenderness |
| Subcutaneous emphysema | Odynophagia |
| Hemoptysis | Pain with tongue movement |
| Bony crepitance | |
| Neck pain | |
| Laryngeal/tracheal pain | |
| Ecchymosis over thyroid cartilage | |

## LITERATURE REFERENCE

### Blunt carotid injury

In one the largest series on patients with blunt carotid injury (BCI), Biffl et al. collected a case series over 6 years and then prospectively identified patients for 3 more years in an effort to generate a classification scheme for these injuries that would also have prognostic and therapeutic implications **[Biffl et al. *J Trauma* 1999;47(5):845–853].** Their grading system is as follows:

1. Grade I: intimal flap with less than 25% luminal narrowing
2. Grade II: an intraluminal thrombus, raised intimal flap, a dissection, or intramural hematomas that compromised more than 25% of the lumen
3. Grade III: Pseudoaneurysms
4. Grade IV: vessel occlusions
5. Grade V: complete vessel transection with free contrast extravasation

During the prospective period of the study, they used digital subtraction angiography to actively screen patients who had any of the following risk factors for carotid injury:

1. Mechanism of severe cervical hyperextension/rotation or hyperflexion, (especially those resulting in patients with displaced midface, complex mandibular fracture, or closed head injury consistent with diffuse axonal injury)

2. Near hanging
3. Anterior neck soft tissue injury (e.g., seat belt abrasion) resulting in significant swelling
4. Basilar skull fracture involving the sphenoid or petrous bone extending into the carotid canal
5. Cervical vertebral body fracture

Although the overall incidence of BCI was 0.38% of blunt trauma admissions, the incidence during the screening arm was 1.07%. The majority (61%) of all their BCI were Grade I injuries; however, 3% of these led to stroke. Almost half of the patients had bilateral carotid injuries.

Only 1 patient required operative repair, although 14 patients with 18 injuries received endovascular stenting. Patients were anticoagulated with heparin if they had no contraindications, treated with antiplatelet agents and low molecular weight heparin if they had a relative contraindication to anticoagulation (e.g., solid organ injury or pelvic fracture), or no anticoagulation if they had a strong contraindication (e.g., intracranial bleeding). Of the Grade I injuries, 70% resolved with anticoagulation therapy compared with 63% without it. Of note, some injuries did progress when viewed on repeat angiography.

## KEY POINTS

- The neck contains a high density of vital structures that are relatively unprotected from external forces
- Management of penetrating neck trauma evolved from mandatory exploration to selective management
- Platysma violation defines superficial versus deep wounds
- Neck anatomy is divided into three zones with implications on management
  - Zone I—Clavicles to cricothyroid membrane
  - Zone II—Cricothyroid membrane to the angle of the mandible
  - Zone III—Above the angle of the mandible
- The neck also divided into anterior and posterior triangles
  - Carotid artery and the jugular vein located in space between these triangles

- All hemodynamically unstable patients go to OR regardless of zone of injury
- Zone II injuries with hard signs of injury go immediately for operative exploration
  - Stable zone II injuries without hard signs undergo ED workup for operative planning
- Zone I and III injuries with hard signs undergo ED workup if possible to guide surgical approach
- All patients with platysma violation are admitted for observation regardless of negative workup
- Consider blunt carotid injury in blunt neck trauma.
  - Concern is subsequent risk of stroke
- Strangulation injuries and near hanging involve primarily vascular and airway obstruction
  - C-spine injuries are rare

## PENETRATING NECK TRAUMA

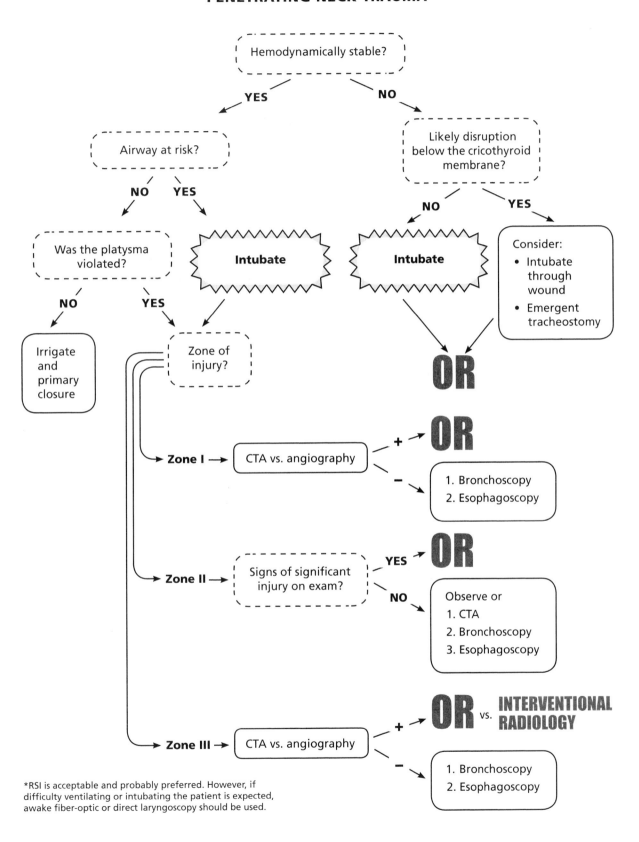

*RSI is acceptable and probably preferred. However, if
difficulty ventilating or intubating the patient is expected,
awake fiber-optic or direct laryngoscopy should be used.

# CHAPTER 6

# Cervical, Thoracic and Lumbar Spine Injuries

## CASE SCENARIO

A 48-year-old male presents to the ED with a chief complaint of neck pain after a motor vehicle crash that occurred the previous night. He was an unrestrained driver who slid across a patch of ice and struck a tree at about 40 mph. He was driving an older model vehicle without airbags. He sustained significant front-end damage but was able to drive away from the scene of the crash. He developed neck pain immediately after the accident, and it has persisted. His vital signs are normal, and he has no past medical history.

1. What is the first thing you do?
   a. Examine the patient and evaluate for midline c-spine tenderness
   b. Order a c-spine CT scan
   c. Order plain films of the c-spine
   d. Administer oral analgesics and discharge home with primary care physician follow-up

In this patient the ABCs are obviously intact, so the next step is to go to the secondary survey, which includes palpation of the c-spine. The fact that this patient sustained his injury the previous night should not lower your suspicion for serious injury. It is to your discretion whether or not the patient needs imaging of the c-spine and, if so, what type of imaging. Clinical decision rules have been developed to help decide who needs imaging. Factors that should influence you to obtain images include a major mechanism crash, significant midline cervical tenderness, significant pain with neck range of motion, intoxication or altered mental status, or abnormal neurologic exam or neurologic complaints. In many EDs, CT is replacing plain radiography for the evaluation of c-spine fractures in patients with a high suspicion for fracture.

Your examination reveals significant upper c-spine midline tenderness along with an obvious swelling above his left clavicle.

2. What is the next step in your management?
   a. Take the patient to CT scan immediately
   b. Administer oral analgesics
   c. Place the patient in a hard cervical collar
   d. Perform a detailed neurologic exam

Although neurologic sequelae of c-spine injuries can manifest immediately, they can be delayed as well. Additionally, all c-spine injuries, even those with potential for spinal cord impingement, do not automatically result in neurologic compromise. Therefore, if based on the mechanism and presentation, you are concerned enough, an appropriate imaging test should be ordered, and the c-spine should be protected.

3. In this patient, what is the most appropriate imaging modality to evaluate for c-spine injury?
   a. Plain radiographs
   b. Computed tomography
   c. CT myelogram
   d. MRI

Radiographs have a higher incidence than CT scan of missing osseous injury. In patients with concerning mechanism or clinical examination, those with altered mental status or concomitant injuries, it is best to proceed with a CT scan.    Answers: 1-a; 2-c; 3-b

## BACKGROUND

Cervical, thoracic, and lumbar spine injuries are common and can be devastating when the spinal cord is damaged as well. Although there is hope in the future for the ability to regrow CNS nerve tissue, currently spinal cord injury is essentially irreversible and permanent. In the acute setting, the emphasis is on making a diagnosis of spine fracture and spinal cord injury and preventing further neurologic compromise. The majority of spine injuries occur as the result of a blunt mechanism (MVCs and falls) and alcohol is often involved.

Spine trauma can result from injury by a number of mechanisms. In the c-spine, vertical compression, hyperflexion, hyperflexion with rotation, hyperextension, hyperextension with rotation, lateral bending, and distraction are all possible mechanisms. In the thoracolumbar spine, the main mechanisms of injury are flexion compression and flexion distraction. Injury can result from any of these mechanisms either alone or in combination. Having an understanding of the mechanism along with knowledge of the c-spine anatomy can help in the diagnosis of certain injury patterns.

## CLINICAL ANATOMY

The vertebral column consists of 7 cervical, 12 thoracic, and 5 lumbar vertebrae, with cartilaginous discs separating each vertebral body from its neighboring vertebra. The sacrum and coccyx technically contain five and four vertebrae respectively, but these are fused and not separated by intervening discs.

The spine must be simultaneously stable enough to support the body and flexible enough to allow intricate movements. The structure of the vertebrae varies throughout the spinal column, but the basic blueprint entails a *vertebral body* located anterior to the spinal cord, with a posterior arch (Figure 6-1). The arch is composed of two *pedicles* and two *laminae*. The laminae come together to form the *spinous process* in the midline, forming the posterior aspect of the spinal canal. A *transverse process* and an *articular process* extend off the anterolateral aspect of the arch. The transverse and spinous processes serve as sites for attachment of the muscles of the back. The articular surfaces (or facets) help provide flexibility needed for motion. The intervertebral discs, which are sandwiched in between the vertebral bodies, aid in absorbing vertical compression applied to the spinal column.

There is an intricate group of accompanying ligaments that also add stability to the spinal column. The *anterior spinal ligament* runs along the anterior aspect of the vertebral bodies, while the *posterior spinal ligament* runs along the posterior aspect of the vertebral bodies. The *ligamentum flavum* connects the laminae of the vertebrae. The *interspinal ligament* runs between the spinous processes, while the *supraspinal ligaments* extend posteriorly down the spine along the tip of the spinous process.

The guiding principle of spinal stability can be understood by conceptualizing the spine as three individual columns. The *anterior spinal column* consists of the anterior aspect of the vertebral body, the anterior spinal ligament, and the anterior half of the annulus fibrosis (intervertebral disc). These structures collectively resist extension forces. The *middle spinal column* consists of the posterior half of the vertebral body

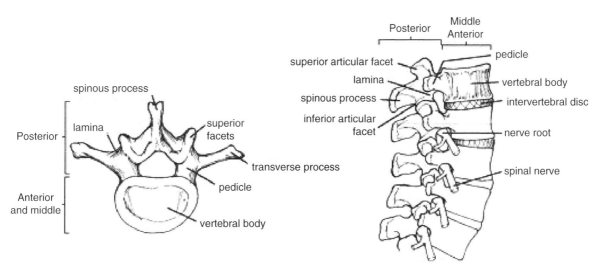

**FIGURE 6-1** Cervical vertebra and vertebral column

and annulus and the posterior spinal ligament. The components of the *posterior spinal column*, which together resist flexion forces, include the vertebral arch, the ligamentum flavum, the capsular ligaments, and the interspinous and supraspinous ligaments. Any injury in which two of the three columns are completely or partly disrupted is considered unstable.

## PRIMARY SURVEY

Spine injury should *always* be considered in the setting of trauma. It is well documented that a c-spine fracture may not always be obvious and can often be overlooked, especially in the presence of multiple injuries that distract from the c-spine. This is certainly true for thoracic and lumbar spine (TL spine) injuries as well. Therefore, a c-spine collar should be placed on all victims of blunt trauma where a c-spine injury is possible (Box 6-1). Additionally, patients should be maintained on log roll precautions until injury has been excluded. This is especially true for patients in high-speed MVCs, falls from greater than 6 feet, and those who are intoxicated, have altered mental status, neurologic symptoms, or painful distracting injuries (e.g., femur fracture). Suspicion should be even higher in elderly patients who often have osteoporotic bones and calcified cervical ligaments.

Although palpation of the c-spine is part of the secondary survey, gross assessment of neurologic function can be done at the end of the primary survey. In the ABCs, this can be considered D for disability. If conscious, the patient should be asked to squeeze both hands and to wiggle his or her toes. This is useful information because it is reassuring that no major spinal cord injury has occurred. In patients who have altered mental status or who are unconscious, withdrawal to pain in all four extremities should be assessed.

### BOX 6-1  How to protect your patient's spine

Cervical collars alone reduce flexion and extension movement but are inadequate to prevent lateral movement. All patients with the possibility of spine trauma must be placed on a long spine board to prevent secondary cord injury. Athletes wearing helmets and shoulder pads at the time of injury should be immobilized in their equipment (removal should occur after imaging has taken place). Moving a patient onto or off a spine board involves a log roll. One person maintains the head and neck in neutral position while at least two others gently roll the patient. The clinician holding the head and neck directs the others to avoid asynchronous movements.

## SECONDARY SURVEY

The secondary survey should include palpation over the entire spine for point tenderness. Extremities should be examined for strength and sensation. The best way to test sensation is to compare sharpness on both sides. The rectal exam is crucial in suspected spinal cord injury to assess for rectal tone and perianal sensation. The rectum is innervated by the lowest portion of the spinal cord, the S5 nerve root, via the pudendal nerve. Decreased rectal tone or sensation suggests spinal cord injury. Priapism is also seen in association with spinal cord injury. Also, in acute spinal cord injury, reflexes will be absent. Over time, reflexes will return and become hyperreflexic because of lack of inhibition from above. In the presence of spinal cord injury with paraplegia, it is important to assess the bulbocavernous reflex, as its absence precludes drawing conclusions about return of neurologic function, as explained later. During the secondary survey, it is important to log roll the patient and palpate the vertebrae along the entire length of the spine. Tenderness to palpation or the presence of a step-off raises concern for fractures and indicates the need for imaging. Unconscious patients with a significant mechanism should receive a CT scan of the head, c-spine, chest, and abdomen, stability allowing, with TL reconstructions to assess for vertebral fractures even in the absence of findings on physical exam. The patient should be kept on strict log roll precautions until the spine can be cleared both radiologically and clinically (requiring the patient to be conscious).

## IMAGING

Cervical imaging should be performed for cases involving high-mechanism accidents (e.g., high-speed MVCs, fall from greater than 6 feet), c-spine tenderness, significant pain, neurologic deficits, altered mental status or intoxication, or significant distracting injuries. There has been a great deal of effort to study the indications for c-spine films; however, the overall utility of plain films of the spine can be debated. An adequate c-spine series consists of three views: AP, lateral, and odontoid. The lateral must include the C7–T1 junction. If not, a swimmer's view is required, which is taken with one arm extended over the head and aimed through the axilla in order to see the C7–T1 junction. For the thoracolumbar spine, lateral and AP films are obtained if there is significant pain or tenderness.

Interpretation of the c-spine series is an important skill that can be remembered by the ABCs, which are also applied to interpreting the TL series as well (Table 6-1). A is for alignment. On an AP film, look at

## LITERATURE REFERENCE

# NEXUS and the Canadian c-spine rules

The question of whether imaging is relevant in patients who are stable, lack obvious neurologic deficits, and have not suffered major mechanism trauma is highly debated. Imaging all stable and alert patients, who complain of posterior neck pain regardless of mechanism, would result in millions of unnecessary and wasteful radiographs. The National Emergency X-Radiography Utilization Study (NEXUS) Low-Risk Criteria (NLC) and the Canadian C-Spine Rule (CCR) have been proposed as guidelines to determine which stable and alert trauma patients require plain radiographs (Tables 6-1 and 6-2). The results of these studies indicate that simple clinical criteria can be used to exclude fracture safely without imaging in many low-risk subjects. The CCR also identifies patients at high risk for c-spine injury. The CCR includes evaluation of range of motion as a final criterion in patients who could otherwise be cleared clinically. There have been attempts to compare the two decision rules. Results suggest that the CCR is superior to the NLC in terms of both sensitivity and specificity for c-spine injury—these decision rules pertain to the use of plain radiographs and do not address CT scanning **[Stiell, et al. *N Engl J Med* 2003; 349:2510–2518]**.

Stiell et al. conducted a prospective cohort study in nine Canadian EDs compare the two decision rules. The rules were applied by almost 400 physicians for patients before radiography was performed. Of the 8,283 patients studied, 169 of them had clinically significant c-spine injuries. After 845 patients were excluded from final analysis (range of motion was not assessed), it was shown the CCR was more sensitive than the NLC (99.4% versus 90.7%) and more specific (45.1% versus 36.8%). Furthermore, the use of CCR would have yielded a lower radiograph rate (55.9% versus 66.6%) **[Knopp et al. *Ann Emerg Med* 2004; 43(4): 518-520]**.

**TABLE 6-1   Things to look for on the c-spine series**

| | |
|---|---|
| AP | Alignment of spinous processes and lateral masses<br>Uniform intervertebral disc spaces<br>Cord foramen 10–13 mm |
| Lateral | Alignment of anterior and posterior margins of vertebrae<br>- Allowed C2–C3 subluxation of 3 mm in adults and 5 mm in children<br>Alignment of spinolaminar line and spinous processes<br>Examine each body, pedicle, lamina, and spinous process for fracture<br>Predental space <3 mm in adult and 5 mm in children<br>- Space between dens of C1 and vertebral body of C2<br>   Retropharyngeal space <6 mm at C2 and 22 mm at C6<br>- Larger in children, 1/2 to 1/3 the width of the vertebral body<br>Assure uniform vertebral body height, looking for compression fracture |
| Odontoid | Alignment of lateral masses of C1 and C2<br>Symmetrical spacing of lateral masses around dens<br>Look for dens fracture |

**TABLE 6-2   NEXUS versus Canadian low risk criteria to preclude imaging**

| NEXUS[a] | Canadian[b] |
|---|---|
| 1. No midline tenderness | 1. Absence of high risk factors |
| 2. Not intoxication |    Age <65 years |
| 3. Normal mental status |    Low mechanism |
| 4. No focal neurological deficits |    No extremity paresthesias |
| 5. No painful distracting injuries | 2. Factors that allow range of motion testing<br>   Simple rear end collision<br>   Sitting position or ambulatory<br>   Delayed onset of pain<br>   Nontender midline |
| | 3. Able to rotate neck<br>   45° each direction |

[a]All criteria must be met to avoid x-ray.
[b]Must meet all criteria in 1; meet any in 2 to move on to 3; and meet 3; otherwise x-ray required.

## LITERATURE REFERENCE

## Will you miss fractures with x-rays?

C-spine x-rays have traditionally been used to assess for c-spine fractures. The questions are: "How sensitive are the x-rays?" and "Will significant fractures be missed?" Griffen et al. looked at 1,199 trauma patients who received both a c-spine series (AP, lateral, odontoid, plus swimmer's view if C7–T1 not visualized) and CT scan. C-spine series missed 35% of fractures identified by CT scan, the majority of which needed only immobilization with a hard collar. However, nine patients required immobilization with a halo device, and three required surgery **[Griffen et al. *J Trauma* 2003;55(2):222–226; discussion 226–227].**

Spiral CT scan of the chest and abdomen with reformatting of the spine is now being used to diagnose TL fractures. Hauser et al. prospectively looked at 222 consecutive patients with high-mechanism trauma and an indication for TL imaging (point tenderness, neurologic deficits, and altered mental status), of which approximately 13% had a fracture. All patients were imaged with both plain films and CT. The sensitivity for CT was 97%, while that of plain films was only 58%. However, neither modality missed an unstable fracture **[Hauser et al. *J Trauma* 2003;55(2):228–234; discussion 234–235].** Sheridan et al. looked at more than 1,900 patients in the course of a year, 79 with thoracic and lumbar fractures. CT had a sensitivity of 95% and 97% (for thoracic and lumbar fractures, respectively) compared with a sensitivity of 62% and 86% for TL x-rays **[Sheridan et al. *J Trauma* 2003;55(4):665–669].** Traditional CT scan is not as sensitive in the diagnosis of compression fracture, but this has increased with reformatted images that provide a three-dimensional image.

the alignment of the spinous processes and lateral masses along the spine, and look for a vertebra that is not contiguous with the one above and below it. On the lateral c-spine x-ray, there are four regions of alignment: the anterior margin of the vertebral bodies, the posterior margin of the vertebral bodies, the spino-

laminar line, and the tips of the spinous processes (C2 to C7). B is for bones. It is important to have a systematic approach to looking for fractures, looking at each vertebral body, pedicle, lamina, and spinous process. The lateral view is the most sensitive for diagnosing fractures, with about 90% of fractures seen on this view. It is important, however, to closely examine the odontoid view for a dens or lateral mass fracture. C is for cartilage, which is evaluated by looking for uniform space between vertebral bodies. Reduced intervertebral space would suggest disc rupture. Finally, the S is for soft tissues. Inspecting the soft tissues is extremely important as it can give clues to a fracture that is otherwise not plainly apparent. The most common finding associated with fracture is retropharyngeal space swelling. The retropharyngeal space is easily visualized on the lateral x-ray, and it should be no more than 6 mm at C2 and 22 mm at C6.

CT scan is a superior modality to plain x-rays, and it should be utilized if there is a high suspicion for fracture or an abnormality on x-rays. In the past decade, CT has become universally available, and it should be used in patients with a high-mechanism injury, altered mental status, or neurological deficit. It should also be used in elderly patients in whom plain x-rays of the spine are usually abnormal and difficult to interpret because of normal degenerative disease of aging.

## MANAGEMENT

If adequate radiographic studies show no evidence of fracture and the patient has a normal neurologic exam, the patient should be re-examined with the intent to clear his or her neck and back, allowing him or her to have the collar taken off and to be removed from log roll precautions. For this to occur, the patient must have a normal mental status, no focal neurologic deficit, no distracting injury, and must be sober. If these criteria are met, then the collar can be removed while holding the patient's neck in manual midline stabilization. The c-spine vertebrae are individually palpated. If no tenderness is present, the patient is asked to look to the left and to the right (turning the head at least 45 degrees in either direction) and then to touch the chin to the chest and tilt the head backward. The patient's head should *not* be passively moved by the examiner. If none of this elicits significant pain, then the collar can be removed.

It is important to remember that even a normal CT scan does not exclude the possibility of ligamentous injury, with the subsequent possibility of neurologic compromise if not properly immobilized. Patients with severe cervical pain or tenderness require immobilization with a hard collar and follow-up within a week. If tenderness persists, then further imaging is indicated. Traditionally, lateral x-rays with the patient in flexion and extension (flexion–extension views) are obtained 1 to 2 weeks after acute injury. An abnormal gap between the anterior vertebral bodies (in extension) or the spinal processes (in flexion) suggest ligamentous injury, which would require long-term immobilization. An MRI is indicated acutely if there are neurologic deficits with or without acute fracture on CT scan. An MRI is also indicated for patients with abnormal flexion–extension x-rays at follow-up.

If a fracture is found on plain films, further workup is required. If the fracture is located in the c-spine, the entire c-spine should be imaged with CT, because there is a high rate of coincident fractures. Similarly, TL spine fractures seen on plain film also require a CT of at least the vertebrae in close proximity to the fracture. Next, the stability of the fracture and the presence of canal impingement by bone fragments should be determined (Table 6-3 and Box 6-2). If there is canal impingement or an unstable fracture, immediate consultation with a spine surgeon is warranted. If the patient has an isolated transverse process or spinous process fracture with a normal neurologic exam and without other injuries, they can be seen in close follow-up with a spine surgeon. Any patient with a stable cervical fracture should be discharged only in consultation with a spine surgeon with a hard collar and explicit follow-up instructions.

### Complete Spinal Cord Injury

A complete spinal cord injury is defined as total loss of motor function and sensation distal to the site of a spinal cord insult. Before making this diagnosis, several things must be considered. First, any evidence of minimal cord function, such as sacral sparing must be sought. *Sacral sparing* includes perianal sensation, normal rectal sphincter tone, or slight toe flexor movement. The presence of any of these indicates a partial cord lesion, and the patient has a chance for a marked improvement in function. Second, spinal shock can mimic a complete spinal cord lesion. *Spinal shock* is a result of concussive injury to the cord and results in a temporary loss of function distal to that site. Spinal shock can last up to 24 to 48 hours after injury. It should be considered in the absence of the bulbocavernosus reflex (Box 6-3). The return of this reflex after injury, typically within 24 hours, indicates that spinal shock

has resolved, and the prognosis for neurologic recovery can be better estimated. The use of steroids to improve outcome from spinal cord injury has undergone a good deal of scrutiny. There are several spinal cord syndromes that can result from traumatic injury, which are summarized in Table 6-4.

Aside from spine stabilization and prevention of further injury, there is little to do in the ED in regard to acute management for spine injury. It has become a standard of practice to administer high-dose steroids to acute spinal cord injury within the first 8 hours in hopes of improving neurologic outcomes. In theory, steroids can prevent secondary neuronal injury by inhibiting release of inflammatory mediators that result in local vasoconstriction and ischemia. This has been clearly demonstrated in animal models, but its utility in humans is an area of great controversy given the potential serious complications of high-dose steroids, and the questionable neurologic benefit.

### SCIWORA

In children and sometimes in adults, a syndrome referred to as spinal cord injury without radiographic abnormality (SCIWORA) needs consideration. As the name suggests, imaging does not reveal a vertebral fracture. During injury, the neck ligaments stretch, resulting in the cord stretching as well. This leads to neuronal injury and, in some cases, complete severing of the cord. Although symptoms may be present on arrival to the ED, up to one-third of these patients have a delayed onset of neurologic deficits. Symptoms may not develop until 5 days after injury. Thus it is important to warn parents to be alert for developing signs or symptoms. Most children with SCIWORA recover completely, especially those with delayed symptom onset.

### Neurogenic Shock

Neurogenic shock can result from severe spinal cord injury because of loss of vasomotor tone and lack of reflex tachycardia from disruption of autonomic ganglia. Classically patients will be hypotensive and bradycardic. Other sources of hypotension should be sought, however, because hemorrhagic shock is a much more common etiology of hypotension in the trauma patient. Neurogenic shock is usually mild and self-limited, responding to IV fluids alone. Occasionally, a peripheral vasopressor is required to restore vascular tone.

**TABLE 6-3 Spine fractures**

| Injury | Stability | Mechanism | Description | Radiographic findings | Treatment | Notes |
|---|---|---|---|---|---|---|
| Anterior subluxation | Stable | Hyperflexion | C-spine is hyperflexed and posterior ligamentous structures are disrupted | Widening of the spinous processes | Variable | Unstable if anterior ligament complex is disrupted |
| Clay shoveler's fracture | Stable | Hyperflexion | Avulsion of spinous process of lower cervical vertebrae (typically C7) | Avulsion of C7 spinous process | None | — |
| Wedge fracture (Compression fracture) | Stable | Hyperflexion | Most of force is absorbed by vertebral body with posterior ligament complex remaining intact | Diminished height and increased concavity of anterior border of vertebral body and increased density of body | Hard collar if >50% height loss, then surgical stabilization | Potentially unstable if vertebral body height decreased by >50% or multiple contiguous wedge fractures |
| Flexion teardrop fracture | Unstable | Hyperflexion | Fracture through the anterior–inferior aspect of a vertebral body with disruption of both anterior and posterior longitudinal ligaments | Teardrop-shaped fracture of inferior aspect of a vertebral body | Surgical reduction | — |
| Bilateral facet dislocation | Unstable | Hyperflexion | Disruption of ligamentous structures —>inferior articulating facets of the upper vertebra dislocate over the superior facet of the lower vertebra. Results in anterior displacement of superior vertebra | Vertebra is dislocated to at least 50% of its width | Surgical reduction | — |
| Chance fracture | Unstable | Hyperflexion | Posterior ligamentous tear, extending through spinous process and into vertebral body | AP: lucency on medial aspects of pedicles. Horizontal through tranverse process | Closed or open reduction | Occurs with MVC when passenger used only lap belt. High coincidence of bowel injury, especially in children. Highest incidence at L2, possible from T12–L4 |
| Atlanto-occipital dislocation | Unstable | Hyperflexion | Occiput is dislocated from atlas | Malalignment of occiput on C1 | Cervical traction | Traction is generally light and exact positioning depends on injury type; usually devastating injury |

*(continued)*

**TABLE 6-3** Spine fractures *(continued)*

| Injury | Stability | Mechanism | Description | Radiographic findings | Treatment | Notes |
|---|---|---|---|---|---|---|
| Unilateral facet dislocation | Stable | Flexion and rotation | Inferior facet on one side becomes displaced anteriorly | AP: spinous process will deviate Lat: vertebral body deviated <50% of its width. | Hard collar or halo; then surgical reduction | In thoracolumbar spine, vertical orientation of facets makes a fracture-dislocation more likely than isolated facet dislocation |
| Rotary atlantoaxial dislocation | Unstable | Rotation | Forced extreme rotational torque of C1 on C2, usually without flexion | Asymmetry of the lateral masses of C1 and odontoid process; unilaterally magnified lateral mass | Halo-vest; cervical traction | — |
| Avulsion of anterior arch of C1 | Unstable | Hyperextension | Avulsion of inferior aspect of anterior C1 arch | Lat: fracture fragment anterior/ inferior to C1 | Surgical stabilization | — |
| Posterior arch of C1 fracture | Unstable | Hyperextension | Posterior arch compressed by base of skull and C2 spinous process during forced extension | Odontoid: no lateral mass displacement. Lat: fracture through posterior elements | Varies depending on degree of instability | Fracture is relatively stable because anterior and middle column generally preserved but classified as unstable because of location |
| Hangman's fracture | Unstable | Hyperextension | Abrupt deceleration causing the skull, atlas, and axis (acting as a unit) to be severely hyperextended Results in bilateral pedicle fractures of C2 | Lat: fracture comes through pedicles of C2 with disruption of posterior cervical line; C2 on C3 anterior subluxation | Variable depending on degree of displacement | Cord injury not common with initial fracture because broken pedicles effectively decompress spinal canal Secondary cord injury possible |
| Extension tear drop fracture | Unstable | Hyperextension | Forced extreme extension causes anterior longitudinal ligament to avulse anterior-inferior aspect of the vertebral body | Variably-sized triangular bone fragment avulsed from base of one of the vertebral bodies | Hard collar | Most common in lower cervical vertebra; seen in diving accidents Potential for central cord syndrome |

*(continued)*

**TABLE 6-3 Spine fractures** *(continued)*

| Injury | Stability | Mechanism | Description | Radiographic findings | Treatment | Notes |
|---|---|---|---|---|---|---|
| Burst fracture | Stable | Vertical compression | Vertebral body shattered outward from vertical load with fracture fragments potentially compromising spinal canal | Lat: comminuted vertebral body, height loss AP: vertical fracture through body; loss of height | Surgical decompression if fracture fragments compromise canal, otherwise hard collar | Occurs in cervical and lumbar regions, which are capable of straightening on impact May result in anterior cord syndrome. |
| Oblique fracture | Stable | Vertical compression | Vertical compression results in oblique fracture line through vertebral body that may extend into the articular pillar | Lat: likely normal. AP: fracture line extending laterally on vertebral body | Hard collar | Fracture line may be vertical as well |
| Jefferson fracture | Unstable | Vertical compression | Occipital condyles compress articular masses of C1, fracturing anterior and posterior arches | Lat: widening of the predental space (>3 mm in adults and 5 mm in children) Odontoid: lateral displacement of lateral masses | Halo-vest (if minimally displaced can use hard collar) | May cause retropharyngeal swelling |
| Odontoid fracture | Type 1— stable Type 2— unstable Type 3— unstable | | Disruption of odontoid and stability of C1 on C2 | Odontoid view: Apical ligament avulsion Fracture through base of odontoid Fracture extends into body of C2 | Hard collar Halo-vest Halo-vest | — |

**BOX 6-2 Specific c-spine injuries from least to most stable**

- Rupture of transverse ligament of the atlas
- Odontoid fracture
- Flexion teardrop fracture
- Bilateral facet dislocation
- Hyperextension fracture dislocation
- Extension teardrop
- Jefferson fracture
- Unilateral facet dislocation
- Anterior subluxation
- Simple wedge compression fracture without posterior disruption
- Pillar fracture
- Fracture of the posterior arch of C1
- Clay shoveler's fracture

**BOX 6-3 The significance of the bulbocavernosus reflex**

Absence of the bulbocavernosus reflex indicates either spinal shock (reversible) or complete spinal cord injury (irreversible), and a prognosis cannot be made until this reflex returns. It is elicited by either squeezing the glans penis in a man or tugging on the Foley catheter in a woman. An intact reflex will result in contraction of the anal sphincter. In the setting of spinal cord injury, the return of this reflex heralds the end of spinal shock, at which time an assessment of permanent neurologic deficit be made. The duration of spinal shock is typically less than 24 hours.

## LITERATURE REFERENCE

 ## Should we be giving steroids to patients with spinal cord injury?

Administration of high-dose corticosteroids to spinal cord injury patients emerged as the standard of care in the past two decades. Based on animal data, which indicated that steroids improved functional outcome in spinal cord injury, the National Acute Spinal Cord Injury Studies (NASCIS I, II, and III) were undertaken to assess the ability of steroids to improve outcomes in human spinal cord injury. These studies compared various doses of methylprednisolone and other agents (e.g., tirlazad and naloxone) to see if any improvement in outcome could be detected. In brief, the investigators concluded that methylprednisolone (30 mg/kg bolus followed by 5.4 mg/kg for the next 24 hours) should be standard treatment within 8 hours of nonpenetrating spinal cord trauma to improve outcome **[Bracken et al. *JAMA* 1984;251(1):45–52; Bracken et al. *N Engl J Med* 1990;322(20):1405–1411; Bracken et al. *JAMA* 1997;277(20):1597–1604].** Although in many centers it is standard of care, this practice is highly controversial because of its questionable benefit in the face of serious adverse effects (e.g., GI hemorrhage, infection, or pulmonary embolism). A major criticism of NASCIS is that the small benefit reported is derived from subgroup analysis and not from the primary outcome of the study. Numerous studies have been designed to investigate the significance of the adverse outcomes associated with high-dose steroid use. Qian et al. studied eight patients with blunt spinal cord injury, five of whom received steroids per NASCIS protocol and three who did not. Muscle biopsy and electromyography showed evidence of muscle damage consistent with acute corticosteroid myopathy in four of five patients who received steroids. None of the patients in the nontreatment group had similar biopsy findings. This suggests that methylprednisolone per the NASCIS protocol may itself induce muscle dysfunction, and the small functional recovery proposed by NASCIS may actually be that from myopathy rather than recovery of spinal cord function **[Qian et al. *Spinal Cord* 2005;43(4):199–203].**

| TABLE 6-4  Partial cord syndromes | | | |
|---|---|---|---|
| **Syndrome** | **Mechanism** | **Exam findings** | **Notes** |
| Anterior cord | Compression or flexion | Loss of motor function, sharp pain, and temperature below level of injury<br>Proprioception, vibration sense intact | Minimal chance of return of function |
| Central cord | Hyperextension | Buckling of the ligamentum flavum into the cord —> contusion of the central portion of the cord.<br>Upper extremity motor deficit > lower extremity deficit | Most common partial cord syndrome<br>More than 50% of patients have return of bowel and bladder control, become ambulatory, and regain some hand function.<br>May present as quadrapelegia with sacral sparing |
| Posterior cord | Variable | Loss of proprioception and vibration sense with preservation of motor function, sharp pain, and temperature | Rare, prognossis generally good, but initially patients have difficulty walking because of proprioceptive loss |
| Brown-Sequard | Hemitransection | Loss of ipsilateral motor, vibration, and proprioception and contralateral pain and temperature sensation | Patients may make significant recovery |

**TABLE 6-4 Partial cord syndromes** *(continued)*

| Syndrome | Mechanism | Exam findings | Notes |
|----------|-----------|---------------|-------|
| Cervical root | Disc herniation<br>Facet dislocation | Isolated nerve root injury; deficit usually entails both sensory and motor function | – |
| Conus medullaris | Canal compromise | Injury located at T11–L1 clinically produces mixed upper and lower motor neuron findings; if isolated may present with loss of bowel and bladder function | Poor prognosis for meaningful recovery |
| Cauda equina | Canal compromise | Located from L1–L5; lower motor neuron deficit involving lumbar and sacral nerve roots<br>Bowel and bladder dysfunction, sensory loss | Prompt surgical treatment may result in good recovery |

## KEY POINTS

- C-spine structure and stability can be considered in three separate columns
  - *Anterior spinal column* from anterior longitudinal ligament to midway through vertebral body
  - *Middle spinal column* from midway vertebral body to posterior longitudinal ligament
  - *Posterior spinal column* from vertebral arches to interspinous ligament
- Disruption of two of the three columns typically constitutes structural instability
  - C1 and C2 fractures have higher likelihood for instability because of fewer supporting ligaments
- Spinal cord injury should always be considered in the setting of trauma
  - C-collar and log roll precautions until radiologically and/or clinically cleared
- Cervical imaging indicated in high-mechanism, midline tenderness or significant pain, neurologic deficits, altered mental status or intoxication, or significant distracting injuries
  - NEXUS and CCR are rules developed to identify patients who do not need imaging.
  - CT should be used if high suspicion, altered mental status, abnormal x-ray, or neurologic deficit
- Ligamentous injury can exist even in setting of normal radiographs or CT scan
  - MRI indicated acutely if neurological deficit or abnormal splaying between bones
  - Hard collar and follow-up in 1 week required for those with significant pain or tenderness

- Look for evidence of sacral sparing as this bodes well for return of function
  - Perianal sensation, intact rectal sphincter tone, or slight toe flexor movement
- Spinal shock precludes making conclusions regarding return of function
  - Return of bulbocavernosus reflex at 24 to 48 hours heralds resolution of spinal shock
- High-dose methylprednisolone is a recommended guideline but shrouded in controversy
- Neurogenic shock is hypotension and bradycardia because of loss of autonomic-mediated vascular tone
  - Usually responds to crystalloid resuscitation; vasopressors rarely required

# Chapter 7

# Blunt Thoracic Trauma

## CASE SCENARIO

A 17-year-old male is brought in by EMS after a head-on MVC in which he was the restrained driver. EMS reports that there was significant damage to the car, including steering wheel deformity. On scene the patient was awake and alert with a blood pressure of 100/50, heart rate of 120, respiratory rate of 28, and oxygen saturation 94% on room air. He has no medical history, takes no medications, and has no allergies. He had a large bore IV placed in the right antecubital vein and was immobilized with a c-collar on a long spine board. On arrival to the ED, his repeat vital signs are a blood pressure of 94/42, heart rate of 138, respiratory rate of 32, and oxygen saturation 96% on a nonrebreather (NRB) facemask.

He is answering questions and is alert; you notice a small laceration over the center of his forehead. His anterior neck appears normal, and the trachea is midline. He has cervical tenderness at the level of C4 to C5. He has a thoracic seat belt sign on his chest, his right chest wall moves paradoxically with inspiration, and he has subcutaneous air on the right. He has decreased breath sounds over the right chest and is tender over the sternum. His abdomen is not tender, and his pelvis is stable. He has palpable distal pulses and can move all extremities. He complains of right knee pain and is unable to flex it secondary to pain and swelling. There is an open wound extending across the joint.

The FAST exam is negative, and you order a trauma series. You now notice his oxygen saturation is 90% on an NRB, his repeat blood pressure 88/44, and he is clearly more tachypneic at 38 breaths per minute.

1. What is the next step in this patient's management?
    a. Intubate immediately for airway control
    b. Assess his trachea for midline positioning and repeat the FAST exam
    c. Place a chest tube on the right side in the fifth intercostal space
    d. Apply ice to his knee and encourage deep breaths to prevent secondary pneumonia

This patient has multiple signs of pneumothorax on exam . While it is not unreasonable to assess his trachea and perform a repeat FAST exam, this should not distract from his clinically apparent pneumothorax. Given that he is hypoxic and hypotensive, he may well be developing a tension pneumothorax on the right that requires immediate decompression. Tracheal deviation, while much talked about, is not frequently present in tension pneumothorax, and its absence certainly should not be used to exclude the need for an urgent chest tube.

After placing the chest tube, his hemodynamics improve somewhat. His CXR shows the chest tube to be in good position and a fully expanded right lung. His mediastinum is one-fourth the diameter of his chest at the level of the aortic notch. He has a right scapular fracture. The chest tube initially puts out approximately 800 cc of blood. A repeat blood pressure is 104/64 with a heart rate of 126 bpm.

Given the suspicion for a fractured sternum and the episode of hypotension, your chief resident tells you that this patient needs to go for an aortagram immediately.

2. Is this a reasonable plan?
    a. Yes, a sternal fracture clearly places this patient at risk for blunt aorta injury (BAI)
    b. Yes, chest trauma and circulatory shock make BAI likely
    c. No, a CT scan is adequate to assess aortic injury
    d. No, the patient should be taken directly to the OR given the degree of hemothorax

This patient clearly should not leave the department to get an angiogram. He had a large volume of blood from the chest tube and can decompensate quickly. While an aortic tear is on the differential, sternal and scapular fractures do not necessarily make it more likely that BAI is present. CT scan is generally considered the diagnostic test of choice when evaluating the aorta in a stable patient who needs to be evaluated for other injuries as well.

The patient is sent for CT scans of his head, c-spine, chest, and abdomen. The chest CT shows a small left-sided pneumothorax, multiple right-sided rib fractures, and underlying pulmonary contusion. Injection of his knee joint with methylene blue causes the blue fluid to leak from the laceration, indicating communication with the joint. Orthopedics is consulted because this patient will need to go to the OR for a joint wash-out. In addition, an x-ray of the right knee shows a displaced tibial plateau fracture. His chest tube has now put out a total of 1,000 cc, and his blood pressure is 110/70.

3. What is the next step?
   a. STAT echo to evaluate for cardiac contusion
   b. Placement of a left chest tube
   c. Send cardiac enzymes to evaluate for myocardial injury
   d. A thoracostomy to identify the source of thoracic bleeding

A chest tube should be placed on the left because this patient will receive positive-pressure ventilation in the OR. Myocardial contusion can occur with blunt chest trauma and can cause tachycardia and decreased cardiac output. Great lengths to make this diagnosis are unnecessary unless the patient has unexplained hypotension. There is no specific treatment for myocardial contusion, although an inotropic agent (e.g., dobutamine) may be required to augment cardiac output if hypotension is present.

As the patient is getting prepared for the operating room, your junior resident wants to know if you want the patient to receive continued prophylactic antibiotics to prevent pneumonia.

4. What is your response?
   a. Yes, given his pulmonary contusion he is at high risk for pneumonia
   b. No, there is no role for prophylactic antibiotics in patients with lung contusions
   c. No, but he should undergo bronchoscopy daily for pulmonary "clean-outs"
   d. Antibiotics should be started in 24 hours if repeat CT scan shows worsening contusion

There is no role for prophylactic antibiotics in the patient with a pulmonary contusion. Care is supportive, including oxygen, hydration, and physical therapy with incentive spirometry. Antibiotics are indicated for this patient for the laceration that communicated with his joint space.

Answers: 1-c; 2-c; 3-b; 4-b

## BACKGROUND

Chest trauma, including both blunt and penetrating, accounts for up to a quarter of all trauma deaths. For the purposes of this chapter, we define blunt chest trauma as any injury to the thoracic cage, front or back, that does not result in a missile or other object entering the thorax. Motor vehicle accidents are the most common mechanism. The severity of injuries seen in blunt chest trauma is quite variable, for example, the rare case of blunt esophageal rupture (Box 7-1), but even seemingly minor injuries can have significant complications (e.g., isolated rib fractures in an elderly patient). Although death in the field can occur with

---

**BOX 7-1  Blunt esophageal rupture**

Blunt esophageal rupture is quite uncommon and thus has not been well studied; however, it is clear that when this injury is unrecognized, it is usually fatal. This is largely because the esophagus lacks a serosal covering, allowing rupture anywhere along its course to seed the mediastinum with bacteria and oral and gastric secretions. While the mediastinal pleura initially contains the rupture, the resulting inflammatory response rapidly breaks down this barrier. The negative intrathoracic pressure generated by respiration then spreads the esophageal contents across the thorax. As with Boerhaave's syndrome, the weak wall of the left posterior distal esophagus is generally the site of rupture.

blunt chest trauma, those patients who survive to the ED have a good chance of survival. As such, many of the injuries we will discuss will be diagnosed early in the primary survey since they are part of the B and C of the ABCs. Furthermore, significant blunt chest trauma is usually associated with abdominal injuries and, therefore, one should strongly consider aggressive workup for potential abdominal pathology in patients who have significant blunt chest trauma.

## CLINICAL ANATOMY AND PHYSIOLOGY

The thorax is unique in that it is designed to expand and contract constantly from birth to death, undergoing changes in volume that are not seen anywhere else in the body. Additionally, it houses multiple critical organs and blood vessels. Thus, it must be both flexible and sturdy, allowing the organs within it to function freely yet still be relatively sheltered from injury. When the thorax is disrupted by trauma, physiologic changes take place that alter its function and can result in distress.

The flexibility and strength of the chest wall are products of the costal facet joints, whereby the ribs articulate with the vertebral column. Anteriorly the ribs are continuous with the costal cartilages that are inserted into the sternum. This provides an encompassing shield around the heart and lungs that expands as the ribs articulate superiorly during inspiration. When part of the chest wall moves abnormally, such as in flail chest, severe derangements in the physiology of breathing can result, leading to problems with oxygenation and ventilation. The heart, being so well shielded, is in fact vulnerable to force applied anteroposteriorly, which can cause compression between the sternum and vertebral column and result in myocardial contusion or rupture.

## PRIMARY SURVEY

Significant chest trauma will often be apparent in the primary survey as it will likely impact breathing and circulation. The most important aspects of the primary survey in blunt chest trauma are auscultation while watching for symmetrical rise and fall of the chest wall, chest palpation, and vital signs. The anterior neck should also be quickly visualized for swelling, tracheal deviation, or distended neck veins. The latter would indicate either tension pneumothorax or pericardial tamponade. Breath sounds are often difficult to hear in the trauma bay; therefore, close attention must be paid for signs of respiratory distress such as tachypnea or labored breathing. Palpation during the primary survey should involve placing both hands over the anterior chest and

---

> ### BOX 7-2 Antibiotics after chest tube placement
>
> There is extensive literature on this topic; however, there is still a large amount of controversy regarding whether or not it is necessary to administer prophylactic antibiotics to patients who receive a chest tube. If the chest tube is placed under controlled conditions with proper attention to sterile technique, antibiotics are probably unnecessary. If the tube is placed emergently under less ideal conditions, it is probably reasonable to give a single dose of a first generation cephalosporin, such as cephazolin (Ancef). It seems unlikely that more than a single dose is useful in any of these cases.

feeling for crepitus, flail segments, or points of significant tenderness. A more thorough exam should be saved for the secondary survey. Vital signs can indicate circulatory shock or hypoxia, both of which should raise the concern for significant chest trauma.

Two questions answered during the primary survey are: Does this patient need intubation? and Does this patient need a chest tube? Intubation should be performed immediately in the setting of respiratory distress, hypoxia, or circulatory collapse. A quick assessment of the need for tube thoracostomy is also necessary, as intubation and positive-pressure ventilation can turn a simple pneumothorax into a tension pneumothorax. In the setting of acute respiratory distress with a suspicion for chest trauma, chest tubes should be placed as the patient is being intubated. It will usually be apparent as to which side to place the tube based on chest wall contusion, flail segment, crepitus, or decreased breath sounds. If the patient is deteriorating quickly, intubation with bilateral chest tubes should be performed. See Box 7-2 regarding antibiotic administration after chest tube placement.

The FAST exam in blunt chest trauma is important for detecting a pericardial effusion that may indicate myocardial injury and impending pericardial tamponade. The experienced eye can also gauge cardiac output or global cardiac function. Additionally, ultrasound can be used to detect a significant pneumothorax or hemothorax. In a supine patient, this can be evaluated by placing the probe in the midaxillary line at the level of the sixth through eighth ribs or just below the nipple line. Air or blood will be seen as a black stripe outside the lung parenchyma.

## IMAGING

### Trauma Series

The CXR of the trauma series for blunt trauma is typically obtained with the patient in the supine position, and thus a small pneumothorax may be difficult to see because the extrapulmonary air will track anteriorly, allowing the lung to expand to the margins of the chest wall. In some cases, a pneumothorax will only be visible as a deep sulcus sign in which the costophrenic angle is long, narrow, and pointed. Additionally, there may be evidence on x-ray of subcutaneous emphysema, which suggests a possible occult pneumothorax or other injury to the aerodigestive system. Another important finding on AP CXR is unilateral haziness of an entire lung, which indicates layering of blood behind the lung (i.e., hemothorax). It is also important to look at the mediastinum, which on the AP view should not be more than one third the diameter of the chest. Important but often forgotten is to look at the bones, specifically looking for rib, scapula, or clavicle fractures. Keep in mind, however, that the portable CXR is not sensitive for thoracic injuries, and further workup should be obtained if the suspicion is high.

### CT Scan

A CT scan should be obtained for patients with a significant mechanism along with chest pain, tenderness, or abnormal vital signs, provided of course that the patient is hemodynamically stable. Studies have shown that CT is not only superior diagnostically, but it also alters management in a significant number of patients. This is especially true when the CXR is abnormal but not diagnostic. A chest CT is probably most useful for evaluating the aorta and detecting other mediastinal injuries, as mediastinal structures are difficult to evaluate otherwise. CT scan detects injuries that are often not apparent by plain radiography, including pulmonary contusions, rib, or sternal fractures, or pneumo- or hemothoraces. Furthermore, CT scans also provide detail of the thoracic spine and the cervical–thoracic junction that is far superior to that of plain radiography.

### EKG

Some trauma centers obtain routine EKGs on all major trauma patients. While this test does not often change management, it is cheap, easy, and quick. There have been several case reports of blunt chest trauma inducing coronary artery occlusion leading to myocardial infarction; albeit they are rare. More commonly, trauma and the resulting catecholamine surge can induce myocardial ischemia in elderly patients. In patients with multiple medical problems, an EKG may provide information about medications to be avoided (e.g., haloperidol in patients with a prolonged QT interval). An EKG can also provide clues to certain drug overdoses (e.g., prolonged QT or QRS intervals in TCA overdose). Therefore, it is prudent to obtain an EKG in patients with significant trauma, altered mental status, or who complain of chest pain.

## MANAGEMENT

The crucial question after initial stabilization in the management of blunt chest trauma, as in all trauma, is whether the patient needs to go to the OR. Injuries specific to thoracic trauma that require operative care include aortic tears and significant hemothoraces (more than 1,000 cc initially or persistent output of 200 cc per hour with hemodynamic compromise). For stable patients, time can be spent in the ED characterizing the extent of injury (e.g., obtaining CT scans or other studies). Specific thoracic injuries will be covered from outside to inside, including chest wall, pulmonary, and cardiac injuries. Aortic injuries are covered in a separate chapter that is really an extension of the discussion of blunt thoracic injury (see Chapter 9).

### Injury to the Chest Wall

Chest wall injuries themselves may not be life-threatening, but they are an indicator of significant underlying injury. Given that the chest wall functions as a respiratory bellows in addition to its function of protecting vital organs, it is no surprise that chest wall injury can have a significant effect on breathing. The most dramatic example of this is in *flail chest* where multiple consecutive ribs (at least three) are fractured in at least two locations, resulting in a mobile segment of chest wall that moves paradoxically with inspirations (as the chest expands in inspiration creating negative intrathoracic pressure, the flail segment is sucked in). In addition to extreme pain, this injury will result in respiratory compromise, and the majority of these patients will require intubation. Even if the patient seems to be managing initially, the high incidence of underlying pulmonary contusion will likely lead to worsening respiratory status as the lungs become more edematous and lung compliance decreases.

Seemingly simple injuries, such as isolated rib fractures or contusions, can be significant because of splinting. Splinting refers to the inability to take a deep breath because of pain. This is especially a problem in the elderly or in those with underlying pulmonary disease, who have a high likelihood of developing pneumonia. Some of these patients may even warrant admission overnight for observation, pain control, and incentive spirometry to maintain lung expansion. When sending a patient home with a rib fracture, it is important to emphasize deep breathing, at least once per hour, to prevent atelectasis and secondary pneumonia. It is also important to discharge patients with adequate narcotic analgesia to prevent splinting. Incidentally, a former practice of chest taping or braces has fallen out of favor as it tends to prevent deep breathing. See Box 7-3 regarding other fractures to consider in the thorax.

**BOX 7-3 Ribs are not the only bones in the chest that can break**

In addition to ribs, fractures of the clavicle, sternum, and scapula must be considered in blunt thoracic trauma. Clavicle fractures are usually seen with a fall onto the shoulder, (e.g., a fall from a bike) and are less common in MVCs. They typically occur at the junction of the middle and distal thirds of the clavicle, and they require no specific treatment other than a sling. Injury to the underlying subclavian artery and vein should be considered for depressed fractures or those sustained during high-speed MVCs. Sternum fractures are not uncommon, especially in unbelted drivers in MVCs where direct impact with the steering wheel is sustained. Other than causing significant pain, sternum fractures require no specific treatment, but they should raise the suspicion for underlying cardiac contusion or aortic injury. A sternum fracture, however, should not necessarily mandate the search for these injuries as studies have never shown a clear association between the two. Scapular fractures require a high-energy mechanism and are usually associated with other injuries. It was previously believed that a scapular fracture should mandate the search for aortic injury, but this dogma has been refuted. Fractures to the body of the scapula are most common, although fractures to the acromion or coracoid process, scapular spine, and glenoid fossa are possible as well. A thorough neurovascular exam should be performed on the ipsilateral arm to look for associated brachial plexus or axillary arterial injuries, especially with injury of the acromion process. Management for scapular fractures is usually conservative.

## Pulmonary Injury

Lung injuries consist of either lacerations, causing a pneumothorax or hemothorax, or contusions. A simple pneumothorax is common with blunt chest injury and is defined as a pleural air collection without mediastinal shift or communication outside the chest wall. A pneumothorax is most often the result of isolated alveolar rupture because of the surge of intrathoracic pressure associated with injury. Less commonly, a pneumothorax can be the result of laceration from a penetrating rib fracture or tracheobronchial disruption. The decision about whether to place a chest tube is clinical (based on respiratory effort, rate, and oxygen saturation), and not necessarily based on its size on x-ray. However, the bigger the pneumothorax, the less likely it is to spontaneously re-expand with oxygen therapy alone. It is common practice to place a chest tube in patients who are mechanically ventilated regardless of the size of the pneumothorax, given the risk of tension pneumothorax with positive pressure. Other methods of decompressing a pneumothorax have been used with varying success, including placement of a pigtail catheter and other smaller, less invasive means. The problem with these methods is that they are ineffective in draining a hemothorax, which is often associated with a traumatic pneumothorax. A small, asymptomatic pneumothorax can simply be observed overnight while the patient receives supplemental oxygen (results in high blood oxygen saturation that promotes reabsorption of nitrogen-rich pneumothorax).

After a chest tube is placed, it is hooked to a suction device that utilizes a reservoir of water to detect air being drawn from the thoracic cavity through the chest tube (causing bubbling in the reservoir), indicating an air leak internally. If this air leak is large, tracheobronchial injury should be suspected, and bronchoscopy is indicated. Smaller air leaks can result from pulmonary lacerations, an inadequate seal between the tube and the chest wall, or leaks in the tubing connections or apparatus.

Pulmonary contusions are more insidious, being more difficult to diagnose, and can be more difficult to manage. A pulmonary contusion is a blunt injury to pulmonary parenchyma that results in cellular damage, capillary leak, and alveolar exudates. This injury can be detected by a nondistinct haziness on CXR that will often initially appear innocuous and then "blossom" several hours after injury. Symptoms will include respiratory difficulty, tachypnea, and decreased oxygen saturation due to the V/Q mismatch that occurs with pulmonary exudates. Pulmonary contusions are clearly seen on chest CT, which can demonstrate the size of the contusion. This is useful information in predicting the patient's course, as large contusions invariably result in respiratory compromise requiring intubation and mechanical ventilation. Treatment for pulmonary contusions is supportive with close attention paid to respiratory effort, especially in elderly patients. Aggressive pain control, avoidance of overhydration, and chest physical therapy are all recommended. This is important given the high incidence of pneumonia. Prophylactic antibiotics are not recommended for patients with pulmonary contusion.

## Blunt Myocardial Injury

While any significant blunt chest trauma can cause blunt myocardial injury, most cases result from high-speed MVCs. Given its more anterior position, the right ventricle is more frequently injured than the left. There is a spectrum of blunt cardiac injury, with the most benign form being cardiac contusion and the most fatal being cardiac rupture. Injuries can include those to heart valves, traumatic coronary artery occlusion or dissection, or traumatic rupture of the chordae tendinae. Blunt cardiac rupture is usually lethal on impact, but there are case series in the literature describing patients surviving to ED arrival with septal or free wall ruptures. Given a patient in extremis after blunt thoracic trauma, this diagnosis can be made during the primary survey in the presence of circulatory shock, distended neck veins, and pericardial fluid on FAST exam. This should prompt immediate transfer to the OR for open thoracotomy or ED thoracotomy if the patient loses vital signs en route or on arrival to the ED. However, the outcome for patients with traumatic arrest following blunt trauma is generally grim.

More often cardiac contusion will be a consideration in the ED for patients with blunt thoracic trauma. There is no way to definitively make this diagnosis, and there is frankly no treatment; therefore, it is a clinical diagnosis with debatable significance. Pathologically, it involves contused myocardial tissue, cell damage, and exudates into the myocardium (essentially a bruise of the myocardium). The result can be decreased cardiac output, tachycardia, and, less commonly, arrhythmias (Box 7-4). Myocardial dysfunction is typically transient, and most patients make a full recovery without specific intervention. Rarely, a cardiac contusion can result in myocardial dysfunction to the degree that cardiac out-

put is compromised. Trauma patients in circulatory shock should first be assumed to have hemorrhage, pericardial tamponade, or tension pneumothorax. Cardiac contusion can be considered after these have been ruled out. Dobutamine, a β-receptor agonist, can be used to augment myocardial contraction in this case.

---

**BOX 7-4  Complications of cardiac contusion**

- Arrythymias
- Conduction abnormalities
- Cardiogenic shock
- Ventricular wall rupture
- Valvular insufficiency
- Ventricular aneurysm (late complication)
- Constrictive pericarditis (late complication)
- Ventricular arrythmias from scar tissue (late complication)

---

## LITERATURE REFERENCE

 ## Do we need to diagnose or observe blunt cardiac injury?

There have been a myriad of studies attempting to determine which patients with blunt chest trauma can be sent home without extended observation for possible cardiac injury. It would seem logical that cardiac biomarkers (e.g., CPK, CK-MB, and TnI) could be used to look for cardiac injury, just as they are in the patient with suspected acute coronary syndrome. However, early studies that looked at the use of CPK and CK-MB showed that these biomarkers are neither sensitive nor specific for cardiac contusion as defined by echocardiography. Many are looking to TnI, given its known sensitivity and specificity for myocardial infarction.

Bertinchant et al. looked at 94 consecutive patients with blunt chest trauma and no symptoms referable to blunt cardiac injury. They underwent serial enzyme evaluation, EKG, and echocardiography. Twenty-six patients ultimately were diagnosed with blunt cardiac injury by echocardiography. CPK, CK-MB, and CK-MB index were not shown to correlate with the presence of cardiac injury. TnI and TnT were associated with myocardial injury but had very low sensitivities. The specificity of troponins was nearly 100%, meaning

that a negative troponin assured lack of myocardial injury. However, given the lack of sensitivity, a positive troponin result added little to the evaluation **[Bertinchant et al. *J Trauma* 2000;48(5):924–931].**

On the other hand, Salim et al. found that serial TnI measurements were quite useful in conjunction with serial EKGs. When both tests were abnormal, the positive predictive value was 62%; and, if both were normal, the negative predictive value was a 100% **[Salim et al. *J Trauma* 2001;50(2):237–243].** A subsequent study looked at 333 patients with blunt thoracic injury, and it showed that clinically significant cardiac contusion is excluded with a normal EKG and TnI at 0 and 8 hours **[Velmahos et al. *J Trauma* 2003;54(1):45–50; discussion 50–51].** Based on this, it can be argued that the standard algorithm for high-energy mechanism thoracic trauma (e.g., ISS > 15, steering wheel deformity, or associated thoracic injuries such as pulmonary contusion, flail chest, and hemothorax) should include a period of observation with cardiac monitor, serial EKGs, and TnI measurements.

## LITERATURE REFERENCE

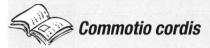 *Commotio cordis*

*Commotio cordis* (also referred to as myocardial concussion by some authors) is an episode of ventricular fibrillation, that is triggered by an innocent-appearing chest blow that leaves no evidence of external chest trauma or evidence of cardiac injury on autopsy. This condition seems to occur most frequently in children and adolescents, but it has been reported in patients up to age 50. The mechanism entails a direct blow to the chest centered over the cardiac silhouette and must occur during a vulnerable aspect of the cardiac cycle just prior to the peaking of the T-wave. Approximately 85% of these patients will not have a return of spontaneous circulation, although early defibrillation seems to improve outcomes **[Maron et al. *J Am Coll Cardiol* 2005; 45(8):1371–1373].**

It seems reasonable to develop an algorithm that identifies patients at risk for complications (e.g., arrhythmias requiring treatment) from cardiac contusion. The first question is whether symptoms such as tachycardia or hypotension are because of blunt cardiac injury, as discussed previously. The second question is whether asymptomatic victims of high-mechanism thoracic trauma are at risk for complications of blunt cardiac injury and require observation or a workup for this. It is certainly reasonable to obtain a 12-lead EKG to look for evidence of myocardial ischemia and to keep the patient on a cardiac monitor. However, it is well established that significant cardiac arrhythmias are extremely rare after the first minutes of the injury, as occurs in *commotio cordis*. A common practice is to obtain cardiac enzymes and use positive results as an indication to admit a patient for observation or to obtain echocardiography. The utility of this practice has never been scientifically validated. Similarly, the role for echocardiography in the management of suspected cardiac contusion is also unclear, with the exception of blunt thoracic trauma, circulatory shock, and no clear reason other than possible cardiac injury.

## KEY POINTS

- The anatomy of the thorax plays important protective and physiological roles
  - Armor for heart, lungs, and great vessels
  - Mechanical bellows for respiration
  - Maintains negative intrathoracic pressure that facilitates cardiac venous return
  - The heart is the source of all forward blood flow
  - The lungs provide a mechanism for blood oxygenation
- Injury to the thorax can affect any of these vital functions
- B and C of the primary survey are critical in thoracic trauma
  - Intubate if inadequate ventilation
  - Chest tube if respiratory difficulty and any evidence of pneumothorax or hemothorax
  - Large-bore IVs and crystalloid resuscitation, followed by type O blood if in shock
- FAST exam to evaluate pericardium for potential tamponade
  - May require pericardiocentesis or thoracotomy if unstable
- Trauma series CXR to evaluate mediastinum and lungs
- Chest CT if stable and potential for significant injury, especially aortic injury
- Flail chest will compromise ventilatory function, often requiring intubation
- Pulmonary contusions will compromise tissue oxygenation
- Elderly with simple rib fractures are at high risk for pneumonia
- Myocardial contusion should be considered in high mechanism
  - May initially cause arrythmias, but most typically sinus tachycardia
  - Usually of little clinical significance
  - Normal EKG at 0 and 8 hours essentially exclude this diagnosis
  - May result in decreased cardiac output, rarely requiring dobutamine

# CHAPTER 8

# Blunt Abdominal Trauma

## CASE SCENARIO

A 32-year-old restrained driver who struck a telephone pole at about 55 mph is transported to the ED. He had reportedly fallen asleep at the wheel and veered off the road. He has no recollection of the accident and complains of discomfort in the right lower chest region that is worse when he breathes. His pulse is 126, blood pressure 86/50, respiratory rate of 28, and oxygen saturation 92% on oxygen. The primary survey reveals an intoxicated man with a patent airway, normal neck anatomy, equal bilateral breath sounds, and palpable femoral pulses. Two large-bore IVs are quickly established, and normal saline is started through both. On secondary survey, he is extremely tender over the 9th to 12th ribs on the right side; you feel crepitus. He has mild RUQ tenderness without guarding or rebound. The focused abdominal sonography in trauma (FAST) exam shows no obvious free intraperitoneal fluid. After the first liter of fluid, a repeat blood pressure is 84/48.

1. What is the next most important step?
    a. Obtain a trauma series
    b. Expedite transport to CT scan
    c. Type and cross 4 units of PRBCs immediately
    d. Place a right-sided chest tube

This patient is tachypneic, hypotensive, and hypoxic. Given his right-sided tenderness and crepitus, he likely has a right-sided hemothorax or pneumothorax, despite the fact that his breath sounds are equal. This diagnosis cannot wait for a confirmatory x-ray given the patient's instability. It is appropriate to order 4 units of PRBCs after placing the chest tube. In fact, uncrossmatched blood should be obtained for a trauma patient who is persistently hypotensive after a rapid 2 L fluid bolus.

A right-sided chest tube is placed with return of 600 cc of blood. You hook up the chest tube kit to an autotransfuser to recycle the blood. A trauma series is obtained that shows right-sided rib fractures, the chest tube ending in the superior aspect of the lung, and a small residual pneumothorax. The pelvic x-ray is normal. In the meantime you administer a unit of uncrossmatched blood.

2. What type of blood should be used?
    a. Type A, Rh−
    b. Type B, Rh+
    c. Type O, Rh−
    d. Type O, Rh+

Type O blood is universal donor blood, and it will not result in transfusion reactions in type A, B, AB, or O recipients. Women of childbearing age should receive type O, Rh− (type O−) blood in order to prevent development of anti-Rh antibodies in case they are Rh−. If this is the case, then any future pregnancy is in jeopardy if the fetus is Rh+. Men and older women can and should receive type O, Rh+ (type O+) blood.

The chest tube has not drained any more blood, and a second unit of blood is being transfused. Repeat vitals include a pulse of 112, blood pressure 100/62, respiratory rate of 20, and oxygen saturation of 98% on oxygen. He still complains of severe right-sided pain.

**3.** What is the most appropriate next step?

 **a.** Obtain CT scan of head, c-spine, and abdomen
 **b.** Obtain CT scan of abdomen only
 **c.** Perform diagnostic peritoneal lavage (DPL) given hypotension
 **d.** Repeat FAST exam

Given that his vital signs have improved with the chest tube and administration of blood, he can now be transported to CT scan. The FAST exam can also be repeated, but even a positive finding in the setting of improving hemodynamic status would not discourage from obtaining a CT scan to characterize the injury. Given his intoxication and scalp contusion, a CT scan of the head and c-spine should also be done. The CT scan of the abdomen reveals a liver laceration with hemorrhage into the hepatorenal recess. He is taken to the OR for an ex-lap.

Answers: 1-d; 2-d; 3-a

## BACKGROUND

The abdomen is notorious for hiding significant injury in blunt trauma. For this reason, the abdomen is a major focus when evaluating blunt trauma victims. The abdomen contains solid vascular organs (e.g., spleen and liver) that when lacerated can lead to significant intra-abdominal hemorrhage. The abdomen can hold 2 to 3 liters of blood or up to half the circulating blood volume. Missed diagnosis of intraperitoneal blood can be lethal; therefore, the detection of free intraperitoneal blood is the primary objective in the evaluation of blunt abdominal trauma. This can be accomplished via the FAST exam, DPL (in grossly unstable patients), observation and serial abdominal examinations (in low-risk patients), or CT scanning.

## PRIMARY SURVEY

An abdominal exam is not part of the primary survey, but it is a major focus of the secondary survey.

### BOX 8-1   Focused abdominal sonography in trauma (FAST) exam

Ultrasound has emerged as an integral part of traumatic evaluation. Its primary objective of detecting free intraperitoneal blood or fluid is accomplished by the focused abdominal sonography of trauma (FAST). This examination includes views of Morrison's pouch, the pouch of Douglas, the splenorenal recess, and the pericardium. Ultrasound is portable and thus can be performed in the trauma bay simultaneously with evaluation of the patient. Additionally, it is noninvasive, can be performed within a few minutes, and does not deliver ionizing radiation. Essentially, it allows a quick determination of whether hemoperitoneum is present. Its main disadvantages include the fact that it is operator-dependent, limited by body habitus and overlying bowel gas, and likely will not identify solid organ parenchymal damage if there is no associated free fluid.

The abdomen should be considered when assessing vital signs. Tachycardia or hypotension should prompt a search for blood loss, and the abdomen is a common source in blunt trauma. The FAST exam is performed by a member of the trauma team shortly after the primary survey is completed. Its primary purpose is to detect free intraperitoneal blood (Box 8-1).

## SECONDARY SURVEY

The abdominal exam occurs during the secondary survey and can provide important clues to injury. In the setting of hypotension or critical injury, visible contusions or abdominal distention can be evidence of significant intra-abdominal blood. In this case, a FAST exam or DPL should be the priority in order to make a diagnosis of hemoperitoneum. The physical exam should focus on the presence of tenderness, guarding, or rebound. A rigid, tender, abdomen with rebound is itself an indication for ex-lap. It should be remembered that low anterior chest tenderness may signify rib fractures with underlying liver or splenic injury. Bowel sounds are of little use in the exam for trauma. The presence of gross blood in the stool should prompt a workup for an abdominal injury as well.

## MANAGEMENT

### Consider Mechanism

Mechanism must be considered when deciding how aggressively to work up potential intra-abdominal injury. The most common mechanism for this injury is an MVC. It is useful to talk with EMS personnel about the mechanism of the crash (e.g., head-on, rear-end, or T-bone) and the degree of vehicular damage (e.g., amount of driver's side intrusion, bending of the steering wheel, or broken windshield). Evidence of a significant mechanism should always prompt a thorough evaluation for abdominal injury.

Other injuries should also influence the suspicion for significant abdominal injury. For example, pelvic or femur fracture should prompt investigation of abdominal injury. Likewise, a mechanism forceful enough to cause broken ribs or a pneumothorax can also cause splenic or liver injury. Trauma patients with altered mental status because of head injury or intoxication require thorough evaluation of the abdomen, typically with a CT scan when the mechanism is concerning.

Alternatively, consider isolated intra-abdominal injury in patients who receive direct blows to the abdomen. An example is a sports injury such as football or soccer, where the injury is a helmet or shoulder blow to the abdomen. Falls onto hard objects can also cause isolated splenic or liver lacerations. It is important to realize that ambulatory patients who otherwise look well can still have significant intra-abdominal injury.

### Let the Vital Signs Guide the Workup

Patients with evidence of shock may require early aggressive operative management. Hypotensive trauma patients in extremis are often otherwise young, healthy patients, and hypotension in these patients is usually a precursor to death. There is no time to take these patients to the CT scanner. If the FAST exam reveals hemoperitoneum, the hypotensive patient should be taken to the OR for exploratory laparotomy. If the FAST exam is negative, a source of hypotension must be sought. Common sources include hemothorax, hemoperitoneum, retroperitoneal bleeding, pelvic fractures, and femur fractures. Even in the setting of a negative FAST exam, hemoperitoneum must be considered, as its sensitivity is low for free blood volumes of less than 500 ml.

For unstable patients with a negative FAST exam, a diagnostic peritoneal lavage (DPL) should be considered. This procedure involves placing a catheter into the peritoneal space and aspirating for blood or intestinal contents (Box 8-2). The first step is aspiration of free peritoneal fluid; if gross blood or gastric contamination is recovered, the procedure is complete. Aspiration of 10 ml or more of blood is highly suggestive of intraperitoneal injury; some studies cite a greater than 90% positive predictive value with this amount of aspirate. In the absence of hemoperitoneum, the peritoneal cavity is instilled with 1,000 ml of normal saline and then allowed to drain back out. This fluid is sent to the lab for cell count. A yield of greater than 100,000 RBCs per ml in lavage fluid is considered positive for intraperitoneal injury in the setting of blunt abdominal injury. Unstable patients with evidence of intraperitoneal injury require exploratory laparotomy.

---

**BOX 8-2 Procedure—diagnostic peritoneal lavage (DPL)**

Always prep the infraumbilical area with Betadine and prepare a sterile field. Anesthetize the area using lidocaine with epinephrine. A *closed DPL* involves inserting a needle two finger-breadths below the umbilicus. A guidewire can then be inserted into the abdomen and the peritoneal lavage catheter inserted over the guidewire. The catheter should be directed inferiorly toward the pelvis to place the tip in the retrovesicular space. The problem with this method is the risk for bowel perforation with the needle. An *open DPL* is done with a vertical skin incision one third the distance from the umbilicus to the symphysis pubis. Alternately, patients with pelvic fractures or pregnant patients should have the incision made supraumbilically. The linea alba is identified, pulled up, and divided. The peritoneum is then entered directly through a small incision in the peritoneal lining, through which the catheter is placed. Many employ the *semi-open DPL*, in which an incision is made down to the linea alba, which is then knicked with a scalpel. Pulling the tissues up, a trocar, through which the DPL catheter is threaded, is used to pop through the peritoneal lining. After completing the procedure, the fascia and skin can be reapproximated with sutures.

---

Patients who are hemodynamically stable are generally safe to go for CT scan. The major advantage of CT scan is its high-definition image of intraperitoneal and retroperitoneal organs. It is sensitive in detecting hemoperitoneum and solid organ injury. It is also sensitive for detecting extraluminal free air, which is indicative of hollow organ injury. Despite its superior characteristics, injuries to the small bowel, mesentery, diaphragm, and pancreas may be missed with CT scan. An IV contrast is often administered, which increases sensitivity for detection of solid organ, bowel wall, and vascular injury. A concern with IV contrast administration is acute renal failure, and its use should be withheld if the creatinine level is greater than 1.5. Special caution should also be taken with elderly patients or those with comorbidities such as diabetes and hypertension.

CT scan should not be delayed for the administration of oral contrast. The addition of oral contrast helps evaluate the bowel wall and can increase sensitivity in demonstrating bowel rupture with extravasation of contrast or duodenal hematomas. Oral contrast is not necessary for the detection of solid organ injury, free intraperitoneal blood, or retroperitoneal injury. In centers where oral contrast is administered, the scan should still be done emergently, as the contrast only needs to be in the proximal digestive tract. It is important to realize that CT scan is not a perfect test; and, despite a normal reading, the patient still may have bowel wall contusion, a small hollow organ perforation, or diaphragmatic injury (Box 8-3). This emphasizes the importance of

---

**BOX 8-3  Pancreatic and duodenal injuries can be insidious**

Diagnosis of retroperitoneal injury can be difficult. A high index of suspicion based on mechanism of injury is critical in detecting these injuries. Pancreatic injuries occur in the setting of rapid decelerating and falls from heights. There are no radiographic or laboratory findings that conclusively support pancreatic injury. Amylase elevation may result from injury to a number of organs, including small bowel and ovaries. These injuries may initially be completely asymptomatic, and initial CT scan may be normal as well. Symptoms may develop days later as leakage of enzymes from the injured organ results in autodigestion. Duodenal injuries may also be asymptomatic early on. Duodenal wall hematomas can result in gastric outlet obstruction, producing abdominal pain with vomiting. Duodenal injuries are often caused by rapid increases in intraluminal pressure, as with high-speed vertical or horizontal decelerating trauma.

---

**BOX 8-4  Simplified grading system for blunt liver and spleen injuries**

The traditional grading systems for liver and spleen injuries are difficult to remember, and hence the variation in grading used by different physicians. At our institution, a slightly simplified system, based on the grading system established by the American Association for the Surgery of Trauma, is used to make communication easier and standardized.

Grade I: less than 1 cm laceration or less than 10% subcapsular hematoma

Grade II: laceration 1 to 3 cm or subcapsular hematoma 10% to 50% of the surface

Grade III: more than 3 cm laceration or more than 50% hematoma

Grade IV: hilar laceration

Grade V: total damage (macerated or avulsed)

---

observation and re-examination when the mechanism is significant or when the physical exam is concerning.

## SPECIFIC INJURIES

### Stomach and Small Bowel Injuries

Gastric perforations that occur in blunt abdominal trauma are usually accompanied by significant intra-abdominal soilage, leading to peritoneal signs on exam. Small bowel injuries can also be picked up on exam. Although it is not sensitive enough to exclude small bowel injury, the presence of a seatbelt sign (ecchymosis across the lower abdomen) increases the odds of having a small bowel injury fivefold. CT scan is not sensitive for identifying these injuries. Thus, patients with a negative CT scan but good mechanism for hollow viscous injury and persistent abdominal tenderness, should be admitted for serial exams. Pancreas and retroperitoneal duodenal injury can also pose a diagnostic challenge (Box 8-3).

### Solid Organ Injuries

Of the solid organs of the abdomen, the liver and spleen are the most likely to be injured in blunt traumatic mechanisms. In general, grading systems are used to describe the amount of damage to solid organs. While there are multiple grading systems for the liver, spleen, and kidneys, the basic system outlined in Box 8-4 is a good rule of thumb. The trend in blunt solid organ injury is toward nonoperative management, with the main indications for ex-lap being hemodynamic instability despite appropriate resuscitation or peritonitis. The threshold to operate on splenic

injuries is generally somewhat lower than that for liver injuries; the spleen can be removed to stop bleeding, whereas the liver can only be packed or cauterized, with lobar resection rarely, if ever, performed. Angiography with embolization is another method that should be considered in patients with suspected arterial injuries to these organs.

---

**LITERATURE REFERENCE**

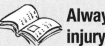 **Always consider diaphragmatic injury**

Diagnosis of diaphragmatic injury is often delayed. This can result in morbidity and even mortality for the patient. This delay is primarily because of the limitations of imaging to identify an injury. The right hemidiaphragm is protected by the ivier, hence the left hemidiaphragm is injured three times more frequently. The most common presenting symptom is nonspecific abdominal pain. Both CT scan and ultrasound have poor sensitivities for detecting this injury. Laparoscopy is often necessary to make the diagnosis. As MRI use is becoming more widespread, its ability to accurately diagnose diaphragmatic injury is being studied. Barbiera et al. performed a retrospective review studying the CT, x-ray, and MRI findings of patients diagnosed with diaphragmatic injury after blunt abdominal trauma. In all cases, MRI revealed both site and size of the rupture. Its sensitivity surpassed that of CT scan **[Barbiera et al. *Radiol Med (Torino)* 2003;105(3):188–194].**

## LITERATURE REFERENCE

## Can most solid organ injuries be managed nonoperatively?

It is clear that unstable patients with intraperitoneal blood because of solid organ injury generally require operative repair. Nonoperative management, however, has been established for patients who are hemodynamically stable. The question remains as to which stable patients require an operation regardless. Several studies have established that blood transfusion requirement is an independent predictor for required surgery in the setting of blunt solid organ injury. Velmahos et al. performed a prospective observational study at a high-volume Level I trauma center to determine if grade of injury dictates the need for operative intervention. Doctors offered 78 patients nonoperative management for liver injury, regardless of grade. Patients with hemodynamic instability or concomitant hollow viscous injury were excluded. Of those, 23 patients were operated on immediately but only 12 because of their liver injuries. Of the remaining 55 patients, 8 patients eventually required surgery but none because of liver injury. The authors concluded that nonoperative management of liver injuries is safe and successful regardless of grade in the setting of hemodynamic stability

[Velmahos et al. *Arch Surg* 2003;138(5):475–480; discussion 480–481].

The presence of a contrast blush on CT scan has been associated with an increased failure rate of nonoperative management for blunt splenic injury. Thus, several studies have examined the role of angiography and embolization in the nonoperative management of splenic injuries. Dent et al. performed a retrospective review to test the hypothesis that including selective splenic arteriography and embolization in the nonoperative management algorithm for blunt splenic injuries results in higher success rates. They compared all 168 patients with findings of splenic injury over a 24-month period at a Level I trauma center to the data from a previously published series from the same institution that studied 251 patients. The current group had a higher success rate for nonoperative management of their splenic injuries (82% versus 65%, $p < 0.01$). They concluded that selective use of arteriography and embolization in patients with blunt splenic injury is a useful adjunct to nonoperative management [Dent et al. *J Trauma* 2004;56(5):1063–1067].

## LITERATURE REFERENCE

## Is splenic contrast blush significant in children as well?

It is always said that children are not just small adults. Therefore, the management of abdominal solid organ injury in this population has been investigated and compared to treatment of similar injuries in adults. The issue of contrast blush in the presence of splenic injury on CT scan has been the focus of a number of studies in children. Lutz et al. performed a review of 133 children with blunt splenic injury in a 4-year time period at a Level I pediatric trauma center. A single radiologist retrospectively

reviewed all CT scans to confirm grade of injury and the presence or absence of contrast blush. They found that the contrast blush was associated with higher grades of splenic injury but did not necessarily require embolization or surgical intervention. This is in contrast to the significance of splenic blush in adults. Management should be determined based on physiological response to injury rather than specific radiographic findings [Lutz et al. *J Pediatr Surg* 2004;39(3):491–494].

## KEY POINTS

- Abdominal organs are at high risk in blunt trauma because of lack of shielding
  - Solid organs (liver and spleen) can tear and cause significant intraperitoneal bleeding
- The peritoneal cavity can hold 2 to 3 L of blood
- Circulatory shock should prompt a search for intraperitoneal free blood
  - FAST exam is sensitive for detecting 500 cc or more of blood
- Hollow organs (bowel, bladder, and gallbladder) can rupture because of increased pressure
  - Spilled bowel contents will result in peritonitis
- Unstable patients with peritonitis or a positive FAST exam require immediate ex-lap
- DPL is useful for unstable patients with a negative FAST exam and no other obvious source of injury
- CT scan is indicated for stable patients where there is a suspicion for injury
  - Abdominal tenderness, even in the setting of seemingly minor trauma
  - High mechanism but altered level of consciousness (unreliable exam)
  - Useful in visualizing abdominal and retroperitoneal injuries
  - Not sensitive for bowel wall contusion, hollow organ perforation, or diaphragmatic injury
- There is a role for conservative observation for stable intraperitoneal injuries

# BLUNT ABDOMINAL/PELVIC TRAUMA

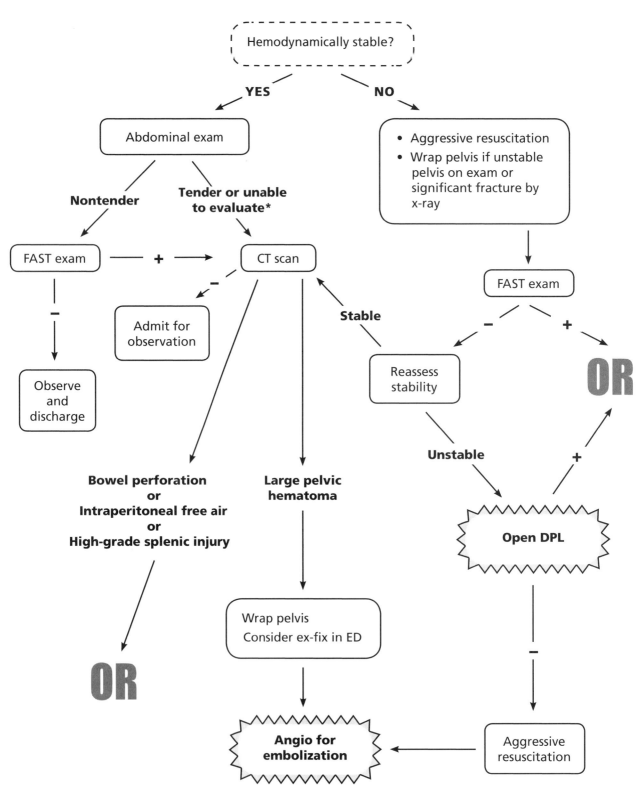

*Unable to evaluate if:
- Altered mental status
- Severely intoxicated
- Intubated and sedated
- Distracting injury

# CHAPTER 9

# Aortic Injury

## CASE SCENARIO

An 18-year-old male is brought to your trauma center via EMS after the front end of his car was crushed by the rear wheels of a tractor–trailer truck that swerved into his lane on the highway. He underwent a prolonged extrication and was transiently hypotensive in the ambulance. On arrival his vital signs include a pulse of 120, blood pressure of 110/58, respiratory rate of 22, and oxygen saturation of 100% on a nonrebreather mask. He is able to talk and complains only of pain in both his legs. The primary survey is unremarkable except for weak femoral pulses bilaterally. The secondary survey is remarkable for a large laceration across his anterior left ankle with exposed bone but minimal active bleeding, and a deformed lower leg with an open fracture. Two large-bore IVs are obtained, and the patient is placed on oxygen by a facemask.

1. What is the next priority in management?
   a. Call an orthopedic consultant to take patient to the OR for open fractures
   b. Obtain a trauma series
   c. Intubate the patient for airway control
   d. Clinically clear the patient's c-spine

Based on mechanism of injury, high-speed MVC with rapid deceleration, the concern for a life-threatening injury is high. Once the ABCs are addressed, the next step is to obtain a trauma series in the bay. This is to assure there are no major injuries that need to be addressed before the patient leaves for CT (e.g., displaced cervical fracture, pneumothorax, or unstable pelvic fracture). At this time the patient is alert, cooperative, hemodynamically stable, and maintaining his airway; therefore, intubation is not necessary. His orthopedic injury will require a wash-out and reduction in the OR; however, the focus now should be on other potentially life-threatening injuries. The c-spine should not be cleared at this point clinically because of the distracting orthopedic injury; the c-spine must be imaged.

The trauma series shows no cervical fracture, a normal mediastinum with a distinct aortic knob, clear lung fields, and no evidence of pelvic fracture. A FAST exam is performed in the bay, which is normal.

2. Which statement describes your concern for a potential blunt aortic injury (BAI)?
   a. Relatively reassured given the distinct contour of the aorta on CXR
   b. Relatively reassured given the combination of normal mediastinal width and the normal position of the trachea and bronchi
   c. Moderate level of concern, but given his stablility, workup can be conducted after other injuries are treated
   d. Moderate level of concern given mechanism and transient hypotension in field

While findings on x-ray can be suggestive of BAI, a normal CXR can in no way rule out the diagnosis. The specificity of finding a displaced trachea or left mainstem bronchus on chest x-ray is greater than 90% for BAI. However, the sensitivity is less than 10%, meaning that this finding is present in only 10% of cases of BAI. Alternatively, the presence of a widened mediastinum on CXR has about 90% sensitivity for aortic injury. However, the specificity is not that great, meaning that many portable x-rays will show an apparently wide mediastinum where no aortic injury exists. Additionally, given the pulse differential between upper and lower extremities, the suspicion for BAI should remain high. The mortality for this injury is 30% at 6 hours of presentation, if untreated.

**3.** You decide that the patient needs further evaluation for BAI. What is your next diagnostic test?
   **a.** OR thoracoscopy
   **b.** CT angiogram of the chest
   **c.** Aortogram
   **d.** Transesophageal echocardiography (TEE)

While this is a topic of some debate, most clinicians would agree that this patient needs a CT angiogram first, especially in Level I trauma centers where new generation multidetector scanners are often available. Before CT with angiographic capabilities, aortography was the standard for diagnosing BAI. The problems with aortography are that it requires the patient to leave the ED, and it does not provide information about other structures in the chest. TEE is an alternative diagnostic modality for patients who are too unstable to go to CT. TEE would typically be done in the OR to evaluate the aorta while other injuries are being stabilized (e.g., ex-lap to repair a liver or splenic laceration).

Answers: 1-b; 2-d; 3-b

## BACKGROUND

The aorta is the most commonly injured great vessel in blunt trauma. It is responsible for 10% to 20% of MVC-related deaths. These injuries are often misclassified as "traumatic aortic dissection," a condition that is actually quite rare. This term refers to a separation of the media along the length of the aorta, similar to a spontaneous aortic dissection. Blunt aortic injury (BAI) includes aortic transection and aortic rupture. Aortic transection is a circumferential, full-thickness laceration of the aorta; these patients are usually dead at the scene. Aortic rupture refers to a partial laceration of the aorta. The injury usually occurs at the level of the ligamentum arteriosum, which anchors the aorta to the mediastinum, but injuries can occur in any part of the aorta. Greater than 90% of patients with BAI die at the scene. Patients who survive to hospital presentation usually have ruptures that are contained within the adventitia, the outermost layer of the aortic wall. If not diagnosed early, the prognosis for these patients is poor.

## MECHANISM

The classic mechanism of BAI is a head-on motor vehicle collision in which there is a rapid deceleration creating enormous shear forces on the aorta. However, there is literature evidence to suggest that up to half of BAIs occurs in side-impact or T-bone collisions. Any other mechanism that creates a rapid deceleration (e.g., fall from greater than 30 feet, blast injuries, or pedestrian struck by a car) can cause BAI. Finally, there are multiple reports of BAI after minor trauma, so it is important to always keep this diagnosis in mind.

More specifically, there are multiple hypotheses as to how the aorta is actually damaged. First, the aorta is anchored around the level of the ligamentum arteriosum to the posterior wall of the thorax by the intercostal arteries and paravertebral connective tissues, and thus it is less mobile than other structures, such as the heart, to which it is directly attached. As such, a force that tears these structures away from the aorta can induce injury. Second, the aorta may be compressed by the anterior thorax, resulting in a direct injury. Finally, the aorta may experience a pressure surge from either thoracic or abdominal compression, generating high enough wall stress to cause rupture—the so called "water-hammer" effect. The high incidence of injury at the level of the ductus (or isthmus) may be because of inherent weakness of the aorta in this area or to pre-existing tension placed on this section of the aortic wall by the ductus.

## PRIMARY AND SECONDARY SURVEYS

The key to diagnosis begins with suspicion of injury in the context of an adequate mechanism. There is no pathognomonic sign of BAI, and the physical exam findings are neither sensitive nor specific. While some findings are suggestive of aortic injury (e.g., asymmetry between leg and arm blood pressures or pulses and intrascapular murmur), the absence of these findings in no way excludes BAI. The presence of chest or back pain along with hypotension should cause significant concern for this diagnosis. A good deal is made in surgical lore of concurrent injuries that put the patient at higher risk for BAI. The bottom line is that there appears to be no foolproof algorithm to identify all patients at risk for BAI.

**LITERATURE REFERENCE**

## Are other injuries reliably associated with BAI?

1) Scapular fractures **[Brown et al. *Am Surg* 2005;71(1):54–57]**
   - Retrospective 10-year review of 35,541 blunt trauma admissions
   - Scapular fracture in 1.1% and BAI in 0.6%
   - Only 1% (4/392) patients with scapular fracture had BAI
   - Scapular fracture was associated with rib fractures and extremities fractures but not BAI
2) First rib fracture
   a) **Gupta et al. *Cardiovasc Surg* 1997;5(1):48–53**
      - Retrospective review of 730 cases
      - Three percent incidence of vascular trauma if nondisplaced, increased incidence with displaced fractures
      - Presence of first rib fracture with other injuries (head, thoracic, abdominal, or long bone fractures) increased risk of vascular injury to 24%
   b) **Kirshner et al. *Ann Thorac Surg* 1983;35(4):450–454**
      - Study examined association of first and second rib fractures with BAI
      - Patients with BAI equally likely to have no rib fractures, any rib fracture, or first and second rib fractures
   c) Multiple other studies from the early 1980s, most with similar results failing to show an association between isolated first rib fracture and BAI
3) Sternal fractures
   a) **Swan et al. *J Trauma* 2001;51(5):970–974**
      - Ten-year retrospective review of deceleration thoracic injuries
      - Major injury defined as myocardial contusion, BAI, tracheobronchial disruption, flail chest, or sternal fracture
      - Out of 142 MVC patients, 6 of whom had more than one major injury and 33 had BAI, none had both BAI and sternal fracture.
   b) **Hills et al. *J Trauma* 1993;35(1):55–60**
      - Retrospective review of 12,618 trauma patients, of whom 172 had sternal fractures
      - None of these patients had BAI
      - Twenty-two patients seen over same period with BAI, none had sternal fracture

**Trauma Series**

The trauma series CXR should be closely examined for signs of a mediastinal hematoma, which would suggest aortic injury (Box 9-1). The classic sign for aortic injury is a widened mediastinum, defined as greater than one-fourth the width of the thorax or 8 cm at the level of the aortic arch. The aortic knob should also be inspected for distinctness of its borders. Other x-ray findings suggestive of mediastinal hematoma include left-sided apical pleural cap, pleural effusion, and displacement of the trachea, left mainstem bronchus, or NG tube. Therefore, while a CXR will be obtained in all of these patients, it cannot be used to include or exclude the diagnosis of BAI.

The diagnosis of BAI has changed significantly in the past 10 years with the advent of the multidetector CT scanner. The previous gold standard was the aortogram, which entailed taking the patient to an angiography suite, catheterizing the patient through a femoral artery, and injecting dye at the root of the aorta to assess for irregularities in blood flow and aortic anatomy. The disadvantages of this are that a potentially unstable patient must go to the angiography suite, expert angiographers (radiologists) must be available to perform and interpret the test, and the test itself is invasive and carries its own risks.

**BOX 9-1  CXR findings found with BAI**

- Widened mediastinum—greater than one-fourth the width of the thorax
- Indistinct aortic knob
- Left-sided apical pleural cap
- Left-sided pleural effusion
- Displaced trachea
- Displaced NG tube
- Displaced left mainstem bronchus

**TABLE 9-1  CT scan to diagnose BAI**

| Findings | Clinical implication |
|---|---|
| 1. Normal aorta | Aortic injury is excluded |
| 2. Mediastinal hematoma with preservation of the fat plane surrounding the aorta | Aortic injury is excluded |
| 3. Mediastinal hematoma abutting the aorta | Patient needs aortogram |
| 4. Aortic transection | Patient needs immediate operative intervention |

CT angiography is now the standard for diagnosis of BAI in most large trauma centers. It has been shown to have essentially 100% sensitivity and specificity for detecting aortic injury. In contrast to aortography, it provides information about other intrathoracic injuries (e.g., pulmonary contusions, pneumothorax, rib or sternum fractures, and thoracic vertebral column injuries). It is also much less expensive and readily available in the EDs of most Level I trauma centers. Interpretation of various CT results are listed in Table 9-1.

TEE is an alternative modality to making the diagnosis of BAI and can be used in patients who are too unstable to undergo CT angiogram. Its sensitivity to detect BAI is about 85% to 90%, and it is somewhat operator-dependent. The patient must be sedated for the procedure and optimally should be intubated. Hypertension can occur if the patient is not fully sedated, which can exacerbate aortic injury. It also poses a risk for patients with c-spine injury. Despite these disadvantages, it can be useful in unstable patients who are taken to the OR for other injuries (e.g., intracranial hemorrhage, massive hemothorax, or hemoperitoneum) and who are suspected of having aortic injuries as well.

## MANAGEMENT

Management of BAI in the ED, until the patient can be taken to the OR for definitive repair, should focus on reducing the pressure impulse imparted on the injured aorta by systolic cardiac output. Although no randomized control trials have studied the question, it is generally accepted that the main goal is to minimize the change in pressure per unit of time on the aortic wall (dP/dT), hence minimizing wall stress over time. This is accomplished by controlling both heart rate and blood pressure by first using β-receptor blocking agents, followed by nitrates if necessary. Ideal agents for this purpose are esmolol and nitroprusside (Nipride), given their short duration of action. Therefore, if the patient becomes hypotensive, which is common in the setting of blood loss and multisystem trauma, the medications can be turned off with no lasting effects. It is important to avoid using nitroprusside alone, because nitrates cause pure vasodilation with a resulting reflex tachycardia. Therefore, a beta-blocker must always be started first to prevent reflex tachycardia.

IV crystalloid administration should be judicious to minimize coagulopathy and subsequent intraoperative bleeding. If time permits, a radial arterial catheter should be placed, preferably in the right radial artery, to more closely monitor blood pressure. Open thoracotomy is performed via a left lateral chest wall incision; therefore, if central access is needed, a right IJ or subclavian catheter should be placed.

In general, BAI requires operative management. In selected patients, usually those with serious concurrent injuries or medical problems (e.g., sepsis, major burns, or catastrophic head injury), delayed operation may be considered to allow time to optimize the patient's physiological condition prior to surgery. Other more minor injuries (e.g., small pseudoaneurysm) may also be observed. The clamp repair technique is the most common surgical method used today. This involves an open thoracotomy and clamping both the proximal and distal ends of the aorta around the injury. Primary suture repair (without synthetic grafts) is preferred because it decreases the risks of subsequent infection, leakage around the prosthesis, pseudoaneurysm formation, or mural thrombus. A prosthetic graft may be required for more extensive injuries that cannot be sutured primarily. The major complications to this surgery are spinal cord and lower extremity ischemia and renal failure secondary to ischemia. Endovascular repair of BAI has emerged as a viable alternative to open operative repair. This is especially true for elderly patients or those with significant comorbidities who may not tolerate a large operation.

## KEY POINTS

- The aorta is the most commonly injured great vessel in blunt trauma
  - Acceleration/deceleration injury is the most common mechanism
  - Aortic transection results in death at the scene
  - Aortic rupture (partial laceration) may survive to ED

- – More than 90% of injuries occur at the isthmus (e.g., ligamentum arteriosum)
- Suspicion of injury based on mechanism, symptoms, and vital signs
- Chest radiograph can show clues to BAI
  - – Widened mediastinum is most sensitive but not at all specific
- CT angiography for all patients in whom diagnosis is suspected
  - – Limited role for aortography in current practice
  - – TEE can be diagnostic in patients too unstable to go to CT
- ED management focuses on controlling dP/dT
  - – Esmolol first to blunt tachycardic response, then Nipride to vasodilate
  - – Labetolol a good alternative because both β-receptor and α-receptor blockade
- Definitive treatment requires operative repair with open thoracotomy
  - – Clamp technique is most common
  - – Expanding role for endovascular stenting

# CHAPTER 10

# Pelvic Fractures

## CASE SCENARIO

A 47-year-old male is brought to the ED from the scene of a high-speed MVC. He was the unrestrained front seat passenger and was found lying supine approximately 10 ft away from the vehicle. There was extensive damage to the body of the car. At the scene, his vital signs were a heart rate of 112 bpm, blood pressure 86/55, respiratory rate of 20, and oxygen saturation 99% on room air. In the ED, his vital signs are essentially unchanged. He is awake but amnesic to the event and is complaining of lower abdominal pain. The trauma captain determines that his airway is intact and that he has equal breath sounds.

1. What is the most appropriate next step?
   a. Roll the patient to look for possible scalp or back trauma
   b. Rock the patient's pelvis to determine stability
   c. Oxygen, 2 large-bore IVs, aggressive crystalloid resuscitation, cardiac monitor
   d. Perform a FAST exam searching for free intra-abdominal blood

In the setting of hypotension, an expedient search for the source must be performed. However, the primary survey takes priority. Simultaneous with the primary survey (ABCs) is IV–$O_2$–monitor. The patient should be placed on oxygen by a nonrebreather facemask, which is especially important given his likely circulatory shock. Airway and breathing are already accounted for. Circulation has already been partially addressed by the fact that the patient was hypotensive in the field and remains so in the ED. You check for a radial pulse, and it is thready. Large-bore IV access is obtained, and initial crystalloid is administered. As part of the assessment of circulation you call for 4 units of O+ blood to be brought STAT.

As the IV crystalloid is being infused the patient's blood pressure increases to 95/60. You move on to the secondary survey as another physician performs a FAST exam. Significant findings include a 4 cm laceration to his right scalp, a contusion on his right chest, bilateral lower quadrant abdominal tenderness and guarding, and crepitus with application of pressure over the pelvis. Your colleague finds no fluid in either Morrison's pouch, the splenorenal space, or behind the bladder.

2. What is the next step in this patient's management?
   a. Expedite transfer to OR for ex-lap
   b. Obtain a trauma series
   c. Tie a bedsheet around the pelvis
   d. Perform a DPL

The pelvis should be stabilized as quickly as possible given the crepitus on exam and hypotension. This must be presumed an unstable pelvic fracture with retroperitoneal bleeding. A quick and effective way to accomplish stabilization is to tie a bedsheet around the pelvis. This brings displaced fragments back together and helps tamponade the bleeding. Part of the trauma series is a pelvic x-ray that will detect significant fractures or dislocations. Simultaneously, the search for other causes of hypotension should take place. A CXR will evaluate a large hemothorax, and the FAST exam has demonstrated the absence of large-volume hemoperitoneum. Prior to the availability of the FAST exam, DPL was used to exclude hemoperitoneum. It can still be performed in this setting where the patient is too unstable to go to CT scan or to aid in the decision of whether to go to the OR or to angiography. Looking further for sources of bleeding, the patient does not appear to have a femur fracture, another source of significant internal blood loss. Therefore, the only potential space for a significant hematoma is the pelvis and retroperitoneum.

In this case, the x-ray reveals bilateral pubic rami fractures and a vertical fracture of the sacrum. The patient's blood pressure is now 84/56, and his heart rate is 120.

3. What is the next most appropriate intervention?
   a. Immediate operative internal fixation of the pelvis
   b. Immediate exploratory laparotomy to ligate the bleeding vessels
   c. Administration of vasopressors to support blood pressure
   d. Transfusion of PRBCs

In the setting of pelvic fractures and signs of shock, blood should be transfused early and rapidly to maintain tissue oxygen delivery. Bleeding from pelvic fractures can be quite significant, and providing only crystalloid is insufficient. If the patient's status does not respond to blood transfusion or the transfusion requirement is large (greater than 4 units PRBCs over a period of an hour), angiography or another definitive modality of treatment should be performed.

This patient receives 2 units of blood, and his blood pressure improves to 110/72; his heart rate decreases to 100 to 105 bpm. He is stable enough to transfer to the radiology suite for CT scans. A CT scan of the pelvis with contrast shows a contrast blush around the external iliac vessels. After returning to the resuscitation bay, his blood pressure is 102/74.

4. What is the most appropriate course of action?
   a. Arrange angiography for his presumed venous bleed
   b. Arrange angiography for his presumed arterial bleed
   c. Continue blood transfusion and observation
   d. Exploratory laparotomy to ligate arterial bleeding

The presence of contrast blush on CT scan is indicative of arterial bleeding. Hemodynamic instability and the presence of active bleeding are indications for angiography. Venous bleeding may be difficult to control because of extensive collateral flow in a valveless system. Conversely, arterial injuries are well controlled via angiography and embolization. Laparotomy may be necessary in the presence of intraperitoneal bleeding, but it is not the preferred management to control hemorrhage caused by pelvic fractures.

Answers: 1-c; 2-c; 3-d; 4-b

## CLINICAL ANATOMY

The pelvis is composed of the sacrum, the coccyx, and the right and left innominate bones (Figure 10-1). The innominate bone is formed by the ilium, ischium, and pubis on each side. Stability is provided by the ring structure formed by the innominate bones and posterior ligaments. The lumbosacral, sacrococcygeal, and sacroiliac joints, along with the pubic symphysis, allow slight movement. The acetabulum (the socket for the femoral head) is derived from parts of the pubis, ilium, and ischium. A single break in the ring will produce a stable injury, while two or more breaks render the pelvis unstable and prone to displacement.

The pelvis has a rich blood supply, which can result in significant hemorrhage (Figure 10-2). Occasionally a retroperitoneal hematoma may erupt into the abdominal cavity causing rapid fatal blood loss. Patients with pelvic fractures who are hypotensive have a high mortality rate. Bleeding secondary to pelvic fractures is particularly difficult to control because these vessels are not easily accessible surgically. The most efficient access to these sites of bleeding is via intra-arterial catheterization, thus the importance of angiography and embolization.

The posterior arch, derived from the lumbar and sacral plexuses, is a bundle of nerves that runs adjacent to the posterior wall of pelvis. This plexus of nerves is vulnerable to injury with displaced pelvic fractures. This may result in dysfunction of bowel, bladder, or genitalia, as well as lower extremity neurological deficits.

## SECONDARY SURVEY

The most important aspect of the secondary survey of the pelvis is gross stability, which is evaluated by compressing the iliac crests together medially. Patients with a grossly unstable pelvis must be externally stabilized. Initially this is as simple as wrapping the pelvis with a sheet. An unstable pelvis should

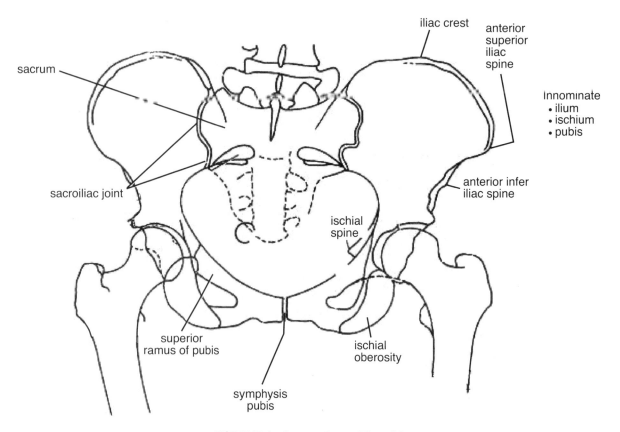

FIGURE 10-1   Bony anatomy of the pelvis

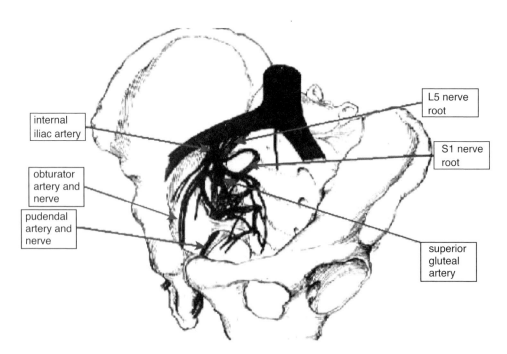

FIGURE 10-2   Vascular anatomy of the pelvis

not be re-examined as to prevent further displacement and hemorrhage. If the pelvis is stable, range of motion of the hips should be checked to rule out hip dislocation, which would require prompt reduction. Other signs of pelvic fracture include perineal or scrotal hematomas. A displaced coccyx fracture can sometime be appreciated on rectal exam.

## MECHANISM

The Young's classification system divides pelvic injuries based on mechanism (Table 10-1). There are three main types of force that cause pelvic injury—lateral compression, anteroposterior compression, and vertical shear forces (Box 10-1). Up to 25% of pelvic fractures result from a combination of injury patterns. The mechanism involved can help predict the likelihood of both mechanical and hemodynamic instability. Lateral compression (LC) injuries do not place the pelvic vessels in tension and thus are not as often associated with significant vascular injury, unless caused by bone fragments. The hallmark of an LC injury is an oblique pubic ramus fracture, oriented horizontally rather than vertically. Anteroposterior compression (APC) injuries place stress on the symphyseal ligaments, sacrotuberous and sacrospinous ligaments, and

---

**BOX 10-1  Mechanisms of pelvic fractures**

- *Lateral compression* injuries account for close to half of all pelvic fractures. Horizontal fractures, sacroiliac joint diastasis, and crush fracture of the sacrum all suggest lateral compression. Mortality is lowest for injuries resulting from a lateral compression mechanism.
- *Anteroposterior compression,* which result in open book fractures, account for almost one-fourth of all pelvic injuries. Head-on motor vehicle accidents are the classic example. Severe anteroposterior compression injuries carry a mortality rate of approximately 25%.
- *Vertical shear* injuries are the least common and the most severe. They are caused by falling or jumping from a height. Radiographically, fractures are vertically aligned with vertical displacement of bony fragments.

---

anterior sacroiliac ligaments. The result is an open book pelvis, sometimes in the absence of an actual bone fracture. Another result is stretching of internal iliac vessels and their tributaries, and the incidence of significant vascular injury is high.

The Tile's classification is based on the stability of the pelvic ring itself (Table 10-2). Tile considers stability as rotational and vertical. Any disruption of the ring

---

**TABLE 10-1  Young's classification of pelvic fractures—based on mechanism of injury**

| Lateral compression (LC)[a] | Transverse fracture of pubic rami, ipsilateral, or contralateral to posterior injury |
|---|---|
| | I—Sacral compression on side of impact |
| | II—Crescent (iliac wing) fracture on side of impact |
| | III—LC-I or LC-II injury on side of impact; contralateral open book injury |
| **Anteroposterior compression (APC)[a]** | **Symphyseal diastasis and/or longitudinal rami fractures** |
| | I—*Slight* widening of pubic symphysis and/or anterior sacroiliac (SI) joint; stretched but intact anterior SI, sacrotuberous, and sacrospinous ligaments; intact posterior SI ligaments |
| | II—Widened anterior SI joint; disrupted anterior SI, sacrotuberous, and sacrospinous ligaments; intact posterior SI ligaments |
| | III—Complete SI joint disruption with lateral displacement; disrupted anterior SI, sacrotuberous, and sacrospinous ligaments; disrupted posterior SI ligaments |
| **Vertical shear (VS)[a]** | **Symphyseal diastasis or vertical displacement anteriorly and posteriorly, usually through SI joint, occasionally through the iliac wing and/or sacrum** |

[a]LC-I and APC-I injuries are usually treated with bedrest followed by protected weight bearing. LC-II and III, APC II and III, and VS injuries usually require open reduction and internal fixation within 2 weeks of injury.

| TABLE 10-2  Tile's classification of pelvic fractures |
| --- |
| **Type A: Stable pelvic ring injury** |
| A1: Avulsion fractures of the innominate bone |
| A2: Stable iliac wing fractures or stable minimally displaced ring fractures |
| A3: Transverse fractures of the coccyx and sacrum |
| **Type B: Partially stable pelvic ring injury (rotationally unstable, vertically stable)** |
| B1: Open book injury—unilateral |
| B2: Lateral compression injury |
| B3: Bilateral type B injuries |
| **Type C: Unstable pelvic ring injury—vertical shear (rotationally and vertically unstable)** |
| C1: Unilateral |
| C2: Bilateral, one side type B, one side type C |
| C3: Bilateral type C lesions |

resulting in an open book fracture is considered rotationally unstable (type B). A vertically displaced (vertical shear, or type C) injury is considered rotationally and vertically unstable.

## DIAGNOSTICS

As part of the trauma series, an AP plain film is indicated in the resuscitation bay if there is any suspicion of significant pelvic fracture. This test can be skipped if the patient is alert, does not have abdominal or back pain, and has a nontender pelvis and a nonsuggestive mechanism. The AP view identifies most fractures and dislocations, although it may not accurately estimate the extent of bony displacement. Look for signs of displacement. Diastasis at the symphysis pubis should not exceed 5 mm and at the sacroiliac joint should not exceed 2 to 4 mm. Overlapping at the symphysis pubis results from a severe crushing force and is always abnormal. An avulsion fracture of the fifth lumbar transverse process can be a clue to sacroiliac joint disruption or a vertical sacral fracture. In operative planning, inlet or outlet views may be helpful. An inlet view demonstrates posterior and cephalic displacement of posterior arch fractures. An outlet view demonstrates sacral fractures and sacroiliac joint disruptions.

CT scan is superior to plain x-rays in diagnosing pelvic fractures and assessing the extent of displacement. Moreover, it will also assess for other intra-abdominal, retroperitoneal, or pelvic injuries that commonly coexist with pelvic fractures. CT with IV contrast can also demonstrate extravasation indicative of vascular injury.

**LITERATURE REFERENCE**

## Utility of the portable AP pelvis x-ray

The traditional trauma series was previously a mainstay of initial trauma evaluation to help guide further management of the patient. This of course was germane in an era prior to the availability of rapid CT scanning. A trauma series seldom provides information that requires immediate intervention in the hemodynamically stable trauma patient who will be going for CT scans. Stewart et al. conducted a retrospective investigation of multiple trauma patients to compare sensitivities of portable pelvis films with CT scan. The portable pelvis film missed 21% of pelvic fractures. This modality was particularly poor for detecting sacral and iliac fractures. No injuries were missed by CT scan that were detected on plain x-ray **[Stewart et al. *Emerg Radiol* 2002;9(5):266–271].** Vo et al. conducted a similar study in which plain x-rays failed to detect pelvic fractures on 8 of 60 patients (25%) with fractures on CT scan **[Vo et al. *Emerg Radiol* 2004;10(5):246–249].**

## MANAGEMENT

### Is the Patient Hemodynamically Stable?

The classification of pelvic fractures is complicated. During resuscitation a rapid assessment of pelvic tenderness and stability is important to consider the possibility of a fracture and its potential source of internal hemorrhage. In subsequent management, the most important distinction to make is whether or not the patient is hemodynamically stable. In unstable patients the emphasis is on vascular injury and stabilizing the pelvis as opposed to definitive repair.

Hemorrhage from pelvic fractures can be rapidly fatal because the injured vessels are noncompressible. Up to 4 L of blood (two-thirds of the circulating blood volume) can collect in the retroperitoneal space before tamponade occurs. Prompt transfusion of untyped PRBCs should be initiated in the setting of pelvic fractures and signs of shock (e.g., tachycardia, hypotension, or altered mental status).

The key to controlling hemorrhage with displaced pelvic fractures is to restore stability and provide compression. The principle is to close bleeding fracture surfaces and allow a primary clot to form. This can be initiated in the trauma bay by wrapping a bedsheet around the pelvis and tying it as tightly as possible. Military antishock trouser or pneumatic antishock garment can be used to tamponade bleeding, although these devices are typically reserved for the prehospital setting. Their use is controversial because they prevent visibility of the abdomen, compromise blood flow to the lower extremities, and have been associated with abdominal compartment syndrome. Orthopedics should be consulted for the possible placement of an external fixator device. The device should be applied in such a way that access to the abdomen is not compromised and fracture fragments are not displaced posteriorly. True open book fractures with an intact posterior ring benefit most from anterior external fixator placement.

Laparotomy for hemodynamically unstable pelvic fracture is not recommended unless there is evidence of intra-abdominal bleeding or intestinal perforation. The presence of free fluid on a FAST exam, along with hemodynamic instability, is of course indication for laparotomy. In the setting of hemodynamic instability, a DPL is often necessary to assess for intraperitoneal blood and the need for exploratory laparotomy. If this procedure is performed intraumbilically as it typically is, it can be falsely positive because of pelvic hemorrhage tracking up into the abdominal fascia. A supraumbilical approach should be employed instead. Some argue that exploratory laparotomy in the setting of an unstable pelvic fracture decreases the ability to tamponade the pelvic bleeding because of the exposure required to access the abdomen. However, others believe that, in the correct setting, applying internal tamponade, or abdominal packing, via laparotomy is an effective means of controlling pelvic bleeding.

Angiography and embolization can definitively treat bleeding from pelvic fractures. Arterial bleeding can be effectively controlled via this method. In contrast, venous bleeding can be difficult to control because of extensive anastamoses and collateral flow in a valveless system. Small branches of the external iliac artery are often responsible for significant bleeding in pelvic fractures. Angiography is indicated for patients with pelvic fractures and hemodynamic instability, those with continued shock after application of external fixator devices, and those whose CT scans demonstrate contrast blushing indicative of arterial bleeding. A large retrospective review of trauma patients showed that the incidence of arterial injury amenable to angiography is about 75% in the setting of pelvic fracture and hypotension refractory to 2 units PRBC transfusion.

---

**LITERATURE REFERENCE**

 ## When to call the OR for unstable pelvic fractures

Should all hemodynamically unstable patients with pelvic fractures go straight to the OR? Several studies have been designed to answer this question. Ruchholtz et al. prospectively studied patients presenting to an ED with high-trauma mechanisms. Patients with pelvic ring fractures, hemodynamic instability, and free fluid on bedside ultrasound were taken to the OR. Retroperitoneal bleeding from pelvic fractures can pass intraperitoneally, causing a false-positive ultrasound. Hemodynamically stable patients underwent further imaging. Of the 31 patients who underwent laparotomy, only one patient had a retroperitoneal hematoma that tracked into the peritoneum. Therefore, confirmed intra-abdominal free fluid by FAST exam is usually from an abdominal source rather than the pelvic fracture. The conclusion is that patients with unstable pelvic fractures and evidence of intra-abdominal free fluid should undergo operative intervention for control of intra-abdominal bleeding **[Ruchholtz et al. *J Trauma* 2004;57(2):278–285; discussion 285–287].**

Heetveld et al. formed a multidisciplinary consensus committee to develop guidelines for management of hemodynamically unstable pelvic fractures, following standard scientific methodology, comprehensive Medline searches, and level of evidence grading. They recommended that the presence of intra-abdominal hemorrhage be assessed by diagnostic peritoneal aspiration and/or FAST exam. The presence of intra-abdominal fluid requires immediate laparotomy and pelvic stabilization. Additionally, angiography for arterial bleeding is indicated. In the absence of intra-abdominal blood, noninvasive pelvic stabilization and angiography should be performed **[Heetveld et al. *ANZ J Surg* 2004;74(7):520–529].**

**TABLE 10-3  Various types of pelvic fractures**

**Ischial tuberosity**

May be caused by forceful hamstring contraction

Treatment: pain medications, rest, crutches, partial weight bearing

**Pubic or ischial ramus**

Most commonly from falls and in the elderly

Treatment: analgesics, crutches

**Ischial body**

Require significant force (fall in the sitting position)

Pain increased with hamstring movement

Treatment: rest, analgesics, doughnut-ring cushion, crutches

Follow-up in 1–2 weeks

**Iliac wing (Duverney fracture)**

May cause abdominal muscle spasm, causing concern on exam

Treatment: analgesics

**Sacrum**

Transverse fractures do not involve the pelvic ring; vertical fractures do

Nerve injury is common with upper sacral fractures

Fractures without neurological symptoms treated with rest and analgesics

Nerve injury may require surgery

**Coccyx**

Most common from direct trauma

Straining at stool or trying to stand may exacerbate pain

Abnormal coccygeal motion may be found on rectal exam

Do not need confirmatory x-rays

Treatment: rest, stool softeners, sitz baths, doughnut cushion, analgesia

**Acetabulum**

Account for up to 20% of all pelvic fractures

Usually occur with other lower extremity fractures

Posterior fractures are most common

May cause chronic pain and sciatic nerve damage

Consult orthopedics

Admit patient

Treatment: Displaced fractures—operative

Nondisplaced fractures—analgesics, rest

### Is the Fracture Mechanically Unstable?

Even patients who are hemodynamically stable may have mechanically unstable fractures and require invasive intervention. As discussed previously, Tile's classification is used to categorize pelvic fractures based on the degree of mechanical stability. Mechanism and fracture site are extremely helpful in suggesting possible operative repair as well (Table 10-3). Mechanically unstable fractures require surgical intervention. As long as the patient is hemodynamically stable, operative repair can be delayed up to 2 weeks. Patients with pelvic fractures that are both mechanically and hemodynamically stable are managed conservatively with limitations on ambulation, comfort measures such as crutches, and adequate analgesia.

## KEY POINTS

- Pelvic stability is provided by innominate bones and posterior ligaments
  - Single break in the pelvic ring will produce a stable injury
  - Two or more breaks render the pelvis unstable and prone to displacement
- Rich blood supply to pelvis can result in significant vascular injury and hemorrhagic shock
- Check for pelvic stability during secondary survey
- Trauma series of AP pelvis in blunt mechanism and suspected injury
- Anterioposterior compression (APC) is more prone to vascular injury than lateral compression (LC)
- The first consideration in management is hemodynamic stability
  - Early and aggressive blood transfusion indicated with signs of shock
  - If hemodynamically unstable, wrap pelvis with a bedsheet
  - Unstable plus intra-abdominal blood requires exploratory laparotomy
- Angiography should be considered
  - Hemodynamic compromise
  - Signs of arterial bleeding
  - Ongoing transfusion requirements

## BLUNT ABDOMINAL/PELVIC TRAUMA

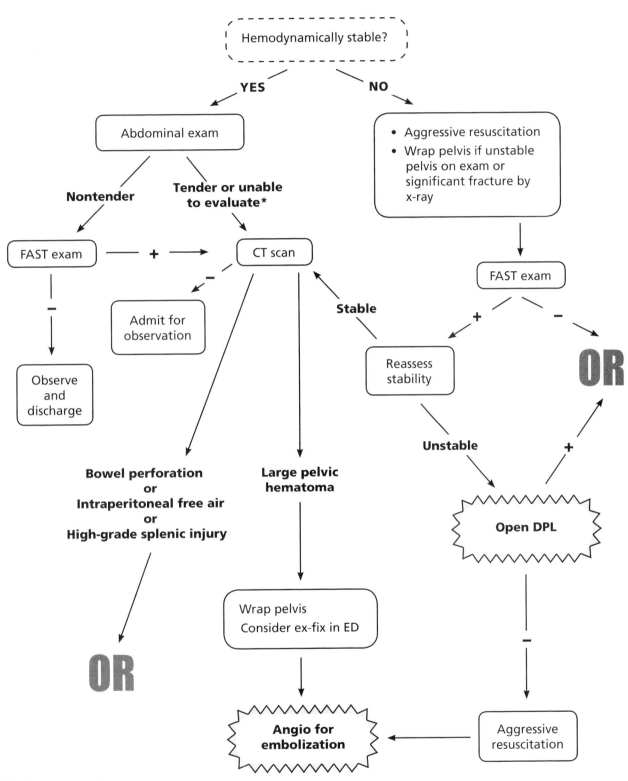

*Unable to evaluate if:
- Altered mental status
- Severely intoxicated
- Intubated and sedated
- Distracting injury

# CHAPTER 11

# Genitourinary Trauma

## CASE SCENARIO

A 46-year-old male is brought to the ED after a fall from 20 feet. At the scene, he was found to be confused and unable to give a history. He repeats every question he is asked without answering it. His initial vital signs in the ED include a pulse of 110, blood pressure 90/60, respiratory rate of 18, and oxygen saturation 99%. IV access is established immediately, and crystalloid fluids are hung. The primary survey reveals an open airway, equal bilateral breath sounds, and strong distal pulses. A repeat blood pressure returns at 120/72, and he becomes more alert. He complains of abdominal and back pain. The secondary survey is remarkable for tenderness along the pubic symphysis, lumbar tenderness, and a drop of blood at the urethral meatus. The patient has normal rectal tone and a firm prostate. The medical student prepares to place a Foley catheter.

1. What is the most appropriate response?
   a. Place the catheter and send sample for urinalysis
   b. A high-riding prostate is not a contraindication to Foley placement
   c. Urethral injury must first be evaluated before placing a Foley catheter
   d. A Foley catheter is unnecessary as blood pressure has normalized

Contraindications for placement of a Foley catheter in trauma are blood at the meatus, a high-riding boggy prostate, and scrotal hematoma. These are signs of urethral injury, and placement of a Foley may create a false passage for the catheter into the soft tissues or result in total disruption of the urethra. However dramatic blood from the urethra may appear, the patient's altered mental status and transient hypotension are concerning for more serious injuries and should be addressed first.

A trauma series is done in the bay and includes a lateral c-spine, AP chest, and AP pelvis, the latter of which shows bilateral pubic rami fractures. You decide to obtain CT scans of the head, c-spine, chest, and abdomen because of the significant mechanism, hypotension in the field, and the fact that he has altered mental status. The CT scan is performed with intravenous contrast. The patient's blood pressure remains stable throughout.

2. What is the most appropriate course of action regarding genitourinary tract imaging?
   a. The CT scan with IV contrast is adequate for excluding urethral injury
   b. Specific urethral imaging is not indicated; patient should be explored in the OR
   c. A retrograde urethrogram should be performed to assess for urethral injury
   d. Urology should be consulted for cystoscopy

A retrograde urethrogram (RUG) is a study to evaluate the integrity of the urethra. Blood at the meatus indicates a possible urethral laceration. Placement of a Foley in this setting may result in creating a false lumen or result in total transection of the urethra. A high-riding prostate on rectal exam indicates total transection of the urethra, which requires operative management.

The RUG shows no evidence of urethral disruption, and a Foley catheter is placed with return of bloody urine. CT scan reveals a liver laceration without evidence of renal injury; there is a small amount of intraperitoneal free blood. It also shows bilateral pubic rami fractures with minimal displacement. There is no deterioration in the patient's hemodynamic status.

3. What is the most appropriate next step?
   a. Arrange an angiogram to assess for renal vascular injury
   b. Admit the patient for observation and serial hematocrit levels

    **c.** Consult urology for further management

    **d.** Perform cystography looking for bladder perforation

A CT scan with IV contrast is insufficient in diagnosing bladder injury, as the contrast does not reach the bladder in time. The bladder is a vascular structure, and rupture or laceration will result in hematuria. This injury should always be considered in the setting of pelvic fractures as well. In this case a cystogram is indicated, which involves injecting about 500 cc of contrast through the Foley catheter and obtaining an AP x-ray. This is followed by a wash-out film after the bladder has been emptied and irrigated with saline. This will show any contrast that has extravasated outside the bladder.

**4.** The RUG shows an extraperitoneal bladder rupture. What do you tell the patient's family about the management of this injury?

    **a.** Operative repair is indicated

    **b.** Management is conservative with a Foley catheter for 14 days and re-evaluation with cystoscopy

    **c.** Requires bilateral nephrostomy tubes

    **d.** Requires cystoscopy and sclerosis if the laceration is small

Bladder rupture can be either intraperitoneal (ruptures into peritoneum) or extraperitoneal (ruptures into soft tissues). The former results in unobstructed flow of urine from the bladder into the peritoneal space, this requires an exploratory laparotomy and surgical bladder repair. The latter represents a contained rupture and typically does not require surgical intervention. Treatment is conservative with Foley catheter placement for 14 days and repeat cystogram to assure healing.    Answers: 1-c; 2-c; 3-d; 4-b

## BACKGROUND

The majority of injuries to the genitourinary (GU) system occur via blunt mechanisms. Their presentation can be subtle; therefore, a high index of suspicion is necessary to avoid missing these injuries. Almost 80% of such injuries involve the kidney, and 10% involve the bladder. Urethral injuries, which are relatively rare, are more frequently caused by penetrating trauma. They are more common in males and are often associated with pelvic fractures. Patients with pre-existing anatomic abnormalities (e.g., tumor) are at greater risk for injury. Fortunately, almost all injuries to the genitourinary tract are not life threatening. Nonetheless, the presence of some GU injuries, such as bladder rupture, require great force and are often accompanied by other injuries that may be life threatening. Nonetheless, other life-threatening injuries should be worked up before focusing on the GU system.

## CLINICAL ANATOMY

The GU system can be divided into three components—external genitalia, lower tract (urethra and bladder), and upper tract (ureters and kidneys). The workup of injury is conducted from an outside-to-inside fashion; therefore, the anatomy will be considered in that order as well. Injury to the external genitalia is not covered in this text. The male urethra can be divided into three parts: the prostatic urethra, the membraneous urethra (the shortest part extending from the prostate to the bulb of the penis), and the spongy urethra (located within the corpus spongiosum). Note that while it is considered part of the lower tract, the bulk of its length is located within the penis. The female urethra is much shorter and thus less susceptible to injury.

The bladder is characterized by its strong muscular walls and distensibility. It is located within the lower pelvis, posterior and slightly superior to the pubic bones. When it is full, it may extend to the level of the umbilicus. The stress on the wall of the bladder increases as it distends, making it more prone to rupture. In females, the uterus is located posterior and superior to the bladder, with the vagina extending from the perineum to uterus. Thus, the pouch of Douglas (the low point of the pelvis in the supine patient) is bordered by the posterior uterus and the sigmoid colon in the female. In the male, the low point is the retrovesicular pouch, bordered by the posterior bladder and the sigmoid colon. The urethra exits the bladder at the apex of the trigone of the bladder. The ureters enter the bladder at the angles of the trigone.

The ureters exit the bladder and course along the lateral wall of the pelvis external to the parietal perineum and anterior to the internal iliac arteries. They pass over the pelvic brim and become retroperitoneal as they course along the psoas muscle and ascend to the renal pelvis. The renal pelvis, formed by the confluence of renal calices is surrounded by fat, giving it a distinctive appearance on ultrasound. The kidneys themselves are also retroperitoneal, located against the psoas major muscles, alongside the vertebral column. The right kidney is slightly more caudad than the left.

## SECONDARY SURVEY

The GU system is not assessed in the primary survey. As part of the secondary survey, a close inspection of the perineum should be performed. First, the external genitalia should be assessed for ecchymosis, bleeding, or other evidence of injury. In females, an external exam should be done to look for blood at the vaginal introitus as well as labial lacerations and hematomas. These findings raise the concern for open pelvic fractures and associated urethral or bladder injuries. Even in the absence of external findings, a bimanual exam should be performed to assess for occult pathology if suspicion is high. In the male, the meatus should be assessed for the presence of blood, which may indicate a urethral injury. In all patients, the folds of the buttocks should be opened to look for lacerations or ecchymosis, which may be indicative of significant pelvic fractures and associated urethral or bladder injury. Perineal lacerations should not be probed as this may dislodge clots and result in significant retroperitoneal bleeding. Rectal examination includes evaluation of sphincter tone, prostate gland position, and gross blood in the stool. A high-riding or boggy prostate denotes disruption of the membranous urethra with subsequent retropubic venous hematoma displacing the organ.

## MANAGEMENT

The workup of GU trauma can best be conceptualized as proceeding from external to internal, or from the urethral meatus to the renal cortex. Injury to external genitalia is assessed first, followed by lower tract pathology, and finally upper tract pathology. Assuming no evidence of urethral injury is found on the secondary survey, a Foley catheter should be placed in all victims of major trauma. If any of the signs of potential urethra injury is present in the male, Foley catheter placement should be delayed until a RUG is performed (Box 11-1). Because the female urethra is significantly shorter, a RUG is not useful. Instead, in the presence of blood, Foley placement is attempted and aborted if there is significant resistance. The inability to pass a Foley catheter in a young, premenopausal woman suggests urethral injury and suprapubic urinary drainage may be necessary.

Once a Foley is successfully placed, the next question to be is answered is whether or not hematuria is present. Gross hematuria (urine looks bloody) has clinical significance that will be discussed further; however, keep in mind that Foley placement can result in a small amount of hematuria initially that does not necessarily imply significant urethral injury. In the absence of urethral injury, gross hematuria implies

bladder injury, and this diagnosis must be pursued. There is extensive data to show that microscopic hematuria in the absence of hypotension is clinically insignificant. However, it is common practice to send urine for microscopic analysis. The question inevitably arises of what to do if there is a moderate amount of microscopic blood. The data support doing nothing acutely and to have the patient follow up in 1 to 2 weeks to assure the hematuria has cleared. Despite common practice, this is also reasonable in children as well.

**LITERATURE REFERENCE**

**Gross hematuria must be significant to be detected by clinicians**

Gross hematuria is an indication for radiographic evaluation in patients with blunt trauma. But how good are clinicians at identifying gross hematuria? Peacock et al. conducted a prospective, randomized, controlled study to determine the ability of clinicians to assess gross hematuria. They were asked to assess various samples with different concentrations of blood diluted in urine for the presence of gross hematuria. Clinicians were able to detect hematuria in 95% of cases only when samples contained more than 3,500 RBCs per hpf. These interpretations were independent of profession, specialty, and level of training. This conclusion demonstrates the need to determine a cutoff for the lower limit of red cells that suggest significant genitourinary injuries **[Peacock et al. *J Trauma* 2001;50(6):1060–1062].**

LITERATURE REFERENCE

## Is microscopic hematuria significant?

Microscopic hematuria is defined as greater than five red blood cells per high-power field. The differential diagnosis of microscopic hematuria in trauma is broad, and not all injuries are clinically significant. Formerly, all patients with microscopic hematuria underwent imaging; however, firmer imaging guidelines exist now and are used to drive practice. In BestBET review, which is published by the Emergency Department of the Manchester Royal Infirmary, 10 studies were reviewed that considered patients with microscopic hematuria ($n = 2,302$) who all had some form of imaging. Of all of the patients without shock or other major associated injury, only one patient had a significant renal injury. Thus, in the absence of hemodynamic instability or other major injury, such as pelvic fracture seen on plain film, microscopic hematuria rarely signifies severe injury, and imaging is not required **[Mackway-Jone. *Emerg Med J* 2002;19:322–323].**

Consensus dictates that gross hematuria mandates a search for bladder rupture, although its presence is uncommon in the absence of pelvic fractures. This search involved either retrograde cystography or CT cystography (Box 11-2). An upper tract injury should be considered in the event of gross hematuria and a nor-

LITERATURE REFERENCE

## When to worry about bladder rupture

Bladder injuries are usually associated with other major injuries. Thus it is important to identify circumstances in which bladder rupture is most likely to be present in order to avoid missing this injury. Morey et al. performed a study to determine when there should be suspicion for this injury. They conducted a retrospective chart review of patients with blunt trauma and bladder rupture at four institutions over a 4-year period. They found that all 53 patients with bladder rupture had both pelvic fracture and gross hematuria. They concluded that all patients with this combination of findings must undergo cystographic evaluation. This implies that in the absence of pelvic fracture, search for bladder rupture may be unnecessary even in the face of gross hematuria **[Morey et al. *J Trauma* 2001;51(4):683–686].**

mal cystogram. In most trauma patients with a blunt mechanism and hematuria, a CT scan is obtained to evaluate for significant intra-abdominal, retroperitoneal, and pelvic injuries. This will also diagnose renal contusions or lacerations (Table 11-1). Delayed scanning with IV contrast will allow time for contrast to travel into the ureters if the suspicion for ureteral injury is high. CT scan is also good for the diagnosis of renal

LITERATURE REFERENCE

## Microscopic hematuria is significant in children, right?

Whereas in adults gross hematuria is used as a threshold of whether to work-up GU injury, in children the traditional dogma has been microscopic hematuria with 50 RBCs per hpf. Santucci et al. recently conducted a study to evaluate this practice. They retrospectively reviewed 720 pediatric patients with suspected renal trauma regarding mechanism of injury, imaging, and final diagnosis. All patients with significant renal injuries either had gross hematuria, hypotension, or a significant deceleration mechanism. This suggests that the imaging criteria for adult management can also be applied to the pediatric

population **[Santucci et al. *J Urol* 2004;171(2 Pt 1):822–825].**

Brown et al. conducted a retrospective medical record review of 1,200 children who sustained blunt abdominal trauma to determine criteria for renal imaging. All children with significant renal injuries had associated injuries of other organ systems. The degree of hematuria did not correlate with the severity of the renal injury. They concluded that children with associated injuries and microscopic hematuria after blunt trauma should undergo radiographic evaluation **[Brown et al. *World J Surg* 2001;25(12):1557–1560].**

**BOX 11-2 The nuts and bolts of the cystogram**

Cystography is accomplished by instilling approximately 300 to 500 mL of contrast media through a Foley catheter using a Tomey syringe without the plunger (contrast drains into bladder under gravity and not forced in). The Foley bag is then reattached and must be held about 2 ft above the patient to ensure adequate intravesical pressure, approximating physiologic voiding pressure, so that extravasation occurs. Failure to generate such pressure may result in a false-negative study. An x-ray is done while the bladder is full. Then the contrast is allowed to drain out of the Foley catheter, and the bladder is irrigated with saline. A repeat x-ray is obtained to look for residual contrast adjacent to the bladder wall, which would signify rupture. A CT cystogram is a feasible alternative and does not require postdrainage reimaging because the high-resolution CT image is able to discern extravasated contrast. This method also requires retrograde contrast administration followed by clamping the Foley.

vascular injuries, which present in the absence of hematuria in 20% to 30% of cases. Renal artery or vein injuries typically result in significant hematoma around the renal pedicle, flank pain, and sometimes hemodynamic compromise. Renal vein injuries are more common and result in greater hemorrhage. Renal artery injury can result in nonperfusion of the involved kidney.

### Penetrating GU Injuries

Penetrating injuries do not follow the same guidelines for workup. The presence or absence of hematuria alone should not drive the decision for radiographic investigation. The location of the wound in relation to the underlying structure should guide this decision. Up to 10% of penetrating wounds with significant genitourinary injury do not produce hematuria.

## SPECIFIC INJURIES

Tables 11-2 and 11-3 provide summaries for specific injuries.

### Urethral Injuries

Urethral injuries in males can be posterior (prostato-membranous) or anterior (bulbous and penile). The two portions are separated by the urogenital diaphragm. If these injuries are undetected, a partial tear may progress to completion. Posterior injuries are commonly caused by pelvic fractures, while anterior disruption results from straddle injuries, falls, gunshot wounds, penile fractures, and self-instrumentation. Partial anterior and posterior urethral tears can be managed with placement of a Foley catheter. Suprapubic catheter placement may be necessary for posterior tears. Complete anterior lacerations require surgical management. Complete posterior injuries are managed with either primary realignment or with suprapubic cystostomy placement. Since females have shorter urethras, lacerations can be repaired over a urethral catheter.

### Bladder

Injuries to the bladder are the second most common type of traumatic injury to the genitourinary system. The main injuries to consider are rupture or contusion.

### TABLE 11-1  Grading system for renal injuries

| Grade | Injury |
| --- | --- |
| I | Contusion (microscopic or gross hematuria, with normal urological study results) Subcapsular, nonexpanding hematoma without laceration |
| II | Parenchyma laceration < 1.0 cm depth limited to cortex, no extravasation Nonexpanding hematoma, confined to retroperitoneum |
| III | Parenchymal laceration > 1 cm depth with extravasation or collecting system rupture |
| IV | Laceration extending through to collecting system Vascular pedicle injury, hemorrhage contained |
| V | Shattered kidney Avulsed hilum (devascularized kidney) |

### TABLE 11-2  Injuries that are usually managed nonoperatively

| | |
| --- | --- |
| Renal contusions | Renal parenchymal ecchymosis, small lacerations, subcapsular hematomas with an intact capsule |
| Renal laceration, minor | Does not involve the medulla or collecting system |
| Bladder rupture, extraperitoneal | Usually results from penetrating pelvic fracture fragment Managed with catheter placement for 10–14 days |
| Urethral injuries, posterior or partial anterior | Posterior injuries commonly caused by pelvic fractures Managed with placement of a Foley catheter |
| Laceration | Suprapubic catheter placement may be necessary with posterior tears |

### TABLE 11-3  Injuries that are usually managed operatively

| | |
|---|---|
| Renal laceration, major | Associated with renal fractures with deep extension<br>Hemodynamic instability is not uncommon |
| Renal vascular injuries | Venous injuries more common. Often cause hemodynamic compromise<br>Arterial injuries cause either bleeding or nonperfusion |
| Renal rupture | Imaging reveals multiple major lacerations, nonperfused kidney, and contrast extravasation<br>Can result in sepsis from continued extravasation of urine retroperitoneally |
| Ureteral injuries | Most frequently caused by penetrating trauma<br>Most commonly occur in the upper third of the ureter<br>Hematuria may be absent if transection is complete |
| Bladder rupture, intraperitoneal | Results from blunt force at the dome of the bladder |
| Urethral injuries, complete anterior laceration | Result from straddle injuries, falls, gunshot wounds, penile fractures, and self-instrumentation |

Bladder contusion causes hematuria, but the cystogram is normal. This condition will resolve spontaneously without intervention. Bladder perforation or rupture can be intraperitoneal, extraperitoneal, or a combination of both. Intraperitoneal rupture results from blunt force at the dome of the bladder, the only area of the organ covered by the peritoneum. Extraperitoneal rupture, which is more common, is usually caused by a bony fracture fragment but can occur in isolation. Clinical signs and symptoms include abdominal pain and tenderness, hematuria, and inability to void. Intraperitoneal ruptures must be operatively repaired. Extraperitoneal ruptures are managed conservatively with catheter placement after urethral injury has been excluded. The catheter remains in place for 10 to 14 days, after which a repeat cystogram is performed to determine if the catheter can be removed.

### Ureter

The least common of all genitourinary injuries, ureteral injuries are most frequently caused by penetrating trauma. Most injuries are located in the upper third of the ureter. Blunt trauma can cause such injury via displaced bony fragments. Flank pain, a palpable flank mass, and hematuria may be present. In the case of complete ureteral transection, hematuria is usually absent. For this reason, stab wounds to the flank should raise the concern for a ureteral injury that requires CT evaluation with contrast and delayed images to ensure the integrity of the ureter. Ureteral injuries are often diagnosed in a delayed manner as patients develop signs and symptoms of infection, sepsis, or urinomas. Ureteral disruption is managed surgically.

### Kidney

Renal contusions are the most common kidney injuries in blunt trauma. CT scan findings include renal parenchymal ecchymosis, small lacerations, and subcapsular hematomas with an intact capsule. Minor lacerations, which do not involve the medulla or collecting system, are managed expectantly. Major lacerations may require surgical repair if accompanied by continued bleeding, hemodynamic compromise, or urinary extravasation. Complete rupture of the kidney will often lead to large retroperitoneal bleeding and instability; therefore, management is operative. Renal pedicle injuries frequently involve laceration or thrombosis of the renal artery or vein, with venous injuries more common, as described previously. Both can cause significant hemodynamic and renal function compromise. Renal pedicle injury can be difficult to diagnose because microscopic hematuria is insensitive, and the pain may not be severe.

### KEY POINTS

- GU system consists of external genitalia, lower tract (urethra and bladder), and upper tract (ureters and kidneys)
- Urethral injury suspected with blood at meatus, scrotal hematoma, or high-riding prostate
  - Foley is contraindicated if any of these signs present
  - RUG required if injury suspected
- Workup progresses from outside to inside

- After ruling out urethral injury, gross hematuria used to prompt further GU workup
  - Bladder injury uncommon without pelvic fracture, even with gross hematuria
  - Degree of hematuria does not correlate with injury severity
- Microscopic hematuria does not require workup *unless*:
  - Hypotension present, even if transient
  - Children with > 50 RBCs per hpf and significant deceleration mechanism
- Retrograde cystography or CT cystography to evaluate for bladder injury
- CT with IV contrast sufficient for diagnosis of renal parenchymal and pedicle injuries
- Hematuria does not guide workup for penetrating injury
  - Workup indicated based on proximity and clinical suspicion alone
- Intraperitoneal bladder rupture requires operative management
- Extraperitoneal bladder rupture is treated with Foley catheter for 14 days
- Renal injuries are nonoperative *unless*:
  - Large retroperitoneal bleeding
  - Hemodynamic instability
  - Urinary extravasation

# CHAPTER 12

# Penetrating Thoracic Trauma

## CASE SCENARIO

A 23-year-old male is brought to the ED after an altercation in which he sustained multiple stab wounds to the left chest. EMS loaded him quickly and sped to the ED. En route, he was moaning and intermittently following commands. His heart rate was in the 90s in the ambulance. He was administered high-flow oxygen, and two large-bore antecubital IVs were started. On arrival to the ED, his heart rate is 110 bpm, and his blood pressure 88/45. His oxygen saturation is 95% on a nonrebreather facemask. Three stab wounds are seen on his left chest wall without any active bleeding. The patient is unable to answer questions and appears sleepy. His jugular veins are somewhat distended, and his breath sounds seem equal bilaterally; there is no obvious chest wall crepitance.

1. What is the first step in this patient's care?
    a. Intubate the patient
    b. Perform an ED thoracotomy to directly control the bleeding
    c. Order a portable CXR to look for pneumothorax or hemothorax
    d. Perform a needle thoracostomy to relieve tension pneumothorax

This patient is in circulatory shock with hypotension and hypoxia, and the first priority is intubation. Simultaneously a reversible cause of shock must be sought and treated. A tension pneumothorax or large hemothorax should be the first consideration, given stab wounds to the chest, although the presence of breath sounds on the left contradict this. However, it would still be reasonable at this point to do a needle thoracostomy on the left because this patient will surely need a chest tube regardless. Also keep in mind that positive-pressure ventilation after intubation can convert a simple pneumothorax into a tension pneumothorax.

He is intubated without complication; there is good purple-to-yellow color change with the $CO_2$ capnometer, and his breath sounds are equal bilaterally. A liter of normal saline and uncrossmatched blood are started. A repeat blood pressure is 84/42, and his radial pulse is weak.

2. What should be done next?
    a. Needle thoracostomy to left side
    b. Chest CT with IV contrast
    c. Perform a bedside ultrasound looking for pericardial fluid
    d. Immediate transport to the OR for exploratory thoracotomy

Restoring adequate circulation starts with identifying the source of volume loss. For this reason, the FAST exam is essentially part of the primary survey, especially in unstable patients. One concern for patients with left anterior stab wounds is myocardial injury and subsequent pericardial tamponade. Simultaneously a left chest tube should be placed, instead of simple needle thoracostomy, because of persistent hypotension. The likelihood that this patient also has a pneumothorax or hemothorax is high, despite the fact that the breath sounds seem normal. The ultrasound shows a large black stripe around the ventricles that are visibly being constricted. At the same time, his heart rate drops below 60 bpm, and he loses his pulse.

3. What should be done next?
    a. Start CPR while placing an IJ central venous catheter for central epinehrine
    b. Start CPR and administer epinephrine 1 mg and atropine 1 mg peripherally

    **c.** Perform ED thoracotomy to relieve tamponade
    **d.** Perform pericardiocentesis

A medical cardiac arrest is treated with epinephrine and atropine, preferably via large central venous catheter above the diaphragm (e.g., IJ or subclavian). However, traumatic arrest is almost always because of blood loss and hypovolemia; therefore, circulation must be restored through blood replacement and control of blood loss. In penetrating chest trauma, restriction of cardiac output must also be considered as an etiology for circulatory shock and arrest. A stab wound to the chest resulting in a witnessed ED arrest warrants ED thoracotomy, otherwise death is certain.

An incision is made on the left from the sternum following the ribs past the midaxillary line one interspace below the nipple line. The intercostal muscles are cut using a large Metzenbaum scissors, and the rib spreaders are placed into the thorax. The ribs are spread apart revealing the pericardium containing a large amount of blood. You nick the pericardium being careful to avoid the phrenic nerve. You then cut superiorly with the scissors to expose the myocardium, which is still beating weakly. A large gush of blood comes out, and you notice a 1 cm laceration in the left ventricle that is pouring blood.

**4.** What do you do?
    **a.** Start internal cardiac compressions, and transfer to OR for repair
    **b.** Suture laceration while administering peripheral epinephrine
    **c.** Perform internal defibrillation to restart cardiac pacemaker
    **d.** Place a Foley catheter in hole, inflate balloon, start CPR, and give blood

The first priority is to stop further bleeding. In this case the primary problem leading to arrest was constriction of cardiac output as opposed to blood loss itself. Therefore, once the bleeding has been controlled, there is a good chance of resuscitating the heart and restoring cardiac output. When blood is pouring from the laceration, the quickest way to stop it is with a Foley catheter. After this is done, administer internal cardiac compressions, administer packed RBCs, and perform internal defibrillation if the heart is fibrillating. For persistent bradycardia, a dose of epinephrine may be warranted now that you know the etiology of arrest is not large-volume blood loss.

One thing you avoided during the procedure was to pull the heart out of its sac and rotate it to look for further lacerations.

**5.** What complication can arise from doing this?
    **a.** Cardiac laceration by the sharp edges of fractured ribs
    **b.** Risk of air embolism
    **c.** Coronary artery tear
    **d.** Displacement of the aorta and esophagus

Introduction of air through a left-sided or posterior cardiac perforation can result in sudden fatal cerebral or coronary air embolism. The risk of this complication is minimized if the heart is not lifted straight up. Despite this, it is sometimes necessary to lift the heart to look for a source if bleeding has not been controlled and the patient is dying.     Answers: 1-a; 2-c; 3-c; 4-d; 5-b

## BACKGROUND

The course of penetrating thoracic trauma can transpire quickly. Often a gunshot or stab wound to the heart will be lethal rapidly, and the patient will die at the scene. Other times, however, a penetrating wound will result in internal bleeding (e.g., pulmonary or subclavian vessel injury), which can be compensated for until a critical moment when cardiovascular collapse occurs. Penetrating thoracic injuries should raise the highest suspicion for lethal injuries, and immediate action should be taken to rule this out (Table 12-1).

## MECHANISM

When evaluating the patient, it can be helpful to know about the weapon or object used to inflict penetrating thoracic trauma. Although often unreliable information, it can be useful to inquire about the length of a

| TABLE 12-1  Possible injuries by penetrating thoracic wounds | |
|---|---|
| Tracheobronchial | - Cervical trachea exposed, usually involved in stab wounds<br>- Dyspnea, hoarseness, hemoptysis, stridor, or subcutaneous emphysema<br>- Pneumomediastinum, pneumothorax, or Hamman's crunch<br>- Suspect if large air leak from chest tube<br>- Intubation required, followed by bronchoscopy<br>- ETT should be advanced past the injury via bronchoscopy |
| Esophageal | - Cervical esophageal injury most common<br>- Severe chest pain or pneumomediastinum<br>- Esophagoscopy needed to diagnose<br>- Broad-coverage antibiotics |
| Great vessel | - Subclavian injuries most common<br>- Can occur with both chest and neck wounds<br>- Can cause massive hemothorax<br>- Early intubation if evidence of expanding neck hematoma<br>- Aortography is test of choice, if stable<br>- OR thoracotomy indicated, if unstable |
| Diaphragmatic | - Left-sided more common due to right-handed attackers and absence of liver<br>- Does not heal because pleuroperitoneal gradient<br>- Difficult to diagnose because often asymptomatic<br>- CT insensitive, look for diaphragm thickening, hemoperitoneum, or hemothorax<br>- DPL with many false negatives, RBC cut-off is 5,000 cells per mm$^3$<br>- Laparoscopy indicated if wound is in the epigastrium or left thoracoabdominal area |

knife blade to gauge the potential depth of penetration. More importantly, keep in mind that the size of the entrance wound does not say anything about the depth of the wound. It is a common mistake to assume a shallow injury when a small entrance wound is present.

It is important to identify all gunshot wounds, both entrance and exit. Entrance wounds tend to be smaller as the force of impact is directed internally. When one wound is identified, always look for another wound, especially on the back side that is sometimes overlooked initially. The gauge and type of firearm can also be useful information. Guns are classified as low velocity and high velocity. Handguns are considered low velocity, with resulting injury limited to the path of the bullet. However, keep in mind that the slower the bullet, the higher the likelihood the bullet will bounce off internal structures, such as bone, altering the path of damage. Hunting rifles and long-muzzled military firearms are high velocity. The much higher kinetic energy associated with these weapons results in more extensive internal blast injuries that can be estimated by looking at the external entrance wound.

## PRIMARY SURVEY

The primary survey in penetrating chest trauma consists of the same assessment of airway, breathing, and circulation. However, unstable patients will require immediate intervention so the primary survey will often include intubation and placement of chest tubes. Intubation is indicated for patients with significant hemodynamic instability, hypoxia, or altered mental status. Tension pneumothorax or hemothorax should be the first consideration in an unstable patient with penetrating thoracic trauma. In this case a needle thoracostomy followed by a tube thoracostomy should be performed in conjunction with intubation.

Often tube thoracostomy is performed without having to intubate the patient. This is common for patients with stab wounds and clinical evidence of a pneumothorax (e.g., dyspnea, decreased breath sounds, or hypoxia), provided the patient is relatively stable, because several minutes will be required to administer adequate local anesthesia for the procedure. The same is true for thoracic injuries from a small caliber handgun; however, there should be a lower threshold for intubating a patient with a gunshot wound because of the higher likelihood of significant internal injury. Clinical evidence of a pneumothorax is often ambiguous because it is sometimes difficult to hear breath sounds. Intervention then should be based on the whole clinical gestalt. The diagnosis can wait for a portable CXR if the patient is stable (e.g., breathing comfortably, normal blood pressure, respiratory rate, and oxygen saturation).

The primary survey should then focus on several areas, and several specific injuries should be considered. The airway should be assessed for significant blood, which may indicate tracheobronchial injury, hemoptysis, and impending airway obstruction. The neck should be inspected for hematomas, distortion of structures (e.g., expanding hematoma or tension pneumothorax), and distended neck veins (e.g., pericardial tamponade). It is important to remember that the thorax is contiguous with the soft tissues of the anterior neck, and a missile to the chest can track into the neck, causing vascular injury or airway compromise. Breath sounds are assessed and the chest palpated for crepitance.

### Trauma Series

The utility of a trauma series may come into question in some trauma resuscitations; however, a portable CXR is critical in penetrating thoracic trauma. It is essential to diagnose and treat a pneumothorax or hemothorax before the patient is sent to radiology for further studies. It is also useful to identify foreign bodies and the location and number of bullets. Evidence of aortic injury can also be seen with a widened mediastinum, indistinct aortic arch, and blunting of the pulmonoaortic angle.

### The FAST Exam

The FAST exam is an important aspect of the primary survey in penetrating thoracic trauma. It is vital to know if there is a pericardial effusion and evidence of tamponade, which is an indication for immediate OR thoracotomy. The probe is placed directly under the xiphoid process and directed toward the patient's left shoulder while pushing into the epigastrium. This will provide a view of the right and left ventricle divided by the septum and surrounded by the pericardium. An effusion will be seen as a black stripe around the ventricles. Evidence of tamponade includes a collapsed right ventricle and decreased myocardial contraction. This should be correlated with clinical evidence of circulatory shock and distended neck veins. The abdominal portion of the exam is also important given that thoracic wounds can extend into the abdomen, especially those in the thoracoabdominal region.

## MANAGEMENT

During the primary survey and once it is complete, the question is whether the patient needs to go to the OR or can stay in the ED for further workup and identification of injuries. This question is answered primarily based on hemodynamic stability. Once the airway is managed, chest tubes placed, and adequate IV access established, unstable patients with penetrating chest wounds need to go to the OR for open thoracotomy. Uncrossmatched type O blood should be immediately available for transfusion. With penetrating thoracic trauma, stopping blood loss is the primary reason for the need to go to the OR. Essentially, if intubation and chest tubes do not fix the problem, then the ED workup is complete, and the patient needs to be in the OR.

### What If the Patient Dies En Route or on Arrival?

There is good data to show that patients found without signs of circulation (unresponsive, apneic, or pulseless) in the field by EMS, whether victims of blunt or penetrating trauma, invariably die. There is data, however, that show that patients with penetrating thoracic trauma who were initially found alive and who subsequently lose signs of circulation either en route to or immediately after arrival to the ED have a chance of living. These patients can be saved with an ED thoracotomy. The most survivable injury is an isoloated stab wound to the heart that has resulted in pericardial tamponade. A thoracotomy kit should be immediately available for this case, especially if there is forewarning that a penetrating chest trauma is expected.

When a patient suddenly loses signs of circulation, the first action taken should be to intubate and to perform bilateral needle decompression and chest tube placement. This relieves a possible tension pneumothorax. Simultaneously the left chest should be prepped rapidly and the incision begun for a thoracotomy (Box 12-1). Once the chest is open, the etiology of death should be apparent. Pericardial blood will be apparent by a deep purple appearance of the pericardium or a tense pericardium. In this case, an incision is made in the pericardium anterior to the phrenic nerve to relieve that blood. The next step is to stop a bleeding cardiac wound by any means possible. This may involve placing a Foley catheter into the wound, inflating the balloon, and applying tension. Otherwise, the laceration can be approximated with horizontal mattress sutures, taking care not to occlude a coronary vessel. The myocardium can also be stapled in a pinch. The only goal is to stop bleeding and restore cardiac output so the patient can go to the OR for definitive repair.

## BOX 12-1  Procedure: Emergency department thoracotomy

ED thoracotomy is a life-saving procedure that is indicated in penetrating thoracic trauma when the patient loses signs of circulation en route to the ED or on arrival. Its goals are fourfold: evacuate pericardial blood and close cardiac lacerations, perform open cardiac massage, control intrathoracic hemorrhage, and cross-clamp the descending aorta to maximize blood flow to the brain and heart. ED thoracotomy is a temporizing measure to restore signs of life and repair lethal injuries until the patient can go to the OR.

After the patient is prepped, an incision is made in the left fifth intercostal space, one interspace below the nipple in males or the inferior mammary line in females. The incision should extend from the edge of the sternum past the midaxillary line laterally, dissecting down to the intercostal muscles. This should be accomplished with two passes of the scalpel. Mayo scissors are used to cut through the intercostal muscles into the pleural cavity. Rib spreaders are inserted (with the handle directed inferiorly) and opened until adequate access to the heart and chest cavity is obtained. If the internal mammary artery is cut and bleeding, it should be quickly clamped. It runs deep and just lateral to the sternum.

Forceps are used to grasp the pericardium. The pericardial sac is opened longitudinally from bottom to top with scissors, anterior to the phrenic nerve. This will evacuate blood and relieve pericardial tamponade if it exists. The right atrium and ventricle are located anteriorly and most often injured. The heart can then be turned laterally and anteriorly for further exposure. Care should be taken to avoid lifting the heart straight up as this may introduce air into a wound, resulting in air embolism. If bleeding, a cardiac laceration should be sought and controlled. This can be accomplished by inserting a Foley catheter and inflating the balloon or with direct digital control. Alternatively, a cardiac laceration can be stapled or whip stitched. Be careful not to ligate coronary arteries. This also allows

for open cardiac massage (internal CPR), internal defibrillation, or intracardiac administration of medications or blood.

Intrathoracic bleeding is quickly identified and clamped, always using pledgets over the tips of the clamps to avoid further vascular injury. Massive intrathoracic injury can be caused by pulmonary hilar and great vessel injuries, and it may be difficult to gain access. In cases of massive hemorrhage and volume loss, the descending aorta can be exposed and clamped in order to divert all circulating blood to the brain and heart. To accomplish this, the lung is lifted, and blunt dissection is performed into the posterior mediastinum. Scissors may be used to initiate this, then the index finger can be used to dissect to the aorta, which lies directly anterior and lateral to the vertebral bodies. It is important to identify the esophagus so it is not clamped. To facilitate this, a nasogastric tube should be placed prior to the procedure. The aorta is isolated and clamped with pledgeted forceps.

When entering the chest, if there is no suspicion for tamponade, the pericardium can be left intact. Internal cardiac massage can also be initiated. One-handed or two-handed techniques can be used, but the fingers should always remain flat under the left ventricle. In the one-handed technique, the heart is compressed upward against the sternum. The two-handed technique involves cupping one hand over the right ventricle while compressing the left ventricle with the other hand. With either technique, fingertip pressure should be avoided at all times. Finally, internal defibrillation can be performed if the heart is in fibrillation, which will be readily visible. Internal paddles are used, placing one on the RV and the other on the LV. The initial shock should be 20 J. If the pericardium was left intact, subsequent shocks can be given as necessary at 40 and 60 J. If the pericardium has been removed, a maximum of 20 J is recommended.

---

If massive thoracic bleeding is present in this setting, the source is often the pulmonary hilum. Bleeding vessels can be clamped with pledgets over the tips of the clamp to prevent further vascular damage. If the wound is in the right chest, then the thoracotomy should be extended across the chest to the right side to repair injuries. During attempts to stop the bleeding, open cardiac massage should be started if the heart is not contracting. If fibrillating, internal cardiac pads should be used to defibrillate the heart. Additionally, uncrossmatched blood can be introduced directly into the heart. During the entire time, any intrathoracic blood should be suctioned and introduced into an autotransfuser.

## SPECIFIC INJURIES

### Pneumothorax

The first thought in a patient with penetrating chest trauma is usually pneumothorax because it is so

common (see Table 12-2 for classification). In fact, a patient with a gunshot wound to the lateral chest should promptly receive a chest tube because pneumothorax is a certainty. There should be a low threshold for placing a chest tube in a patient with a stab wound to the chest. Any signs of difficulty breathing, shortness of breath, tachypnea, decreased breath sounds, crepitance, hypoxia, or hemodynamic instability should prompt immediate chest tube placement. It is a mistake to wait for a patient to become hypoxic before deciding to place a chest tube. Oxygen saturation is not a reliable indicator of a pneumothorax.

For patients who are stable and relatively asymptomatic, a portable CXR can be obtained. Keep in mind that CXR is not 100% sensitive and that a small pneumothorax can be missed. It is common to see a pneumothorax on CT scan that was not seen on CXR. Therefore, a period of observation for 4 to 6 hours before discharge is warranted in patients with a normal CXR and with a wound deemed to be superficial. A pneumothorax can sometimes be detected by bedside ultra-

| TABLE 12-2 Spectrum of pneumothorax | |
|---|---|
| Simple pneumothorax | - No communication outside thorax<br>- No build up of pressure |
| Communicating pneumothorax | - Communicates through chest wound to outside<br>- Sucking chest wound<br>- Lung collapses with inspiration, expands with expiration<br>- Ineffective ventilation<br>- Requires three-sided occlusive dressing until chest<br>  tube can be placed, then needs to be occluded entirely |
| Tension pneumothorax | - Buildup of pressure as air leaks in during<br>  inspiration but is unable to escape during expiration<br>- Shift of mediastinal contents away from the affected lung<br>- Increased intrathoracic pressure reduces return of blood<br>  to the right heart via the inferior and superior venae cavae<br>- Distended neck veins and hypotension<br>- Requires immediate needle decompression/chest tube |

sound. Patients with a pneumothorax require a chest tube, unless it is small and asymptomatic. A small pneumothorax can be treated with supplemental oxygen and overnight admission for observation, followed by a repeat CXR the next day.

### Hemothorax

Penetrating chest wounds that result in a pneumothorax will always have some degree of associated hemothorax. For this reason, when placing a chest tube for penetrating chest trauma, it should be directed superior and posterior. The tip of the tube should end up posterior to the superior lobe of the lung, which is the lowest point when the patient is supine and where blood will pool. Additionally, the tube size should be at least 36 French in order to drain blood adequately; smaller tubes will become clogged. A hemothorax may not be apparent on auscultation of the lungs as the blood pools posteriorly. Similarly, the portable CXR in the supine patient will not appear as an effusion, as would an upright CXR. It appears rather as a diffuse haziness of the whole lung as compared with the contralateral lung. If possible an upright CXR should be obtained, which will show blunting of the costophrenic angle with 200 to 300 mL of intrathoracic blood.

A massive hemothorax in adults is defined as the return of 1,000 mL of blood when the chest tube is placed. If, based on the exam or x-ray, a hemothorax is anticipated, it is wise to have an autotransfuser readily available in order to recycle the blood. Each hemithorax can contain up to 2 L of blood, almost half the circulating blood volume. Therefore, significant hypovolemia can occur with resulting circulatory

shock and even death. Bleeding to this degree will likely be the result of pulmonary hilar vessel or great vessel injury. More commonly, a hemothorax will result from pulmonary lacerations or bleeding from internal mammary or intercostal vessels. The indication to take the patient to the OR for open thoracotomy for control of bleeding is usually quoted as 1,000 cc initial output or 200 cc per hour over 4 hours. This decision is also based on the patient's hemodynamic stability, although continuous output after 1,500 mL should be taken seriously.

### Penetrating Cardiac Injury

Most penetrating cardiac injuries are fatal, but the odds of survival can be good if the patient makes it to the ED alive. Because of its anterior location, the right ventricle is the most commonly injured chamber, followed by the left ventricle, right atrium, and left atrium. Up to one third of penetrating cardiac injuries involve more than one chamber. Precordial and epigastric wounds are more likely to result in cardiac injury than those more lateral.

Cardiac injuries are rapidly lethal since they can cause either massive hemothorax or contained pericardial tamponade. The latter can occur with only 80 to 120 mL of pericardial blood, after which diastolic filling and cardiac output are compromised. Clinical signs include Beck's triad of hypotension, elevated jugular venous pressure, and muffled or distant heart sounds, although these signs are not always present. The FAST exam is probably the most reliable way to make the diagnosis, with the presence of a pericardial fluid stripe, right ventricular collapse, and decreased myocardial contraction.

# Can bedside ultrasound see a pneumothorax?

We use the bedside ultrasound to perform the FAST exam. Can it also be used to detect a pneumothorax with the same accuracy as a portable CXR? Chung et al. compared high-resolution ultrasound and portable CXR for the diagnosis of pneumothorax. The study included 97 consecutive patients who were undergoing transthoracic needle aspiration and biopsy of the lung for other reasons. Immediately after the procedure, both ultrasound and CXR were obtained. A CT scan was done on all patients, showing a pneumothorax in 35 of the 97 patients. As compared to CXR, ultrasound turned out to be more sensitive (80% versus 47%) and more accurate (89% versus 77%) in making the diagnosis. This study suggests that high-resolution ultrasound is a better test than bedside CXR for the detection of pneumothorax **[Chung et al. *Eur Radiol* 2005;15(5):930–935].** Knudtson et al. examined a total of 328 patients to determine the accuracy of bedside ultrasonography in diagnosing pneumothorax. All ultrasounds were performed by surgeons, and results were compared with CXR findings. They found a specificity and accuracy of 99.7% and 99.4%, respectively **[Knudtson et al. *J Trauma* 2004;56(3):527–530].** Kirkpatrick et al. also investigated the utility of ultrasound in diagnosing pneumothoraces in trauma patients. They were particularly interested in the ability of ultrasound to detect pneumothoraces that were missed with portable AP chest radiographs. Their study included 225 trauma patients. Ultrasound results were blindly compared with the results of subsequent radiographic imaging, with CT scan being the gold standard. Both chest x-ray and ultrasound had high specificity (99.6% and 98.7%, respectively). Ultrasound was found to be more sensitive than CXR **[Kirkpatrick et al. *J Trauma* 2004;57(2):288–295].** These studies all demonstrate the utility of bedside ultrasound in the diagnosis of pneumothorax. The question is whether these results can be translated into common practice, where training in ultrasound varies. This modality is only useful in experienced hands, and these data argue for formal training in the diagnosis of pneumothorax by ultrasound.

BOX 12-2 Pericardiocentesis

Traditionally, pericardiocentesis has been used as both a diagnostic and therapeutic tool. Aspiration of even 5 to 10 mL can restore hemodynamic stability by increasing cardiac output. Pericardiocentesis, however, is not a benign procedure. Possible complications include induction of dysrhythmias, precipitation of cardiac tamponade in the presence of simple pericardial effusion, and pulmonary artery or lung injury. Furthermore, this procedure has been shown to have unacceptably high false-negative and false-positive rates. When performing this procedure, if available, it should be done with ultrasound guidance to decrease the risk of complications. When performed successfully, pericardiocentesis can cause stabilization in the setting of small cardiac lacerations. In fact, this procedure may prevent the need for off thoracotomy.

Patients with pericardial tamponade can deteriorate quickly, but the process is also reversible. Stable patients can be taken to the OR for a pericardial window for exploration and repair. Unstable patients require open thoracotomy to evacuate pericardial blood and repair cardiac lacerations. If the patient loses signs of circulation this must be done in the ED. A pericardiocentesis can be performed in the ED in order to evacuate blood as a temporizing measure (Box 12-2). This may buy time until the patient can be taken to the OR.

## KEY POINTS

- Primary survey will often include life-saving procedures
  - Intubation if significant hemodynamic instability, hypoxia, or altered mental status
  - Tension pneumothorax or large hemothorax should be suspected if unstable
    - Needle thoracostomy and chest tube necessary
  - Immediate chest tube for suspected pneumothorax with respiratory difficulty or hypoxia
  - Arrest requires immediate ED thoracotomy
  - Large-bore IV access and type O blood readily available
- FAST exam to evaluate for pericardial blood and tamponade
- Trauma series chest x-ray to evaluate for hemothorax or pneumothorax (upright if possible)
- Unstable patients go directly to OR for thoracotomy
  - Also those with 1,000 cc initial chest tube ouput or 200 cc per hr over 4 hours
- ED thoracotomy if patient loses vitals with EMS or in ED
  - Most effective for penetrating cardiac wounds

## PENETRATING THORAX ALGORITHM

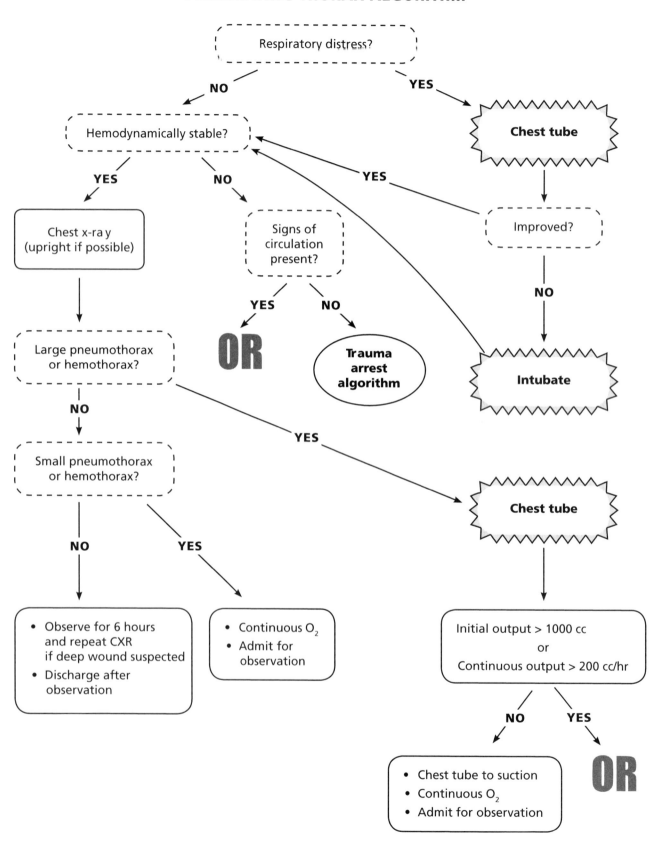

# CHAPTER 13

# Penetrating Abdominal and Back Wounds Trauma

## CASE SCENARIO

A 24-year-old male sustained a stab wound to the left upper quadrant during a gang fight. After the stabbing, the fight dispersed and his friends drove him to the ED. He is taken immediately from triage to a trauma bay in a stretcher.

1. What is your first concern?
   a. Establish IV access, place on oxygen and cardiac monitor
   b. Upright CXR to exclude a pneumothorax
   c. Clinically assess the patient's airway and breathing
   d. Get a set of vital signs

The first priority in this patient, as with all other patients, is to quickly assess the ABCs. In practice this will occur concurrently with establishing IV–$O_2$–monitor and getting a set of vital signs, but the first move is to check airway and breathing. Obtaining a chest x-ray is part of the trauma series that occurs after the primary survey, IV–$O_2$–monitor, vital signs, and FAST exam. Alternatively, chest tube placement should not be delayed until a chest x-ray is obtained if there is clinical evidence of a pneumothorax.

He is alert and oriented with an intact airway, bilateral breath sounds, no chest wall crepitance, and strong symmetrical peripheral pulses. His initial vitals signs are a pulse of 110, blood pressure130/62, respiratory rate of 24, and oxygen saturation of 96% on room air. The secondary survey reveals flat neck veins, normal heart sounds, and no wounds on his neck. His abdomen reveals a 2 cm wound in the left upper quadrant, just under the costal margin, without evisceration of bowel contents. His abdomen is otherwise soft and nontender, although he has focal tenderness just around the wound. No blood is present on rectal exam. A FAST exam reveals normal cardiac contractility without pericardial fluid and no fluid in Morrison's pouch, the splenorenal space, or behind the bladder.

2. What would you do next?
   a. Upright chest x-ray
   b. Arrange for immediate exploratory ex-lap
   c. Local wound exploration to assess for depth and wound tract
   d. Diagnostic peritoneal lavage (DPL)

An upright CXR should be the next step in his management after the primary and secondary surveys, placement of two large-bore IVs, and FAST exam. Immediate laparotomy, after placement of a left chest tube, would be indicated if this patient were unstable. Local wound probing, albeit a common practice, has been shown unreliable in determining peritoneal violation, and it should not be used to exclude peritoneal injuries unless the wound is superficial. A DPL is typically performed in patients with blunt trauma who are too unstable to go to radiology for diagnostic imaging.

The CXR shows no evidence of pneumothorax, and his vital signs and exam remain unchanged. His hematocrit is 39%. A suggestion is made to admit the patient overnight for serial exams and repeat CXR and hematocrit in the morning.

3. What potentially serious injury do you run the highest risk of missing with this strategy?
   a. Diaphragmatic laceration
   b. Pneumothorax

c. Actively bleeding splenic laceration

d. Perforated colon

Diaphragmatic injury should always be considered with penetrating trauma to the upper abdomen or lower chest. The diaphragm is a large structure that spans from the costal margin all the way up to the nipple line with full expiration. Although they often result in hemothorax or hemoperitoneum, lacerations may not be initially significant but can result in herniation of bowel content into the chest, a complication that can occur months or even years later. Although the suggested plan is reasonable to rule out the other injuries listed, given the location of the stab, diaphragmatic injury must be actively sought.

4. What is the best method to diagnose this injury?

   a. DPL

   b. CT scan of the abdomen

   c. Diagnositic laparoscopy or thoracoscopy

   d. Mandatory ex-lap

In the setting of penetrating abdominal wounds, a DPL was previously used to drive the decision of whether to go to the OR for ex-lap. The cut-off for red blood cells in the peritoneal aspirate is 5,000 cells per high-powered field, which is in contrast to the 100,000 cut-off for blunt abdominal trauma. This low cut-off is intended to include diaphragmatic injury in the sensitivity of the test. CT scan is insensitive for detecting diaphragmatic injuries unless the defect is large. However, an abdominal CT scan might be helpful in stable patients with suspected peritoneal violation to assess for solid or hollow organ injuries, hemoperitoneum, hemothorax, or pneumothorax. Laparoscopy is an effective and popular modality for diagnosing diaphragm injuries when the suspicion is high, as with stab wounds to the left thoracoabdominal area. Most would convert to an ex-lap if peritoneal penetration were present on laparoscopy, while some centers would only convert if there were an injury found requiring repair.

Answers: 1-c; 2-a; 3-a; 4-c

## BACKGROUND

Between World War I and 1960, surgery was the rule for all penetrating abdominal trauma. However, there was a high rate of nontherapeutic and negative laparotomies (no injury needing repair or no injury at all, respectively). These surgeries had high associated postoperative complication rates and lengthy hospital stays. Over the years, the trend has shifted toward nonoperative management, with a goal of minimizing unnecessary laparotomies. Today, even some abdominal gunshot wounds are managed nonoperatively. Busy trauma centers, most notably in South Africa, which see a high volume of patients with penetrating trauma have been leaders in developing safe, effective, nonoperative management. The cornerstones of nonoperative management are thorough physical exam, serial re-evaluations of the patient, close monitoring with cooperation and communication between all members of the trauma team.

## CLINICAL ANATOMY AND PHYSIOLOGY

Injury to intra-abdominal organs, as well as retroperitoneal structures, is possible in penetrating trauma to the abdominal wall, flank, buttocks, and back (collectively known as the torso). It is important to know the landmarks of each of the regions of the torso since the workup for penetrating trauma may vary depending on the location of the wound and the type of missile involved (Figure 13–1). The *anterior abdomen* is bordered by the anterior axillary lines from the inferior costal margin to the inguinal crease. The *thoracoabdominal area*, which can house either thoracic organs or abdominal contents, depending on the position of the diaphragm at the time of injury, begins at the nipple line (fourth intercostal space) anteriorly and the inferior scapular tip (seventh intercostal space) posteriorly and extends inferiorly to the costal margins. Generally, wounds in the epigastrum are also considered thoracoabdominal wounds. The *flank* encompasses the area between the anterior and posterior axillary lines from the inferior tip of the scapula to the superior margin of the iliac crest. Finally, the *back* is defined by the posterior axillary lines laterally, the inferior costal margin and the superior margin of the iliac crest (Table 13-1).

### What You Have to Go through to Get to the Important Stuff

Knowledge of the layers of the abdominal wall is important when trying to determine the depth of a

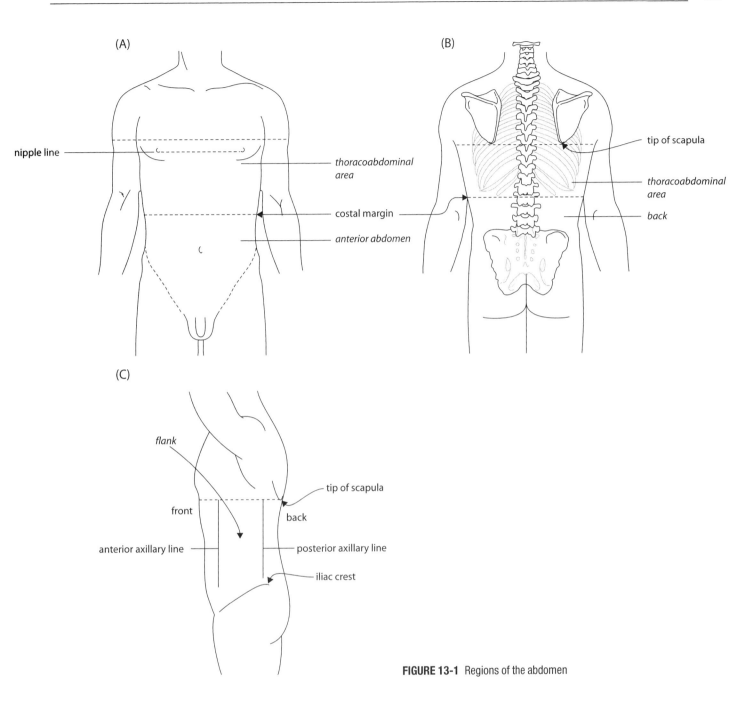

**FIGURE 13-1** Regions of the abdomen

| TABLE 13-1 External borders of the areas of anatomic interest | | | |
|---|---|---|---|
| **Area** | **Superior border** | **Inferior border** | **Lateral border** |
| Abdomen | Costal margin | Inguinal crease | Anterior axillary lines |
| Thoracoabdomen | Fourth intercostal space (anterior) | Costal margin | N/A |
| | Seventh intercostal space (posterior) | Costal margin | N/A |
| Flank | Inferior scapular tip | Illiac crest | Anterior and posterior axillary lines |
| Back | Inferior costal margin | Illiac crest | Posterior axillary lines |

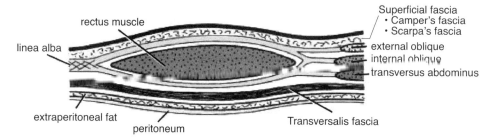

**FIGURE 13-2** Layers of the abdomen
(Adapted from Snell, RS. *Clinical Anatomy*, 7th ed. Philadelphia: Lippincott Williams & Wilkins; 2003.)

wound (Figure 13-2). The layers vary depending on the location on the torso. The first layer of the anterior abdomen is Camper's fascia, a layer containing a variable amount of adipose tissue, below which superficial vessels and nerves are located. Below this is Scarpa's fascia, containing fibrous tissue and little fat. Inferiorly, Scarpa's fascia merges with the deep fascia of the thigh (fascia lata) and perineum (Colles' fascia). Between Scarpa's fascia and the deep fascia of the abdomen, there is a potential space into which blood can track from the pelvis. This accounts for a high false-positive rate for DPLs in the setting of pelvic fractures. Below this is a deep fascial layer that is thin, strong, and attached to the underlying muscle.

The muscles of the anterior abdominal wall lie laterally and insert in the middle into a tough, fibrous aponeurosis, which encases the rectus abdominis, two straplike abdominal wall muscles that lie longitudinally on each side of the midline. The aponeuroses meet in the middle to form the linea alba, a thick, fibrous structure that is a major landmark when performing a DPL. The lateral muscles, from superficial to deep, are the external oblique, internal oblique, and transversus abdominis. The transversalis fascia lies deep to the muscles and is directly adjacent to the parietal peritoneum.

The back is more protected from penetrating injury. First, there are vertebrae that protect the spinal cord. Second, the ribs are thicker in the back, providing more protection to the lungs. It is important to remember that the lungs extend down to the inferior margin of the T10 vertebral body (three intercostal spaces below the scapular tip) and that thoracic injuries should be considered with penetrating back wounds. Thick longitudinal muscles that run parallel to the spine provide another line of protection. It is useful to know that the umbilicus is approximately at the level of the L3–L4 level in physically fit people and that the first portion of the duodenum is at the level of the body of the L1 vertebra.

### Different Types of Abdominal Organs

Differentiation is made in trauma when talking about solid versus hollow organs. Solid organs include the liver and spleen. The significance of these is that they bleed a lot, and injury can cause rapid accumulation of intraperitoneal blood. Hollow organs include the bowel and gallbladder. These are at risk for rupture in blunt abdominal trauma and are at risk for laceration in penetrating trauma. Both result in spillage of intestinal contents into the peritoneal space. The diaphragm is an often forgotten structure in trauma, but it is significant because it separates the thorax from the abdomen. The diaphragm attaches posteriorly to the L1–L3 vertebral bodies, the 6th rib anterolaterally, the 12th posterolaterally, and the xiphosternal junction anteriorly. Small diaphragm lacerations can extend over time to the point where intestinal herniation into the chest occurs. The other sometimes overlooked organ in the abdomen is the bladder. It is important to remember that the superior portion of the bladder is covered by parietal peritoneum and, when full, the bladder can extend up to the level of the umbilicus. Finally, there are many important retroperitoneal structures that can be injured even in the absence of peritoneal violation (Box 13-1).

### MANAGEMENT

Workup depends on hemodynamic stability and presence of peritoneal signs. As in all trauma, however, the initial workup is the same: primary survey, IV–$O_2$–monitor, FAST exam, secondary survey, blood transfusion, and trauma series if necessary. After that, the unifying rule in all penetrating torso trauma is that un-

---

**BOX 13-1  Major retroperitoneal structures**

*Solid Organs*
Kidneys
Pancreas
Adrenal glands

*Vasculature*
IVC
Aorta
Renal arteries
Renal veins

*Hollow Organs*
Ascending colon
Descending colon
Second, third, and fourth parts of the duodenum
Ureters

---

stable patients and those with peritoneal signs, regardless of presence or absence of blood on FAST exam, require laparotomy (see the algorithm at the end of this chapter). Peritoneal signs include diffuse tenderness and rebound (tap tenderness or release tenderness away from the wound). Both intraperitoneal bleeding and spillage of bowel contents can cause this.

## Wounds that Appear Superficial

A certain percentage of patients will present with wounds that appear superficial. In these patients, the first question is: Has the peritoneum been violated? Patients with peritoneal violation will require further evaluation, whether it be ex-lap, CT scan, or simply admission and observation. This question is answered mostly based on physical exam. Local wound exploration (LWE) can be an important aspect of the physical exam to determine whether or not the peritoneum was violated, although this practice is less common today. LWE does not refer to blind probing with Q-tips, instruments, or fingers, all of which are notoriously poor for determining peritoneal violation and can cause further injury. If wounds are to be locally explored, the procedure should be undertaken in standard surgical fashion with proper lighting, sterile conditions, proper instruments, and liberal use of local anesthetic. After the site is prepped and draped, the wound can be extended with a scalpel and the edges retracted to determine the trajectory and depth. When the bottom of the wound is clearly identified and the peritoneum is not violated, the

wound can be irrigated copiously and closed loosely. Drains should not be placed. LWE should not be done for LUQ wounds that could potentially lead into the chest cavity; it also has no utility in flank wounds as it will lead to dissection into the retroperitoneal space.

## Wounds that Definitely or Potentially Violate the Peritoneum

It is now clear that even if a wound is found to violate the peritoneum, the patient does not necessarily need an ex-lap. This is true even in cases of evisceration, especially isolated omental evisceration. There are several options for workup when it comes to hemodynamically stable patients with definite or possible peritoneal violation. The trauma literature has been quite clear for several decades now that patients with stab wounds, who are hemodynamically stable and have no evidence of peritonitis, have no indication for immediate ex-lap. Gunshot wounds, because of the energy of the blast and higher potential for injury, were traditionally taken immediately to the OR. However, over the past 15 years, there has been a large amount of literature from centers that frequently treat gunshot wounds indicating a significant percentage (about 20% to 40%) can be managed nonoperatively.

CT scan has long been recognized as a vital component of the workup for penetrating wounds to the flank and back. However, CT scan has also become an often-utilized modality to assess for intra-abdominal injury in the setting of penetrating thoracoabdominal and anterior abdominal trauma in stable patients. The clear advantage is its sensitivity (greater than 95%) for identifying specific injuries such as solid organ injury, free intra-peritoneal fluid, retroperitoneal vascular injuries, and renal injuries. A triple-contrast (oral, rectal, and IV contrast) is recommended to evaluate both for solid organ injuries (seen with IV contrast) and hollow organ injuries (seen by spilling of oral or rectal contrast). The only limitations are its sensitivity for detecting bowel and diaphragmatic perforation, even given the oral and rectal contrast. A reasonable approach that has developed is to do a CT scan of the abdomen to look for injuries that might require laparotomy and otherwise to observe patients for 24 hours if they have suspected peritoneal violation without definite indication for ex-lap. Some centers advocate observing all patients even if the wound looks superficial on CT. It is likely that as CT technology continues to improve, patients with penetrating abdominal trauma will be managed entirely on the basis of physical exam and CT findings, with role of the FAST exam, DPL, and diagnostic laparoscopy becoming continually more limited.

LITERATURE REFERENCE

## Gunshot wounds as a special case

The role of nonoperative management in the care of patients with torso gunshot wounds (GSW) is slowly gaining acceptance, although the majority of patients will have early indications for ex-lap. The first prospective studies describing nonoperative management of GSW came out of the busy trauma centers of South Africa [**Muckart et al. Br J Surg** 1990;77(6):652–655; **Demetriades et al. Br J Surg** 1991;78(2):220–222]. The arguments that the physical exam was unreliable and that almost all these patients require laparotomy was further debunked by Velmahos et al. in a consecutive case series of 1,856 patients over 8 years. An astounding 38% of these patients were managed entirely nonoperatively. In this study, only 80 patients (11%) of the 705 managed nonoperatively required a delayed laparotomy with five patients having some complication potentially attributable to delayed ex-lap. The authors estimated that at their institution alone over a million dollars were saved annually by using selective nonoperative management principles for gunshot wounds. Nearly half of the laparotomies would have been unnecessary if all patients went for ex-lap. Criteria for ex-lap after a period of observation included unexplained drop in hematocrit or blood pressure and progression of abdominal tenderness from local to deep. Ineligible patients were those intubated, severely intoxicated, and those with head or spinal cord injuries [**Velmahos et al. Ann Surg** 2001;234(3):395–403; discussion 402–403].

LITERATURE REFERENCE

## Penetrating trauma to the pelvis and buttocks

As the nonoperative management of penetrating trauma has become more widely accepted, some have suggested that there are certain wounds that cannot be managed nonoperatively. Examples included transpelvic gunshot wounds and penetrating buttocks trauma. In two consecutive case series, Vemahos et al. attempted to answer this question. The study looked at transpelvic GSWs, which included 37 consecutive patients: 19 went immediately to the OR and 18 were initially managed nonoperatively, with 3 eventually going to laparotomy (all of which were nontherapeutic). Indications for ex-lap were peritoneal signs, gross hematuria, rectal bleeding, or hemodynamic instability. A second study looking at penetrating buttocks trauma included 59 consecutive patients: 40 were managed nonoperatively based on the same criteria. The patients in these two studies were managed primarily based on physical exam findings. While these studies have relatively small numbers, when taken with other studies of nonoperative management of penetrating abdominal trauma, they make a convincing argument that selective laparotomy is feasible [**Velmahos et al. World J Surg** 1998;22(10):1034–1038; **Velmahos et al. Dis Colon Rectum** 1997;40(3):307–311].

The utility of the FAST exam in penetrating trauma is generally limited to assessing the pericardium for presence of effusion or tamponade. Studies looking at its utility in patients who have penetrating trauma generally show that it does *not* affect decision to go to the operating room in a significant number of patients. This is logical, because FAST assesses for the presence of free fluid, which may result from abdominal wall or omental bleeding. Thus, in a patient with a positive FAST exam, who is hemodynamically stable and without peritoneal signs, ex-lap is not mandatory. In this case, CT scan can be done to further characterize injuries that might require laparotomy, or it is also reasonable to observe the patient in the hospital with frequent serial abdominal exams.

DPL was traditionally used as a tool to assess for intraperitoneal injury in both blunt and penetrating abdominal trauma. However, its utility has dropped dramatically with the advent of bedside ultrasound and multidetector CT scanning, given that DPL lacks sensitivity for bowel, diaphragm, or retroperitoneal injuries. Today, in most centers, a DPL would only be performed in a patient with multiple blunt injuries (e.g., head injury and abdominal injury) who is too unstable to go to CT scan. In the 1980s, however, DPL was the next step if LWE was

## CT scan for assessing the patient with penetrating torso trauma

The role for CT in the workup of penetrating torso wounds is increasing significantly with the advent of multidetector CT scanners (MDCTs). There is good evidence to support this approach.

The first question is whether or not CT can be used to determine the trajectory of the wound tracks, allowing patients to be discharged more rapidly if the scan shows a wound track that does not approach any important intra-abdominal structures. A retrospective chart review at a Level I trauma center looked at 50 patients over 6 years who underwent CT scanning to determine trajectory of either a thorax or torso GSW. The review showed that the use of CT allowed the workup for these injuries to be tailored down considerably and limited unnecessary operation, thus making better use of resources **[Grossman et al. *J Trauma* 1998;45(3):446–456].**

Shanmuganathan et al. looked at the use of triple-contrast CT in 200 patients with penetrating trauma to the torso; most were single detector rather than multidetector CTs. The entrance wound was located in the thoracoabdominal area in 42%, abdomen in 18%, flank in 15%, pelvic in 15%, and back in 16% (5% had two wounds).

There was no evidence of peritoneal violation in 132 patients, but 3 of these had evidence of retroperitoneal injury. Of these 132 patients, there were 2 false negatives, both of which had other abnormal findings. One was initially observed, given no obvious indication for laparotomy on CT or on exam. Eventually, the patient developed worsening pain and had a repeat CT showing a mesenteric hematoma and diaphragmatic injury. The other had evidence of thickened diaphragm on CT scan and was taken to the OR and found to have a diaphragm injury. Of the 68 positive CT scans there were 2 false positives, both having no injury on laparotomy. Common positive findings were often as simple as wound tract extending to the organ in question. Of the patients undergoing laparotomy, 93% went on the basis of the CT finding, indicating the reliance on CT in this particular center. Of these patients, less than 15% had a nontherapeutic laparotomy (injury not requiring repair). The overall sensitivity and specificity of CT scan for detecting peritoneal violation were 97% and 98%, with a negative predictive value of 98% **[Shanmuganathan et al. *Radiology* 2004;231(3): 775–784].**

equivocal or peritoneal violation suspected. Grossly bloody aspirate of intraperitoneal contents is considered positive and an indication for laparotomy. If no fluid returns on aspiration, 1,000 mL of saline is infused and drained with the aid of gravity. A positive DPL depends on microscopic analysis of this drained fluid, although there is some debate over the RBC count threshold that constitutes a positive exam. Counts greater than 100,000 RBCs per mm$^3$ are universally considered positive and an indication for ex-lap; but with penetrating trauma, many injuries are missed using this cut-off. For penetrating thoracoabdominal injury where diaphragm laceration is in question, a cut-off of 5,000 RBCs per mm$^3$ is used. Various other cut-offs are used to look for other intra-abdominal injuries.

Another method that has come in and out of favor is the use of laparoscopy. The advantages of laparoscopy are that it is less invasive than ex-lap and thus has a much shorter recovery period and hospital length of stay. The alternative argument, however, is that injuries not apparent clinically or by CT scanning do not require invasive intervention at all, and to undergo such an invasive procedure just to look for a potential injury is of no use. It also has poor sensitivity for small bowel injury, similar to CT scanning, thus decreasing its added benefit over CT. Some studies report as high as a 20% missed injury rate for diagnostic laparoscopy. Therefore, laparoscopy has had a limited role in the general algorithm for penetrating abdominal wounds at most centers. Laparoscopy has gained more utility as a tool for identifying diaphragmatic injuries, for which it has a high sensitivity, in patients with LUQ penetrating wounds who are otherwise stable and have no other injuries found by CT that would require exploratory laparotomy.

## The role of laparascopy in penetrating abdominal trauma

There is a great deal of debate about the role of laparoscopy in management of penetrating abdominal trauma. The known limitations of this technique are that it is not sensitive for detecting injuries to hollow organs and that the extent of damage to the liver, spleen, and retroperitoneum are hard to assess. Leppaniemi et al. looked at the role of laparoscopy versus serial exams in patients with thoracoabdominal SW and an equivocal wound exploration. There were 232 consecutive patients in the study; 79 underwent immediate laparotomy, based on signs of shock or peritonitis. The remainder underwent wound exploration. Of the remaining 153 patients, if peritoneal violation was confirmed by exam ($n = 43$), the patient was randomized to ex-lap versus laparoscopy. If the exam was equivocal ($n = 107$), the patient was randomized to laparoscopy versus nonoperative management. In the group with clear peritoneal violation, 9 of 20 laparoscopies had to be converted to ex-lap, with only one of these ex-laps being negative. The other 11 laparoscopies, however, were all nontherapeutic. There was no difference in morbidity, hospital cost, or LOS. La-paroscopy found mostly minor injuries in the group with equivocal penetration, and this group had a longer LOS. The conclusion was that laparoscopy was no more effective than physical exam or observation in determining significant intra-abdominal injury **[Leppaniemi et al. _J Trauma_ 2003;55(4):636–645].**

The accepted role of laparoscopy in thoracoabdominal injury is in identifying diaphragmatic injuries; however, most studies involving this modality do not focus primarily on the diagnosis of diaphragmatic injury. A recent study by Friese et al. rigorously looked at the accuracy of laparoscopy for diaphragmatic injury by performing both laparoscopy followed by ex-lap or thoracoscopy in all 34 patients. Their results found laparoscopy to be highly sensitive and specific for diaphragmatic injuries **[Friese et al. _J Trauma_ 2005;58(4):789–792].** Thus, given its limitations for intra-abdominal injuries in general, the role of laparoscopy is probably limited to assessing diaphragmatic injury in patients with penetrating thoracoabdominal trauma.

### Think Diaphragm in Left Thoracoabdominal Wounds

The diagnosis of diaphragmatic rupture is quite elusive. While diaphragmatic rents can alter the physiology of respiration and venous return to the chest, as well as cardiac output in serious cases, many patients may be asymptomatic. Physical exam, CXR, and CT scan are known to be insensitive for this injury. CT may show nonspecific findings (e.g., diaphragmatic thickening) or indirect evidence of diaphragmatic rupture (e.g., wound trajectory, hemothorax with liver or splenic injury) but rarely shows any pathognomonic findings (e.g., bowel in the chest) in the acute setting. DPL has been recommended, but there is significant disagreement over the RBC count used as the cut-off. Early case reports show that MRI may be useful; but it is also expensive and not readily available, nor practical, in the acute setting. Several reports in the literature indicate that the presence of diaphragmatic injury, especially in the presence of left thoracoabdominal stab wounds, is quite high. One study found the incidence of occult diaphragmatic injury in this population to be 17%. Therefore, these patients, even when asymptomatic, should generally undergo laparoscopy or thoracoscopy.

### CONCLUSION

The diagnostic algorithm for penetrating torso trauma has been slowly coalescing toward complete reliance on physical exam, vital signs, and CT scan in selected cases (back and flank wounds of any kind and almost all gunshot wounds). In patients with left thoracoabdominal wounds, routine laparoscopy or thoracoscopy should be employed to rule out diaphragmatic injury, and it is important that a FAST exam be done to evaluate for pericardial effusion or tamponade. The different diagnostic and treatment methods are outlined in Table 13-2.

| TABLE 13-2 Comparison of techniques for workup of penetrating abdominal trauma | | |
|---|---|---|
| **Diagnostic manuever** | **Advantages** | **Disadvantages** |
| Serial exams | Performed at the bedside<br>Inexpensive, not including length of stay (LOS)<br>Noninvasive | Operator dependent<br>May miss injuries not causing peritonitis (e.g., diaphragmatic injury)<br>Debatable higher rate of negative ex-lap<br>Requires prolonged observation |
| Local wound exploration | Performed at the bedside<br>Inexpensive | Difficult in obese patients |
| DPL | Performed at the bedside<br>Relatively quick if grossly positive<br>Available in areas with fewer resources<br>Sensitivity is high | Invasive<br>Specificity debated<br>Specific injury not identified<br>Unclear RBC cut-off<br>Misses bowel/retroperitoneal injury<br>Time-consuming if lab analysis required<br>Difficult in obese patients |
| FAST exam | Specificity high (about 90%)<br>Performed at the bedside<br>Easily repeatable<br>Noninvasive<br>Quick | Sensitivity low (50% to 60%)<br>Operator dependent<br>Difficult in obese patients<br>Misses diaphragm/bowel injury |
| Triple contrast CT | Identifies specific injuries<br>Sensitivity and specificity high<br>Relatively quick<br>May allow for earlier discharge<br>Noninvasive | Patients leaves resuscitation bay<br>Contrast is given<br>Misses diaphragm/bowel injury |
| Laparoscopy | Potentially allows repair of injury<br>Generally good for diaphragmatic injury | Operator dependent<br>Invasive<br>Expensive<br>Limited sensitivity<br>Time-consuming<br>Impractical in busy centers |
| Mandatory ex-lap | Identifies specific injuries<br>High sensitivity | Invasive<br>High complication rate<br>Time-consuming<br>Expensive<br>Increases LOS<br>Impractical in busy centers |

## KEY POINTS

- Anatomic region of wound important in workup
  - Anterior abdomen, thoracoabdominal, flank, and back
- Abdominal wounds with peritonitis or hemodynamic instability go directly to ex-lap
- ED workup for stable patients begins with determining peritoneal penetration
  - If base of wound can be clearly identified, then observe for several hours

- Most wounds are not clear or may only seem shallow
  - Local wound exploration (LWE) previously used to determine depth

- Triple-contrast CT scan indicated for definite or possible peritoneal violation
  - If negative, patient should be observed for 24 hours
  - Ex-lap indicated if evidence of bowel spillage, active extravasation, or developing peritonitis

- Trend toward reliance solely on physical exam, vitals, and CT scan
- Back and flank wounds require triple-contrast CT scan
- Diaphragmatic injury must be considered with left thoracoabdominal wounds
  - CT scan has poor sensitivity for diaphragm injuries
  - Laparoscopy or thoracoscopy indicated
- FAST exam should not typically influence management
  - Stable patients can go for CT scan and be observed nonoperatively
- DPL has little utility in penetrating abdominal trauma
  - Lavage fluid cut-off is 5,000 RBC per hpf for diaphragmatic and bowel injury

## PENETRATING ABDOMINAL/BACK WOUNDS

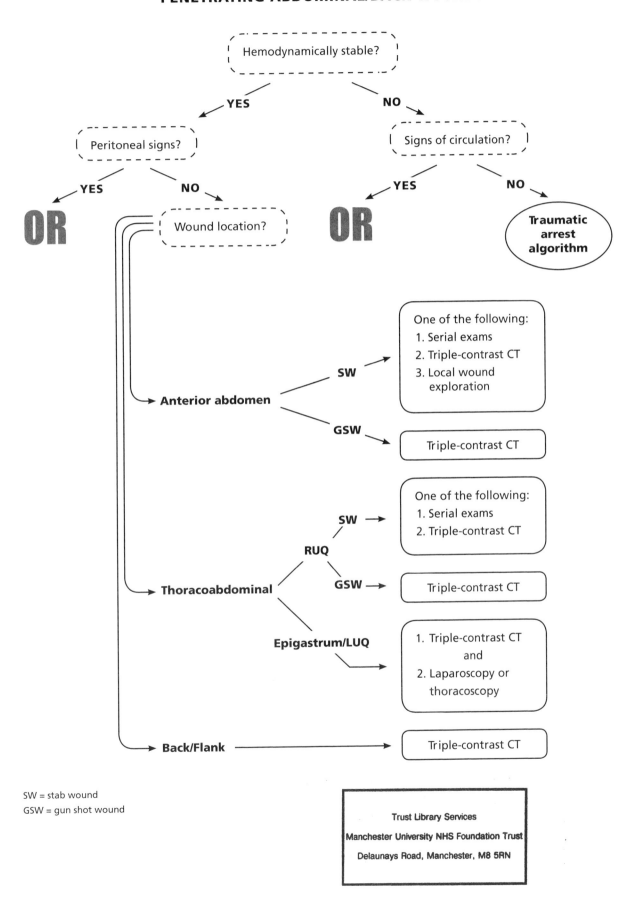

SW = stab wound
GSW = gun shot wound

# CHAPTER 14

# Maxillofacial Trauma

## CASE SCENARIO

A 23-year-old female is about to be transferred to your Level I trauma center from a small rural institution where she presented 1 hour ago after being assaulted. In the field, she was alert and complained of diffuse facial pain. The outside hospital physicians were concerned about her obvious facial deformities, including a possible open globe injury, and arranged for the transfer as soon as they determined her vital signs were normal. Her airway was intact and her respirations normal. C-spine x-rays were obtained while waiting for transport to arrive and were normal.

**1.** As soon as you hear about the transfer, what is your first priority before she arrives?
   **a.** Call ophthalomology for likely emergent operation
   **b.** Call the OR because you think she will likely need emergency surgery
   **c.** Prepare standard rapid sequence intubation medications and equipment
   **d.** Assemble difficult airway intubation equipment and have a cricothyrotomy tray immediately accessible

The grotesque nature of facial injuries can distract the evaluator from the standard trauma assessment. The first step, as always, is airway (the A of the ABCs). Facial trauma poses a unique need for early and aggressive airway management and intervention for two significant reasons. First, distorted facial and airway anatomy, along with soft tissue swelling and hematomas, can make intubation technically difficult. A patient should never be paralyzed unless the ability to use the BVM effectively can be ensured. Facial distortion, however, may compromise the ability to make a tight seal with the mask. Sometimes, a surgical airway is the most appropriate first-line intervention. Regardless, in such patients, equipment for a quick surgical airway should always be easily available. The second fact that mandates aggressive airway intervention is the potential for rapid downward spiral of clinical course. For example, a clot from the oropharynx can become dislodged, resulting in hemorrhage and loss of a patent airway. Therefore, the threshold to secure a definitive airway should be low.

The patient arrives, and you begin your evaluation. Her airway appears to be intact; however, she has some blood in her oropharynx that appears to originate from her right naris. She has a significant nasal fracture with complete lateral displacement of several centimeters. She is breathing without difficulty, and her peripheral pulses are strong. Her vitals include a pulse of 94, blood pressure 132/78, respiratory rate of 18, and oxygen saturation of 98% on oxygen 2 L nasal cannula. You are concerned that oropharyngeal blood may obstruct her airway, but you decide to evaluate her epistaxis before intubating her.

**2.** While you are assembling your equipment for nasal evaluation and packing, what steps can be taken to protect her airway?
   **a.** Insert a nasopharyngeal airway through the left naris
   **b.** Pull her tongue out using a pair of forceps
   **c.** Clear her c-spine if possible, and ask her to sit up
   **d.** Clear her c-spine if possible, and place her in the left lateral decubitus position

Simple maneuvers increase patency in the patient with facial trauma. If c-spine injury is not suspected and other injuries allow, the patient should sit up and lean forward to help open the airway. Mandibular fractures may displace the tongue posteriorly, a situation that may require pulling the tongue anteriorly using forceps or a suture placed through the anterior tongue. You are able to sit her up, and she feels more comfortable. Your examination of the right naris is limited by blood, but you are sure that her grossly deformed nose is the culprit.

**3.** What is the appropriate course of action?
   **a.** Call ENT to reduce her nasal fracture in the OR
   **b.** Reduce her nasal fracture in the ED, assess the need for packing and septal hematoma release, and apply an external splint
   **c.** Cauterize on the bleeding source in the right septum
   **d.** Insert a Foley catheter into the nasopharynx, inflate the balloon, and admit the patient for observation

Nasal fractures cause epistaxis by mucosal injury. Grossly displaced fractures should be reduced. This can be accomplished easily in most cases in the ED. Hemostats can be placed bilaterally in the nares, and outward pressure applied while bringing the bone fragments back to the midline. After reduction, a search for an additional source of bleeding should be performed. Septal hematomas should be drained immediately to prevent saddle nose deformity. Nasal packs are available for both anterior and posterior bleeds. A Foley catheter is generally used to tamponade posterior bleeds. Blind cautery should not be performed because of risk of septal perforation. This patient's fracture is reduced with gradual cessation of bleeding. An external splint is applied.

You now resume your secondary survey. The patient has significant swelling, ecchymosis, and tenderness of her inferior left orbit. The eye itself has a large subconjunctival hematoma with chemosis. The pupil however is round and reactive. She has blurriness out of the left eye as well. She is complaining of double vision when you ask her to look upward. You are concerned about a blowout fracture.

**4.** What is the most appropriate course of action?
   **a.** Obtain a CT scan, and consult plastic surgery for delayed repair
   **b.** Perform an emergent lateral canthotomy to restore normal vision
   **c.** Administer mannitol to reduce intraocular pressure
   **d.** Call ophthalmology for emergent surgical decompression of her entrapped optic nerve

Orbital blowout fractures are caused by blunt trauma to the globe, resulting in increased intraocular pressure that is relieved by fracture of the orbital floor or one of the walls. The orbital floor is extremely thin and thus prone to fracture. Diplopia on upward gaze is caused by inferior rectus muscle entrapment. Orbital blowout fractures are often managed conservatively. Operative repair, delayed 7 to 10 days after injury, is indicated in the presence of persistent diplopia or enophthalmos. Lateral canthotomy is indicated for loss of visual acuity because of sudden rises in ocular pressure, as with a retrobulbar hematoma. Optic nerve damage can be associated with Le Fort III fractures. The subconjunctival hemorrhage, although it often looks ugly, is not in and of itself concerning. The pupils are round and reactive, therefore making the possibility of ruptured globe less likely. Blurred vision can also be the result of traumatic uveitis. However, the patient should also be seen by an ophthalmologist.

Answers: 1-d; 2-c; 3-b; 4-a

## BACKGROUND

Urban centers see more facial trauma caused by penetrating or assault-related mechanisms, while rural centers see more facial injuries resulting from motor vehicle crashes and falls. Facial trauma comprises the majority of ED visits related to domestic violence. In some centers, it has been determined that up to one fourth of women with facial trauma are victims of domestic abuse. Facial trauma is often accompanied by significant injuries in other systems, the search for which should not be deterred by the graphic nature of some facial injuries.

## CLINICAL ANATOMY

The external bony facial skeleton is composed of the frontal bone, temporal bones, zygomas, nasal bone, maxilla, and mandible. These bones form the horizontal and vertical buttresses, bony arches joined by suture lines, that provide stability and support to the face (Figure 14-1). The ethmoid, sphenoid, and lacrimal bones join to form the inner portions of the orbits. Portions of cranial nerves II, III, V, and VI course through the orbital foramina, and disruption of the orbital bones makes these nerves susceptible to damage. The orbital floor and medial wall are as thin as an eggshell, making them prone to fractures.

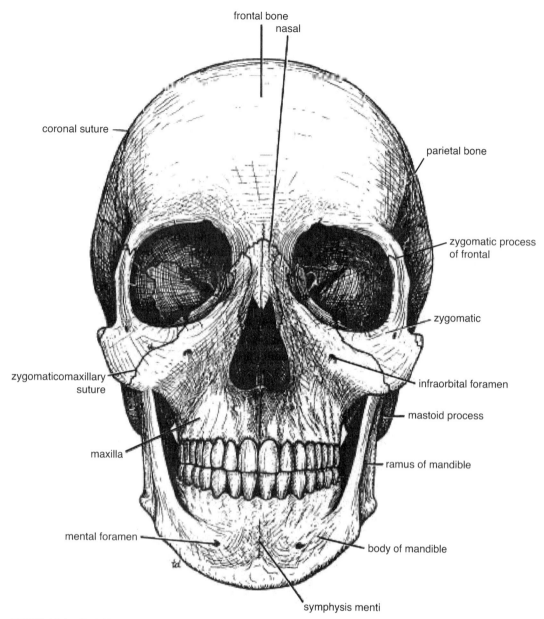

**FIGURE 14-1**   Facial bones
(Adapted from Snell, RS. *Clinical Anatomy*. 7th ed. Philadelphia: Lippincott Williams & Wilkins; 2003.)

## PRIMARY SURVEY

The grotesque nature of some facial injuries should not distract the physician from approaching the facial trauma patient in an organized, sequential manner. Airway management should be aggressive and early because of the potential for rapid deterioration. The mouth is cleared of any foreign body or blood. If the tongue is blocking the airway, a jaw thrust or modified chin-lift should be performed, without neck extension if there is concern for c-spine injury. Mandible fractures may displace the tongue posteriorly and render these maneuvers ineffective. In this case, the tongue should be pulled forward with a towel clip, gauze pad, or large suture placed through the anterior tongue, while preparations for intubation are undertaken.

Facial trauma can make rapid sequence intubation difficult or impossible. This is important, because airway compromise is common and definitive airway management often essential. There are many possible sources of airway compromise that may be apparent (e.g., gross deformity or bloody airway) or may be insidious and progressive (e.g., pharyngeal or neck hematomas that distort airway anatomy). Altered anatomy can make definitive airway placement technically challenging. Having a well thought-out plan with back-up devices is important. Obtaining an effective seal with the BVM can be impossible with loss of bony support structures. Without the ability to bag effectively, a patient should not be paralyzed. If paralytics are going to be administered, always have a surgical airway tray prepared and ready. Fiber-optic and/or awake intubation should be considered as alternatives, if time permits. It may be necessary to go straight to a surgical airway. Cricothyrotomy is possible if the injury is above the level of the larynx. Nasopharyngeal intubation should be avoided because of the risk of cribriform plate disruption and intracranial penetration of the endotracheal tube.

Breathing is usually not a problem in patients with isolated maxillofacial injuries. Hypoventilation is likely due to associated intracranial injury. A CXR should be obtained to rule out concomitant pneumothorax or pneumomediastinum from airway disruption (e.g., larynx or trachea). Facial injuries can have an effect on circulation. Even though the face is highly vascular, signs of shock should always prompt a search for an-

other cause. Direct pressure should be applied to control maxillofacial bleeding; however, blind clamping, which may inadvertently compress important structures such as facial nerves should be avoided. Nasal packing should be used liberally in bleeding that does not cease with pressure alone. If measures to appropriately curtail nasal bleeding are not successful, intubation should be strongly considered.

## SECONDARY SURVEY

The first step of the secondary survey is inspection. Asymmetry or gross deformity points to the injury site. Extraocular movement abnormalities and facial nerve

### LITERATURE REFERENCE

 ## Nasal trauma: How to manage epistaxis and septal hematomas

The most common cause of traumatic nasal bleeding is a mucosal tear, often from a nasal fracture. However, the nose can also drain blood from sinus, maxilla, or basilar skull fractures. In the presence of gross nasal deformity and profuse bleeding, manual reduction should be performed. Nasal reduction and nasal packing are almost always effective in controlling trauma epistaxis. Shimoyama et al. conducted a retrospective review of 521 trauma patients and reported that all traumatic nasal bleeding could effectively be controlled with these two interventions **[Shimoyama et al. *J Trauma* 2003;54(2):332–336].** All patients with posterior nasal packs or bilateral anterior packs must be admitted for airway observation. Septal hematomas must be drained immediately to prevent cartilage destruction and resultant saddle nose deformity.

**Procedure for nasal fracture reduction**—Topical anesthesia is usually sufficient; however, a nasal block with lidocaine (without epinephrine) may also be done. Inject the lidocaine either deep to the nasal fracture by entering intranasally or externally into the fracture site to perform a hematoma block. Bilateral infraorbital blocks may also be performed. Intravenous conscious sedation may be required. Using a scalpel handle or pair of forceps, the depressed nasal bone is elevated in an anterosuperior direction, and the nasal pyramid is manually displaced to the midline. An external splint should be applied for 7 to 10 days.

**Anterior nasal packing**—Compressed sponge (Merocel)—Merocel packing, consisting of compressed polyvinyl acetate, expands on contact with fluid. Trim Merocel foam to

fit through the naris and advance it along the floor of the nasal cavity. Once wet with blood or a few drops of saline, it expands to fill the nasal cavity and tamponade bleeding. The extruding string should be taped to the bridge of the nose.

**Posterior nasal packing**—A 12-French Foley catheter can be inserted through the bleeding naris into the posterior pharynx. The balloon should be inflated with 5 to 7 mL of normal saline. Pull the Foley into the posterior nasopharynx and secure it against the posterior aspect of the middle turbinate. Instill another 5 to 7 mL of normal saline to completely inflate the balloon. An anterior pack is placed in the opposite naris to prevent septal deviation.

**Epistaxis balloons**—Balloons come in anterior (single balloon) or anterior-posterior (double balloon) models. Cover the catheter with antibiotic ointment, insert it along the floor of the nasal cavity, and inflate it slowly with sterile water (approximately 10 cc). Posterior balloons should be inflated halfway, gently pulled anteriorly into the nasopharynx, and then inflated completely.

**Septal hematoma drainage**—Anesthesize the base of the septum bilaterally. Incise the mucosa horizontally over the hematoma. Suction out the clot, and irrigate with normal saline. Excise a small amount of mucosa to prevent early closure and clot reaccumulation. Place a section of sterile rubber band to act as a drain. The nostril should be packed to reapproximate the perichondrium to the cartilage. The patient should be given antibiotics, and follow-up should be arranged within 24 hours.

**TABLE 14-1  Ocular findings and suggested diagnoses**

| Finding | Suggested diagnosis |
|---|---|
| Teardrop-shaped pupil | Globe penetration |
| Abnormal pupil reactivity | Optic nerve or retinal damage |
| Subconjunctival hemorrhage | Orbital fractures<br>Zygomatic fractures (with lateral hemorrhage) |
| Diplopia on upward gaze | Zygomatic or infraorbital floor fractures |
| Enophthalmos (sinking of eye into orbit) | Blowout fracture |
| Proptosis (outward protrusion of eye relative to orbit) | Blowout fracture<br>Retrobulbar hematoma |

dysfunction may occur in association with bony injuries. Look for signs of basilar skull fracture such as periorbital ecchymoses (raccoon eyes) and ecchymosis over the mastoid region (Battle's sign). The entire face should be palpated for bony crepitus, subcutaneous air, tenderness, and step-offs. Subcutaneous air indicates possible nasal or sinus trauma. To assess facial stability, the maxillary arch should be grasped and rocked while the examiner is simultaneously feeling the central face for movement with the opposite hand. Mandibular fracture is suggested by inability to grasp and hold a tongue blade against mild resistance between occluded teeth. Condylar fracture or dislocation causes jaw deviation away from a dislocation or toward a fracture.

The eyes should be inspected carefully. There are several vision-compromising, time-sensitive entities that must be considered and particular physical findings that should be sought (Table 14-1 and Box 14-1). Inspect and palpate the nose. Presence of a septal hematoma mandates drainage to prevent saddle-nose deformity. Clear nasal discharge should alert to the possibility of a CSF leak. The ears should be inspected for hemotympanum, a purple bulging of the eardrum.

## SPECIFIC INJURIES

### Maxillary Fractures

Maxillary fractures should be suspected if there is swelling or tenderness of the midface. It takes significant force to break this bone. The Le Fort classification system is used to describe maxillary fractures (Table 14-2 and Figure 14-2). Airway compromise is most likely with Le Fort III fractures because of disruption of upper airway anatomy and pulling forces on some lower airway structures as the face moves. Blindness can be a devastating consequence of Le Fort III fractures because of optic nerve damage as protective facial structures move. Diagnosis can be made with plain films, although CT scan is the modality of choice

(Box 14-2). Le Fort I fractures with minimal or no displacement may be managed conservatively or with intermaxillary fixation. All other Le Fort injuries are treated with open reduction and internal fixation.

---

**BOX 14-1  Vision-compromising ocular emergencies**

*Globe rupture*—Any penetrating injury has the potential to cause globe rupture. Blunt mechanisms can also cause this injury. Signs and symptoms include shallow anterior chamber, hyphema (blood in the anterior chamber), teardrop pupil, decreased visual acuity, and poor view of the optic nerve on direct ophthalmoscopy. An eye shield, immediate ophthalmology consult, and operative repair are indicated. Tetanus status should be updated. Antibiotics should be given, as the violated globe is prone to infection. Do not measure intraocular pressure if the patient has a confirmed or suspected globe rupture.

*Orbital emphysema causing visual loss*—Orbital emphysema is usually a self-limited, benign condition. However, air may build up under pressure in the orbital socket, causing decreased blood flow to the central retinal artery. To salvage vision, immediate release of this pressure via lateral canthotomy must be performed.

*Retrobulbar hematoma*—This finding may be a complication of blunt trauma to the eye. Patients present with severe eye pain, nausea, vomiting, diplopia, decreased visual acuity, decreased ocular motility, afferent pupillary defect, and proptosis. This can develop over minutes, and the eye must be decompressed with lateral canthotomy immediately. If it develops over hours, conservative management with head elevation, ice packs, and medications to reduce intraocular pressure can be employed. Urgent ophthalmology consultation is important for possible operative decompression.

*Lateral canthotomy*—Orbital pressure can be relieved with a lateral canthotomy. To perform this procedure, a small amount of local anesthetic is injected in the region of the lateral canthal tendon. A straight hemostat is placed in the region between the upper and lower lids. Using scissors, a cut is made across the hemostatic line to the level of the lateral orbital rim. Further orbital decompression is accomplished by performing cantholysis through blunt dissection.

| TABLE 14-2  Maxillary fractures: The Le Fort classification | |
| --- | --- |
| Le Fort I | Transverse fracture that separates the body of the maxilla from the lower portion of the pterygoid plate and nasal septum<br>The hard palate and nasal septum are mobile |
| Le Fort II | Pyramidal fracture of the central maxilla and the palate<br>The nose moves but the eyes do not<br>CSF rhinorrhea is common |
| Le Fort III | Also called craniofacial disjunction<br>Complete facial skeleton separates from the skull<br>The entire face (including the orbits) moves<br>CSF rhinorrhea is common<br>May have significant epistaxis |

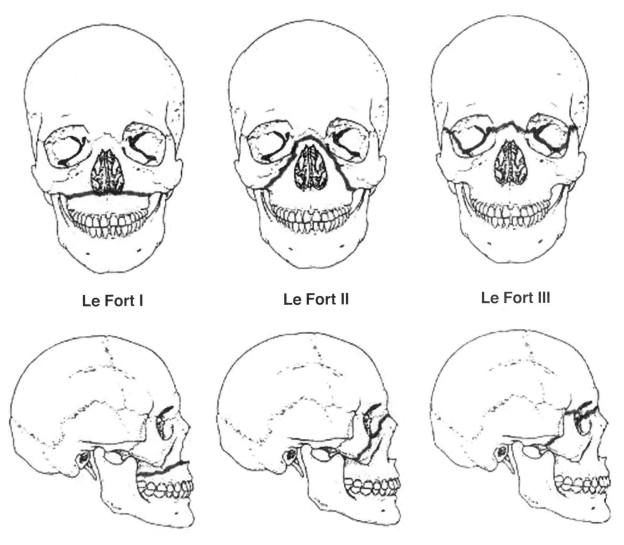

**Le Fort I**          **Le Fort II**          **Le Fort III**

**FIGURE 14-2**   Le Fort classification
(Adapted from Snell, RS. *Clinical Anatomy,* 7th ed. Philadelphia: Lippincott Williams & Wilkins; 2003.)

> **BOX 14-2 Particular plain film views traditionally used to diagnose facial fractures**
>
> *Waters view (occipital-mental view)*—shown to be as sensitive as the entire plain film facial series. It is a PA projection taken with the patient's nose and chin on the film. It evaluates the orbital rims and can diagnose blowout fractures.
>
> *Caldwell view (posteroanterior view)*—taken with the nose and forehead on the film. It allows visualization of bones of the upper face and is most useful for confirming ethmoidal sinus, frontal sinus, and lateral orbital wall fractures.
>
> *Zygomatic arch view (submental-vertex or "jug handle" view)*—shows only the skull base and zygomatic arch.
>
> *Cross-table or upright lateral views*—not helpful. Occasionally, facial elongation, suggestive of Le Fort fractures, can be seen.
>
> *Panorex view*—allows complete visualization of dentition, mandible, and related structures. Often preferred over CT scan for operative planning of mandible fractures.

### Zygomatic Fractures

The zygoma has two major parts: the body (malar eminence) and the zygomatic arch. Fractures of the arch are more common. A tripod fracture involves the infraorbital rim, the zygomatic-frontal suture, and

---

**LITERATURE REFERENCE**

## Do we really need plain films for diagnosing facial fractures?

As CT scan use and availability has become more widespread, are plain films becoming extinct? And if not, should they? Turner et al. studied trends in the use of CT and plain radiography in the evaluation of facial trauma in a Level I emergency department from 1992 to 2002. They concluded that CT scans are more cost effective, less time-consuming, and more comfortable for patients in whom there is a high suspicion of facial injury. They reported that 30% of patients in 1992 had both radiographs and CT scans performed. As the price of CT scanning has decreased tremendously, this modality is now cheaper than the traditional facial plain film series. When plain films detected fractures, CT scan was performed to provide more fracture details. It is preferable to go straight to CT scan if there is sufficient suspicion for facial fractures **[Turner et al. *Am J Roentgenol* 2004;183(3):751–754].**

---

**LITERATURE REFERENCE**

## Do we always have to order dedicated facial CT scans?

Are head CT scans adequate for detecting significant facial fractures in the setting of suspected fracture with facial stability? Lewandowski et al. sought to answer this question. They conducted a retrospective review of patients presenting to a Level I trauma center after blunt trauma. Study patients had both a nonenhanced head CT and a dedicated facial bone or orbit CT. A positive head CT scan included either an air-fluid level within the paranasal sinuses or a fracture of the maxilla, orbit, or zygoma. Intracranial findings were not included. Of the 65 patients with negative head CT scans, none went on to have a positive facial or orbital CT scan. In this study, the sensitivity and negative predictive values of a nonenhanced head CT scan for facial fracture is 100%, concluding that CT scan is an appropriate screening tool for upper facial fractures **[Lewandowski et al. *Emerg Radiol* 2004;10(4): 173–175].**

---

zygomatic-temporal disruption. The most common findings on physical examination with tripod fractures are flatness of the cheek, numbness in the infraorbital nerve distribution, diplopia or disruption of consensual gaze, and depression of the lateral check bone. Arch fractures present with local tenderness, ecchymosis, or edema. Though Waters view x-rays may reveal these fractures, CT scan is again the preferred imaging modality. Surgery may be necessary if there is significant deformity or visual disturbance.

### Orbital Fractures

Orbital fractures are caused by direct trauma to the globe that leads to increased intraocular pressure and decompression by fracture of the orbital floor or walls. The orbital floor is the weakest part of the orbit, making it most susceptible to fracture. Orbital contents most often herniate into the maxillary sinus. Clinical signs include enophthalmos, diplopia (most common on upward gaze because of entrapment of the inferior rectus muscle), impaired ocular motility, and infraorbital hypoesthesia. Plain films may reveal the "hanging drop" sign of herniated contents in the maxillary sinus. CT is much more useful. Acute enophthalmos, which often indicates a significant medial wall fracture and muscular entrapment causing persistent diplopia, require surgery. Surgical repair is always performed 7 to 10 days after the injury to allow for optimal conditions (e.g., decreased swelling, resolving hemorrhage, and more accurate examination). Other fractures are managed conservatively with close outpatient follow-up.

### Mandibular Fractures

Similar to the pelvis, the mandible is a ringed structure. Therefore, it is common to have multiple fractures at sites distant from the point of impact. The condyle is the most commonly fractured part of the mandible. The most common findings on exam include mandibular tenderness, malocclusion, and ecchymosis on the floor of the mouth. Diagnosis can be made with dental panoramic x-rays (panorex). Standard AP and lateral views may miss condylar fractures. Again, CT scan provides more information for possible operative planning. Displaced fractures of the angle and body, bilateral or displaced condylar fractures, and the presence of multiple facial fractures are indications for surgery. Other fractures are usually managed conservatively with wiring of the mandible. These patients may require admission because of the risk of aspiration.

### Frontal Sinus Fractures

Frontal sinus fractures are usually caused by forceful blunt trauma to the forehead. Examination may reveal local tenderness, deformity, or crepitus. CT scan is necessary to evaluate integrity of the posterior wall of the sinus. If this is fractured, a dural tear must be assumed, and the patient must be admitted and treated with intravenous antibiotics. All frontal sinus fractures should be operatively repaired. Isolated anterior wall fractures may be repaired in a delayed manner. Optimal management of sinus fractures, especially regarding antibiotic use, is controversial, and the literature is not compelling one way or the other.

### Nasal Fractures

The nose is commonly injured in trauma because of its location. Nasal fractures can be significantly disfiguring and can compromise ability to breathe easily. A septal hematoma must be sought and treated to prevent cartilage necrosis. Most nasal fractures do not require reduction emergently. Those with gross displacement, airflow obstruction, or epistaxis are candidates for immediate reduction. Nasal films do not determine the need for intervention nor are they indicated for surgical planning. Surgery is indicated to restore cosmesis or repair obstruction to airflow. Patients who are candidates for repair should be referred to an ENT specialist or a plastic surgeon on an outpatient basis. Those with significant deformity or swelling should be evaluated within 7 days.

## KEY POINTS

- Patients with facial trauma should have their airways managed early and aggressively
- Rapid sequence intubation can be difficult or impossible
  - Consider fiber-optic or awake techniques
  - Do not paralyze unless assured that bag ventilation is possible
- Sometimes a surgical airway is the first-line option
- Even though the face is highly vascular, shock is rarely the result of facial trauma
- Nasal packing should be used in significant nasal bleeding
- Once airway is secured, then focus should be on other injuries
  - Specific management for facial fractures is not acute
- Once stable, CT scan is the imaging modality of choice for facial fractures
  - Plain films have limited utility with exception of panorex for mandible fractures
  - Head CT is effective in detecting facial fractures
  - Dedicated facial CT may be necessary to detail orbit fractures
- Be aware of retrobulbar hematoma with exophthalmos and increased IOP
  - Requires immediate lateral canthotomy to prevent optic nerve ischemia
- Maxillary fractures are classified by Le Fort based on facial stability
  - Le Fort II and III require surgery
- Tripod fractures involve infraorbital rim, zygomatic-frontal suture, and zygomatic-temporal suture
  - Often associated with entrapment of lateral rectus muscle and diplopia
  - Surgery required for significant deformity or diplopia
- Orbital fractures usually involve inferior wall followed by medial wall
  - May cause inferior rectus entrapment or endophthalmos
  - Surgery is delayed 7 to 10 days to allow swelling to decrease

# CHAPTER 15

# Penetrating Extremity Injury

## CASE SCENARIO

A 19-year-old male was standing outside a local store "minding his own business," when a fight broke out in the parking lot. He was struck in the right thigh by a stray bullet. The patient collapsed to the ground, and EMS was called by a store employee. En route, two 16-gauge IVs are established and normal saline started. The patient arrives to the ED appearing pale with vital signs including a heart rate of 126 bpm, blood pressure 100/50, respiratory rate of 22, and oxygen saturation of 95% on an NRB face-mask. He has no medical problems, takes no medications, and has no allergies. On primary survey, he is alert and without trauma to the head, neck, or chest. He has clear breath sounds bilaterally. On secondary survey, you note a normal cardiac and abdominal exam and no other signs of trauma except an entrance wound on his proximal thigh (just distal to the inguinal ligament), which is oozing blood. You roll the patient quickly to examine his back and perform a rectal exam. He has no back wounds or blood in the stool. He has a sizeable right thigh hematoma, but there is no pulsating blood coming from the wound. EMS personnel note that it had not changed significantly during the 20-minute transport, and there was not a large amount of blood at the scene. No exit wound is visible. His right DP pulse is present but decreased compared to his left.

1. What do you want to do first?
    a. Go straight to the operating room for exploration
    b. Obtain x-rays of the pelvis and leg, and perform a FAST exam
    c. Intubate the patient
    d. Measure compartment pressures

The patient does not have any of the hard signs of arterial injury and, therefore, a workup in the ED can be performed. Because his airway and breathing are acceptable and you have performed your primary and secondary surveys, it is reasonable to think about a more detailed assessment of the injury. Because there is no exit wound, the location of the bullet must be determined. Additionally, it is reasonable to exclude the possibility of underlying fractures. Therefore, x-rays of the pelvis and leg are appropriate. A FAST exam is also important with gunshot wounds to the pelvis or upper thigh because bullets can often travel upward into the abdomen. If the bullet does not appear on pelvis or leg x-ray, then an abdominal x-ray should be obtained.

You administer fentanyl 50 μgm, and his pain is well controlled. The distal sensation in his lower leg is intact to pain and light touch, and there is no change in his right DP pulse. You are able to flex his knee without causing significant pain. His x-rays show bullet fragments medial to the lesser tuberosity of the femur, just inferior to the inferior pubic ramus. He reports vague chest discomfort. His repeat vital signs are a pulse of 106, blood pressure 120/50, respiratory rate of 22, and oxygen saturation of 95% on oxygen.

2. What is your leading diagnosis?
    a. Venous and soft tissue injury
    b. Occult arterial injury
    c. Compartment syndrome of the thigh
    d. Occult femur fracture

There is no absolute indicator of arterial injury; however, there are certain hard signs that make the diagnosis likely and require swift action. The most concerning signs are a rapidly expanding hematoma or pulsatile bleeding, dusky extremity, or absent distal pulses. Other hard signs include a palpable thrill or audible bruit (both rare), distal motor or sensory deficits (nerves and arteries run together), and pain with passive extension of the muscle compartment involved. Soft signs include a stable hematoma, isolated peripheral nerve deficit, diminished distal pulses, and unexplained hypotension. Soft signs generally indicate a wound to soft tissues or perhaps venous structures.

While you are waiting for the results of the x-rays, he becomes tachypneic, and his blood pressure drops to 80/40 with a heart rate of 160. The oxygen saturation probe is not picking up a reading. A repeat primary survey reveals an intact airway and clear breath sounds, and his thigh looks the same. You look at the back and axilla again to assure you did not miss an injury.

3. What is a plausible explanation for his deterioration?
    a. Occult pneumothorax that has become a tension pneumothorax
    b. Anemia from ongoing occult bleeding
    c. Fat embolism from a femur fracture
    d. Missile embolism to the pulmonary vasculature

Sudden decompensation in this patient is entirely unexpected, and the first thought should be a missed injury. It is important to inspect the entire patient when a gunshot wound is present. It is also important to consider that the internal trajectory of a bullet is not always what is expected. Gunshot wounds to the thigh may travel up into the pelvis or abdomen, but a bullet traversing upward to the thorax would be unlikely. The patient may in fact have a long bone fracture, but it is quite early for a fat embolism to develop. Occult bleeding is a good thought, especially since the thigh can contain upward to 2 L of blood. However, this patient's symptoms appear to be primarily respiratory in nature. Albeit rare, this likely represents a symptomatic missile embolism from a deep leg vein via the femoral vein, common iliac vein, vena cava, and into the pulmonary vasculature (Box 15-1).

4. What is the first priority before the patient travels to the OR, which is on the fourth floor?
    a. Hang 2 units of uncrossmatched blood
    b. Treat the patient with PO azithromycin for likely wound contamination
    c. Intubate the patient
    d. Check compartment pressures in the thigh

The patient is unstable and requires immediate intubation and resuscitation. A portable CXR shows a foreign body located in the proximal portion of the right pulmonary artery. The patient goes to the OR for embolectomy and subsequent leg exploration. A thoracotomy is necessary to gain access to the pulmonary artery. Leg exploration reveals injury to the deep femoral vein with the artery intact.

Answers: 1-b; 2-a; 3-d; 4-c

---

### BOX 15-1  Missile embolism

Missile embolism, defined as the travel of foreign bodies from penetrating trauma through the blood stream, is a rare yet serious complication of penetrating vascular trauma. Often simple x-ray of the extremity cannot exclude this entity given the potential for bullet fragments, shrapnel, or multiple buckshot from a shotgun. Missile emboli can be either arterial or venous, with the former causing distal obstruction and peripheral ischemia (e.g., foot or hand ischemia), and the latter potentially traveling through the right heart into the pulmonary arterial system and resulting in pulmonary embolism. Other complications of central venous emboli can include endocarditis, myocardial injury, or pulmonary infections. Arterial emboli can be removed either with arteriotomy or balloon catheter embolectomy. All centrally-located, symptomatic venous emboli need to be removed either via thoracotomy and direct removal or by percutaneous interventional techniques. Some surgeons will leave asymptomatic missiles in place, which has been shown to be safe.

## BACKGROUND

The management of penetrating extremity trauma, which mostly entails repair of damaged vessels, has evolved rapidly with advances in surgical techniques over the past 50 years. From the 16th century until the 1950s, the only effective surgical technique for acutely injured vessels was ligation, which often resulted in limb ischemia. The first real advances in the field came in the early 1900s when surgeons began publishing large case series detailing repair of chronic vascular injuries, such as pseudoanuerysms and arteriovenous fistulae (AVF). In addition to the vascular injury itself, the other major concern with penetrating injuries to the extremities is infection. Given these wounds are open, they are by definition contaminated. Furthermore, most penetrating injuries, with a few exceptions, are going to have small entrance and exit wounds, making proper irrigation difficult. The use of antibiotics in these wounds will be discussed.

Penetrating extremity injury, along with peripheral vascular trauma, tends to occur in young adult males. It should be noted that of all penetrating extremity injuries, less than 10% will involve vascular damage. Of all vascular injuries that present to the ED, including those to the torso and neck (which have a higher mortality), about half involve the extremities. Of the traumatic vascular injuries to extremities, brachial and femoral artery injury seem to be the most common. Gunshot wounds are the most common cause of peripheral vascular injury, followed by stab wounds and shotgun blasts. It is important to keep in mind that the latter can result in embolization of shotgun pellets. Clearly, when vasculature is damaged, adjacent structures are likely to be injured, sometimes also requiring repair. The most common associated injuries are to adjacent veins and nerves. Also keep in mind the possibility of a fracture, especially in association with gunshot wounds.

## CLINICAL ANATOMY

There are two guiding principles of anatomy to recall when treating penetrating injuries to the extremities. The first is that major nerves tend to follow the course of major arteries. Thus, if one is familiar with the course of the major arteries, the location of important nerves is generally known as well (Figure 15-1). While there are some exceptions to this rule (e.g., the median nerve is not accompanied by vascular structures as it runs through the carpal tunnel), the relationship does hold relatively constant and can serve as an important guide.

The second principle is that, for the most part, extremity musculature is organized into compartments, which are encased by unyielding fibrous fascia. Penetrating injury will often cause bleeding and swelling within a compartment or entirely disrupt arterial flow into the compartment, both resulting in compartment syndrome. When arteries are damaged by penetrating trauma, the pathology can be quite variable, including simple laceration, true or false aneurysms, AV malformation, contusion, creation of an intimal flap, or complete transection. In the case of complete transection, bleeding may be minimal due to arterial vasospasm. With partial lacerations, vasospasm may actually increase bleeding by opening the tear further.

## PRIMARY SURVEY

While it is always tempting in trauma to "go straight to where the money is," a primary survey is warranted before focusing on an extremity wound. This may be as simple as assessing level of consciousness, rapidly inspecting the neck and chest, listening for breath sounds, and obtaining vital signs. If more serious injuries are present (e.g., gunshot to the head, neck, chest, or abdomen), then a profusely bleeding extremity injury can be addressed during the primary survey with a pressure dressing or tourniquet while other life-threatening injuries are dealt with. This is not to imply that peripheral vascular injuries cannot be life-threatening, only that they can usually be controlled with direct pressure while the ABCs are addressed.

## SECONDARY SURVEY

Extremity injuries are examined during the secondary survey, once the patient is stabilized. In assessing circulation, distal pulses should be checked in both the injured extremity and the normal extremity for comparison. The clinical exam in penetrating extremity injury dictates the management and workup, and therefore a systematic approach is critical. The purpose of the exam is to answer the following four questions:

- Has there been an injury to a major artery or vein?
- Has a peripheral nerve been transected?
- Is there evidence of bone, muscle, or tendon injury?
- Is there evidence of compartment syndrome or potential thereof?

The first step in the physical exam is to assess pulses distal to the injury and compare them with the uninjured extremity. It should be remembered, however, that peripheral perfusion may remain intact with arterial lacerations. If pulses are not palpable, a handheld Doppler should be used to confirm their absence. The physical exam can also be supplemented by measuring the arterial pressure index (Box 15-2). Additionally, compare both extremities for color, coolness to touch, and presence of pain with flexion and extension of joints distal to the injury. Arterial insufficiency may also manifest as nerve deficits. Given their high metabolic need and lack of significant glycogen stores, nerves are especially susceptible to ischemia. Distal ischemia also varies, depending on the availability of collateral flow. For example, occlusion of the popliteal artery leads to a high degree of ischemia, and subsequent limb loss, because there are few collateral arteries in this region.

## MANAGEMENT

### Vascular Injury

The hierarchy of decision making in penetrating extremity injury is: (a) When does the patient need to go to the OR, (b) When does the patient need angiography,

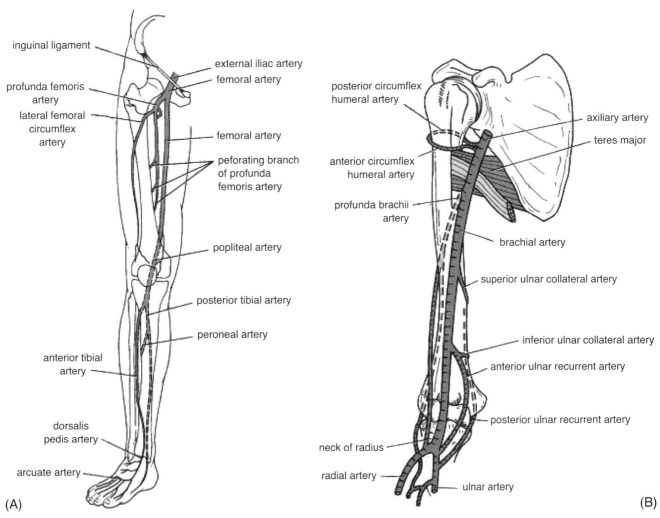

**FIGURE 15-1**  (A) Upper extremity arteries; (B) Lower extremity arteries.
(Adapted from Snell, RS. *Clinical Anatomy,* 7th ed. Philadelphia: Lippincott, Williams & Wilkins, 2003.)

and (c) When can the patient be simply observed and discharged home? See the algorithm at the end of this chapter for a summary of the management of penetrating extremity wounds.

Open wounds (larger lacerations) can bleed profusely, and the first action is to stop the bleeding. Direct pressure to the bleeding site and elevation should always be the first maneuver. The pressure should be placed directly on the injured part of the artery if possible to avoid compression of nearby arteries. If compression alone stops the bleeding from an open wound, then significant vascular injury is unlikely, and the wound can be explored to determine whether major neurovascular structures have been damaged. If ongoing arterial bleeding is present, the bleeding may be difficult to control with direct pressure. In this case, a blood pressure cuff can be used as a tourniquet. Keep in mind, however, that this will result in limb ischemia and subsequent irreversible

---

**BOX 15-2  The arterial-pressure index**

Calculating the arterial pressure index (API) is quite simple and requires minimal equipment. A systolic BP is obtained by inflating a blood pressure cuff proximal to the injury and using a Doppler or even palpation to determine the SBP distal to the injury. Then, the blood pressure is taken in a corresponding noninjured extremity. The ratio of injured to noninjured is then calculated; most authors consider a ratio of 0.90 or less abnormal. Some studies indicate that this cut-off is too low to offer sufficient sensitivity, while others indicate this is a good compromise between specificity and sensitivity. One reasonable approach is to obtain an angiogram or operatively explore all patients with an API less than 0.90 and observe patients with an API of 0.90 to 0.99 for 12 to 24 hours with serial exams. It should also be noted that there are certain arteries (e.g., profunda femoris or profunda brachii) that do not produce distal pulses and thus are not amenable to study by this technique.

tissue necrosis in about 90 minutes, including the time needed in the OR to repair the artery. A tourniquet can also be temporarily applied to inspect the wound and identify the source of bleeding, or to place a procoagulant agent such as Surgicel. While blind ligation of bleeding vessels is contraindicated due to associated nerve damage, small vessel bleeding can often be controlled with an absorbable suture while the tourniquet is inflated. It is important, however, to identify significant arterial bleeding early and transition the patient rapidly to the OR. The importance of rapid repair of injured vasculature has been shown repeatedly in the trauma literature, with more rapid repair times associated with a dramatic decrease in the amputation rate.

In penetrating trauma from gunshots and stabs, the wound is often small, and therefore external bleeding is minimal. This, of course, does not preclude significant arterial injury. In this case, the determination of whether to take the patient to the OR depends on the presence of hard signs of arterial injury (Box 15-3). Traditionally, the presence of any of these signs would warrant surgical exploration for potential arterial injury. In practice, however, this varies depending on the clinical scenario. Absolute hard signs would include a rapidly expanding or massive hematoma, evidence of distal ischemia (e.g., asymmetric pulselessness, dusky or cyanotic appearance), or evidence of compartment syndrome (e.g., pain, paresthesias, or pulselessness). In many cases it is less clear (e.g., hematoma but stable, isolated sensory deficit) or the wound is in proximity to a known large artery without obvious signs of injury, known as "proximity injury." These patients with soft signs can simply be observed without further workup. It has been shown that the incidence of arterial injury is about one-third with the presence of a soft sign, although only a small number of these actually require surgery.

Angiography is considered the gold standard for diagnosing arterial injury, yet other modalities are gaining favor. Radiologic workup is variable among different centers, with some relying more on clinical exam and observation. In general, centers with more experience with penetrating extremity wounds rely more on clinical signs. Otherwise, a radiologic workup is typically undertaken for patients who have a high suspicion for significant arterial injury but may not have hard signs of injury. A good example of this is proximity injury, where the likelihood is high based on the location of the wound (e.g., inner thigh, medial arm). High-velocity, high–kinetic energy wounds may also warrant routine radiographic evaluation, despite, the initial lack of hard signs, due to the extent of blast injury. Our algorithm errs on the side of conservatism. Some may truncate this algorithm by observing those without hard signs except for shotgun wounds (SGWs) or shrapnel wounds. Nonetheless, it has been shown that a careful physical exam has greater than 90% sensitivity in triaging patients correctly to surgery, angiography, or observation.

### Nerve Injury

Determining whether or not a peripheral nerve has been injured can be challenging in the trauma patient because this part of the exam is almost entirely dependent on patient cooperation. As stated previously, knowledge of the course of the major nerves in the upper and lower extremities is crucial (Tables 15-1 and 15-2).

Although protected within the axilla, the brachial plexus can be injured by penetrating trauma. This large network of nerves is responsible for essentially all motion and sensation in the upper extremities. It consists of nerve roots originating from C5–T1 (in the majority of patients) and is divided into five sections: roots, trunks, divisions, cords, and terminal branches. The plexus extends from the c-spine and courses posterior to the clavicle and pectoralis minor, finally giving rise to its branches in the axilla. The trunks occur just proximal to the clavicle and the cords at the level of the insertion of the pectoralis minor. Penetrating trauma to the supraclavicular or infraclavicular region, as well as to the axilla, may damage the nerves of the brachial plexus, leading to dense neurologic deficits in the upper extremity.

Major nerves of the lower extremity arise from the lumbar plexus (femoral) and sacral plexus

---

**BOX 15-3  Hard signs of vascular injury**

- Evidence of active arterial bleeding
  - Expanding or pulsatile hematoma
  - Pulsatile bleeding refractory to compression
- Evidence of arterial disruption
  - Palpable thrill or audible bruit
  - Dusky or cyanotic limb
  - Assymetric absent distal pulse
- Evidence of compartment syndrome
  - Pain out of proportion to appearance
  - Pain with passive ROM
  - Paresthesias
  - Pallor distal to wound
  - Paralysis of distal muscles

Note: The incidence of arterial injury in the presence of any one of these signs is >90%.

LITERATURE REFERENCE

 ## Radiographic study of extremity vessels

**Ultrasound**—Duplex ultrasonography, which combines B-mode (brightness modulation) US with Doppler ultrasound, has been suggested for evaluation of penetrating vascular injuries because of its noninvasive and portable nature. While some studies have reported similar sensitivity to angiography, other studies have questioned this. Additionally, this technology is operator-dependent and not always readily available 24 hours a day. Thus, its role in the evaluation of penetrating extremity trauma is yet to be worked out.

**CTA**—Literature is beginning to emerge regarding the use of CTA in peripheral vascular trauma. The chief advantages of this technique are that it is less invasive, much more readily available, and significantly less time-consuming to perform than angiography. With the advent of multidetector CT scanners and reconstruction of imaged parts, CTA has been replacing conventional angiography for many traditional indications. Busquéts et al. reported their experience retrospectively over approximately 3 years, during which time 97 CTAs were performed on 95 consecutive patients with either blunt or penetrating extremity trauma (30% penetrating). Of the 97 CTAs, 25 were abnormal, with results confirmed either by surgery, angiography, or both. The first 10 patients with negative CTAs,

also underwent angiography, all of which were negative. The authors were able to follow up on 84% of the remaining patients (roughly 8 months postinjury), and no one had a delayed injury. **[Busquéts et al. *J Trauma* 2004;56(3): 625–628; Soto et al. *J Comput Assist Tomogr* 1999;23(2): 188–196].**

There has yet to be a head-to-head comparison of techniques, but experience with CTA in patients with neck injury, combined with the above studies in extremity trauma, indicate that CTA likely has comparable sensitivity. There are some concerns, given the plane of the artery being parallel with the plane of the CT slices, that CTA will miss some subclavian artery injuries.

**Angiography**—This method has been the gold standard for diagnosing arterial injury but is starting to fall out of favor today. Problems include long delay of assembling personnel, the cost, the need to leave the ED, and a small yet not insignificant complication rate of arterial cannulation. Some centers have limited angiographic capabilities in the OR, which seems to have sensitivity comparable to that of formal angiography. There is still much debate, though, over whether or not injuries missed on physical exam, but found on angiography, are likely to be clinically significant.

(sciatic). The lumbar plexus nerves generally supply the motor functions of the thigh, while the sacral plexus generally supplies the lower leg and foot. In general, these nerves are well protected by overlying muscle, with the exception of the peroneal nerve, which is quite exposed at the level of the fibular head.

### Compartment Syndrome

Compartment syndrome is defined as rise in pressure with a compartmentalized group of tissues leading to impaired perfusion, ischemia, and necrosis of muscles and nerves contained within the compartment. Tissue necrosis along with cell lysis can lead to myoglobinemia or hyperkalemia, with subsequent renal failure if left untreated. Although patients with penetrating extremity trauma can present with compartment syn-

drome, it more commonly develops as a consequence of reperfusion after a period of long ischemic time. It can also occur as a late complication of combined arterial and venous injury to a given extremity, as well as in patients who sustain orthopedic injuries or blunt trauma. The lower leg is at highest risk, and compartment syndrome is somewhat common in patients with popliteal artery injury.

The compartments of the lower leg are diagramed in Figure 15-2. Note should be made that the deep posterior compartment contains two of the three arteries that supply the foot, as well as the tibial nerve. The signs of compartment syndrome are typically thought of as the five Ps: pain, pallor, pulseless, paresthesias, and paralysis. However, most of these are late findings. Pain with passive movement of the muscles in the compartment (by extending and flexing the joint below it) is generally considered the most

**TABLE 15-1  Major nerves of the upper extremity**

(Note: Motor and sensory functions are not all-inclusive but are meant to provide an easily testable function and sensation pattern.)

| Nerve | Basic course | Motor function (muscle) | Sensory function |
|---|---|---|---|
| Axillary | Leaves posterior cord at level of pectoralis minor, courses to posterior arm distal to subscapularis, winding around surgical neck of humerus | Lateral rotation of arm (Tm) Abducts arm (Deltoid) | Inferolateral shoulder and adjacent lateral aspect of upper arm |
| Musculocutaneous | Leaves axilla deep to coracobrachialis muscle, pierces it just distal to humeral neck, runs between it and the BB Becomes superficial proximal to the lateral humeral epicondyle, becoming lateral cutaneous n. of forearm | Supinates forearm (BB) Flexes forearm (BB, Br, B) | Lateral aspect of forearm from just distal to elbow to just proximal to wrist |
| Median | Runs on lateral side of brachial artery from axilla, crosses over to the medial side at the mid-arm and runs through the medial aspect of the AC fossa (deep) Stays deep to FDS centrally in forearm, becomes superficial near the wrist, runs through center of carpal tunnel | Opposes thumb to pad of little finger (APB) | Volar tip of index finger |
| Radial | Enters arm medial to humerus between brachial artery and anterior to triceps, coursing laterally at the mid-humerus in the radial groove (with brachial artery) then runs between the BR and Br to the lateral epicondyle of the humerus, divides into deep (terminates in mid-forearm) and superficial (lateral aspect of forearms, where it runs with the radial artery before traversing posteriorly at the distal third of the forearm) | Extends arm at elbow, wrist, and fingers Extends thumbs at MCP joint (thumbs up) | Dorsal first web space |
| Ulnar | Runs along medial aspect of brachial artery, anterior to triceps Passing posteriorly to the medial epicondyl of the humerus and the olecranon before traversing anteriorly again and running medial to ulnar artery and deep to FCU and the anterolateral aspect of the forearm | Abducts fingers | Volar tip of little finger |

Abbreviations: Tm, teres minor; B, biceps; BB, biceps brachii; BR, brachioradialis; Br, brachialis; AC, antecubital; FDS, flexor digitorum superficialis; APB, apponens pollicis brevis; FCU, flexor carpi ulnaris; MCP, metacarpophalangeal joint.

sensitive sign of compartment syndrome. If the diagnosis is suspected, compartment pressures can be measured, although there is much debate about the threshold for compartment pressure that requires fasciotomy. It is generally accepted that normal compartment pressure varies widely from individual to individual, with a broad range of normal being reported in the literature. Most agree that a compartment pressure between 10 to 30 mm Hg below the diastolic blood pressure (about 30 to 40 mm Hg for most people) should be used as a threshold for fas-

ciotomy. The decision to operate is based on a combination of the measured pressure and the clinical exam; however, outcomes are better when the decision to operate is made early.

### Antibiotics in Penetrating Extremity Trauma

Not much can be gleaned from the available literature regarding administration of antibiotics for penetrating extremity wounds, but there are several generally adhered to practice standards. All patients

## TABLE 15-2  Major nerves of the lower extremity

(Note: Motor and sensory functions are not all-inclusive but are meant to provide an easily testable function and sensation pattern.)

| Nerve | Basic course | Motor function | Sensory function |
|---|---|---|---|
| **Femoral** | Exits the pelvis under the inguinal ligament, lateral to the femoral artery, courses through the femoral triangle and divides into terminal branches | Knee extension | Anterior and medial aspects of the knee |
| **Sciatic** | Exits the pelvis inferior to the piriformis and courses laterally to the center of the posterior thigh under the GM and then more inferiorly under the biceps femoris, then divides midway down the thigh into the peroneal and tibial | Dorsiflexes foot Plantarflexes foot | Posterolateral aspect of calf and foot |
| **Tibial** | Splits off sciatic nerve approximately at level of mid thigh and courses through the popliteal fossa just deep to the popliteal fascia and more superficial than the artery or vein and medial to them<br>Courses deep to the soleus and then medially, where it descends under the medial malleolus to the bottom of the foot | Plantarflexes foot | Most of the dorsum of the foot (can check at great toe) |
| **Peroneal (Fibular)** | From the superior aspect of the popliteal fossa it follows the medial border of the biceps femoris, exiting the popliteal fossa superficial to the lateral head of the gastrocnemius<br>Then it passes over the head of the fibula and wraps around the neck (from posterior to anterior) and then divides into the deep peroneal nerve (runs deep to EDL along medial border of fibula, then joins the tibial artery and courses along the lateral aspect of the tibia in the anterior compartment of the leg) and the superficial peroneal nerve (descends deep to peroneus longus muscle and then courses to the medial aspect of the lateral compartment of the leg) | Dorsiflexes foot (deep) Ankle eversion (superficial) | Web space between great and second toe (deep) Distal aspect of lateral shin (superficial) |

Abbreviations: GM, gluteus maximus; EDL, extensor digitorum longus

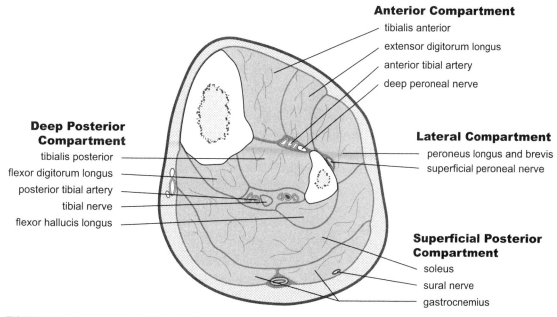

**FIGURE 15-2**   Compartments of the lower leg.
(Adapted from Bucholz RW and Heckman JD. *Rockwood & Green's Fractures in Adults,* 5th ed. Philadelphia: Lippincott, Williams & Wilkins, 2001.)

## Antibiotics in penetrating extremity trauma

The use of antibiotics in penetrating trauma to the extremities has not been thoroughly studied. Schmidt et al. looked at single dose ceftriaxone versus cefoxitin given TID for 3 days. There were a total of 195 patients enrolled. There was no significant difference in the infection rate, and no patient developed a deep tissue infection requiring surgical intervention by posttrauma day 10. Only 5% of patients developed any infection at all. There has not been a randomized controlled trial that looks at single dose antibiotics versus placebo [Schmidt et al. *Chemotherapy* 1999;45:1621–1626].

going to the OR for vascular repair should receive broad spectrum IV antibiotics. Patients who sustain hand or foot penetrating trauma should probably be treated with a short course of oral antibiotics, after a one-time IV dose. For wounds on other areas of the extremities that will be managed nonoperatively, a single dose of IV antibiotics with broad coverage for skin flora is probably sufficient, especially in the case of GSW, SGW, or shrapnel injuries. The case to do so in a stab wound is less compelling, given that antibiotics are not routinely given for lacerations. This of course is provided that the wound is irrigated copiously with sterile saline. Although data is lacking, prophylactic antibiotics should be administered to immunosupressed patients (HIV, chemotherapy, or steroids) or patients with diabetes.

- Hard signs push decision to go directly to the OR for exploration and repair
  - Evidence of active arterial bleed (e.g., expanding hematoma)
  - Evidence of arterial disruption (e.g., distal ischemia or pulseless)
  - Evidence of compartment syndrome (e.g., pain with ROM, paresthesias, or pallor)
- Those with soft signs and proximity injuries can usually be observed
  - About one-third will have injury, few requiring surgery
- Angiography is gold standard for diagnosis of peripheral arterial injury
  - Used when suspicion for injury is high but no hard signs present
  - Used in certain high-energy proximity wounds (e.g., gunshot, shrapnel)
- Venous injury in proximal lower extremities is generally repaired
  - Upper extremity venous injury can generally be ligated due to extensive collaterals
- Peripheral nerve injury should be considered and thorough sensory exam performed
- Pain with passive ROM is most sensitive sign of compartment syndrome
  - Pain out of proportion to appearance or exam is another
  - Pulselessness and distal ischemia are late findings

## KEY POINTS

- Extremities are divided into compartments, containing nerve–artery–muscle bundles
- It is important to know course of major nerves and arteries in extremities
- Apply direct pressure to profusely bleeding extremity wounds as part of ABCs
- Secondary survey includes peripheral pulse, motor, and sensory exam
- Open wounds can be directly explored for major structure injury

# PENETRATING EXTREMITY TRAUMA

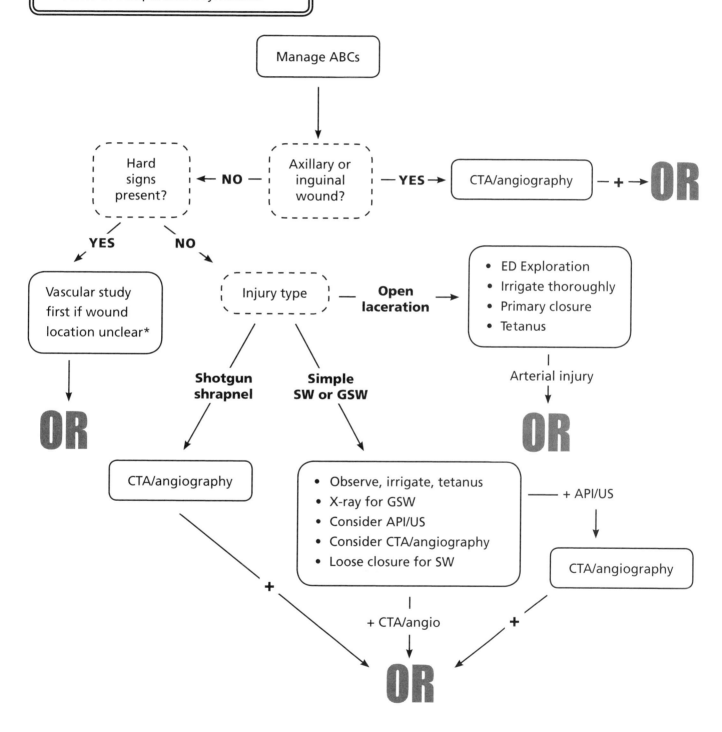

Hard signs:
Rapidly expanding or massive hematoma
Evidence of distal ischemia
Evidence of compartment syndrome

Manage ABCs

Hard signs present? ← **NO** ─ Axillary or inguinal wound? ─ **YES** → CTA/angiography ─ + → **OR**

**YES**      **NO**

Vascular study first if wound location unclear*

**OR**

Injury type ── **Open laceration** →
- ED Exploration
- Irrigate thoroughly
- Primary closure
- Tetanus

Arterial injury

**OR**

**Shotgun shrapnel**      **Simple SW or GSW**

CTA/angiography

- Observe, irrigate, tetanus
- X-ray for GSW
- Consider API/US
- Consider CTA/angiography
- Loose closure for SW

── + API/US

CTA/angiography

+

+ CTA/angio      +

**OR**

+ Positive vascular study = Arterial occlusion/disruption or significant extravasation

* Wound location unclear = Shrapnel, shotgun wounds, wound path parallel to vessel, or extensive soft tissue damage

# CHAPTER 16

# Orthopedic Emergencies

## CASE SCENARIO

A 35-year-old male presents to the ED after being struck by a car while crossing the street. After being hit, he fell onto his right side. He is awake and alert and complaining of severe right knee pain and inability to move his right arm. He is transported by EMS, who establish a 16-gauge IV en route; morphine 4 mg IV is administered. He arrives to the ED alert and oriented. He has no obvious facial trauma, his airway is intact, and he has clear breath sounds bilaterally. He did not black out and remembers the whole accident. He denies medical problems, takes no medications, and has no allergies. His vital signs on arrival are a pulse of 100, blood pressure 145/80, respiratory rate of 14, and oxygen saturation of 100% on room air. A FAST exam is normal. His secondary survey is significant for a "squared-off" appearance to his right shoulder, with an easily palpable acromion process. You notice his right arm is a bit dusky, and you cannot palpate radial, ulnar, or brachial pulses. There is no significant deformity along the course of his humerus or forearm. There is significant swelling around his right knee, with ecchymosis with a valgus deformity below the knee. Although his leg hurts, he does not have increased pain with flexion of his toes or ankle. His DP and PT pulses are symmetric when compared to the left leg. While you were performing the exam, an additional 16-gauge IV was placed, and the patient was given fentanyl 100 μgm.

1. What is the first priority in managing this patient?
   a. Prepare patient for intubation because he will likely go directly to the OR
   b. Trauma series including portable x-ray of right shoulder
   c. Orthopedics consultation for possible compartment syndrome in right calf
   d. Immediate reduction of his dislocated shoulder

This patient's ABCs are intact, and his vital signs are reasonable; intubation is not required. Since immediate life-threatening injuries to the head, neck, and torso are not apparent on primary survey, attention can be focused on the extremities. This patient's extremity exam is concerning given the apparent ischemic right arm. While in most cases a first-time shoulder dislocation should be confirmed with an x-ray, this constitutes an emergency that must be corrected immediately. Compartment syndrome is less concerning given the ability to range the ankle without significant lower leg pain, although it seems obvious that his leg is fractured.

You administer midazolam 2 mg and an additional 100 μg of fentanyl while the patient is on high-flow oxygen and a cardiac monitor. You inject lidocaine 10 cc into the shoulder joint just inferior to the acromion process. Slow traction and slight external rotation results in an easy reduction. You are then able to feel a slight radial pulse, and his arm develops more color. A neurologic exam reveals intact distal strength and sensation. You now more closely examine his right leg and notice he has a tense knee effusion and therefore is unable to range his knee. A trauma series is done, and it shows no obvious abnormality. You order x-rays, including right shoulder, humerus, right knee, and tibia/fibula. You also order c-spine x-rays given that he has mild cervical tenderness that is difficult to assess given his distracting injury.

2. What is the most likely injury sustained to the right leg?
   a. Tibial plateau fracture
   b. Knee dislocation
   c. ACL/PCL rupture
   d. Distal femur fracture

This mechanism is classic for a tibial plateau fracture given the bumper height of most cars. A knee dislocation results in obvious deformity and is often associated with vascular injury. ACL and PCL rupture will also result in hemarthrosis but are less likely given the mechanism. Distal femur fractures are also possible with a direct-impact mechanism such as this; however, this injury is not associated with hemarthrosis.

C-spine films are normal, and the shoulder x-ray shows a reduced shoulder with a fracture of the anterior lip of the glenoid (Bankhart fracture). Knee x-ray shows a displaced lateral tibial plateau fracture, depressed about 0.5 cm. You apply a posterior splint to stabilize the knee. The orthopedist wants to admit the patient for open reduction in the OR in the morning. There are no beds available in the hospital, and the patient stays in the ED overnight. On repeat exam 12 hours later, he has strong DP and PT pulses and a warm foot with intact sensation. He complains of increasing pain when he wiggles his toes or with passive motion of his ankle. You remove the ACE wrap and notice increased leg swelling below the knee; he has significant tenderness of the lateral aspect of the lower leg.

3. What do you need to do now?
   a. Place his leg on three pillows, apply ice, and put the bed in Trendelenberg position
   b. Check compartment pressures
   c. Perform arthrocentesis
   d. Provide analgesia, and repeat his exam in 2 hours

Leg pain with passive leg movement and tenderness over the anterior tibial compartment are signs that should raise suspicion for compartment syndrome, which is plausible given the significant impact injury. Even though elevation and analgesia are indicated, this exam warrants measurement of compartment pressures.

Measurement with a handheld Striker reveals a lateral compartment pressure of 50 mm Hg, which is significant given his diastolic blood pressure is 70 mm Hg. Orthopedics is notified, and arrangements are made for emergent fasciotomy. While waiting for the operation, he becomes tachypneic, and you notice he is confused. You also notice petechiae on his arms and legs, which are new.

4. What is your clinical diagnosis?
   a. Pulmonary embolism
   b. Likely aspiration pneumonia
   c. Fat embolism syndrome
   d. Psychogenic hyperventilation, leading to hypercarbia and change in mental status

This patient is demonstrating the classic signs of fat embolism syndrome. While lower extremity injuries predispose to pulmonary embolus because of immobility, this would not be expected so early. Aspiration is possible but unlikely given that he has been alert and oriented at all times since the accident. Anxiety should be a diagnosis of exclusion, and, in fact, anxiety in the setting of recent trauma should precipitate a survey for clinical deterioration (primary and secondary surveys with repeat vital signs). Incidentally, hyperventilation causes hypocarbia, not hypercarbia.               Answers: 1-d; 2-a; 3-b; 4-c

## BACKGROUND

The vast majority of patients sustaining blunt trauma have some form of musculoskeletal injury. These injuries often cause significant pain and may distract from other more life-threatening injuries. Even though extremity injuries can threaten the long-term function or even survival of a limb, they rarely constitute an acute life threat. Entire textbooks are devoted to the topic of the management of orthopedic trauma, and an exhaustive review of this topic is beyond the scope of this text. This chapter provides a basis for diagnosing and treating orthopedic injuries and focuses on a few specific emergencies that pose more immediate threat to life and limb. See Box 16-1 for orthopedic terminology useful for describing fractures.

## PRIMARY SURVEY

As the primary survey is to identify immediate life threats, orthopedic evaluation should not be part of this survey. It is, of course, impossible to ignore certain orthopedic injuries (e.g., open fractures, amputations, and profusely bleeding extremity wounds) as the patient is rolled into the trauma bay. It is imperative, however, to start with the ABCs by assessing level of consciousness, airway patency, breathing, and ade-

---

**BOX 16-1  Clinically relevant fracture terminology**

When describing a fracture to an orthopedic consultant over the phone, it is imperative that terminology is used that conveys the nature of the fracture. The following are descriptive terms that are used (and in this order) when describing a fracture:

**Open versus closed**—Open fractures have an associated overlying break in the skin. While this is often obvious, it may be as subtle as a small puncture wound in close proximity to the fracture.

**Fracture type**—The fracture line should be described in reference to the long axis of the bone in question. Modifiers include *transverse* (perpendicular to the long axis), *oblique* (at an angle to the long axis), *spiral* (rotational fracture), or *comminuted* (in three or more parts).

**Exact anatomic location**—Both the name of the bone and the area or specific part of the bone fractured (e.g., distal third, surgical neck, condyle).

**Displacement and angulation**—Displacement refers to lateral displacement (away from the axis of the bone) of the distal fracture fragment relative to the proximal fragment. The amount of displacement is described either in millimeters or in relation to the thickness

of the bone (e.g., 3 mm displacement, or 25% displacement). *Angulation* refers to angular deviation of the distal fragment relative to the proximal fragment. *Valgus* indicates deformity in a lateral direction, while *varus* indicates a deformity in a medial direction.

**Intra-articular versus extra-articular**—Mention should be made whether the fracture line enters a joint since this affects management and functional prognosis.

*Other descriptive modifiers are important to include as well.*

**Impacted fracture** is caused by compressive forces, resulting in loss of length.

**Buckle fracture (Torus fracture)** occurs in children and involves a "wrinkling" of the cortex without an obvious break.

**Incomplete fracture (greenstick fracture)** is seen in children and involves a break that does not extend circumferentially around the cortex, and thus on x-ray "one" cortex appears broken while the other is intact.

**Avulsion fractures** occur when a tendon pulls a small fragment of bone off from its insertion site.

**Distraction** occurs when the fracture fragments are separated.

---

quate circulation. Once the patient is stabilized, then attention can be turned to orthopedic injuries.

## SECONDARY SURVEY

Again, examination of the extremities should not precede a thorough evaluation of the head, neck, c-spine, chest, and abdomen. The orthopedic exam should consist of palpation of all extremities and passive range of motion of all major joints so that injuries are not missed. Most potential fractures should be detected by doing this alone. The second component is a neurovascular exam of all four extremities. Motor function, sensation, and pulses should be examined. This is done to assess for complication of fractures or soft tissue injury. A fracture associated with impaired neurovascular function requires immediate attention to preserve long-term function of the limb. In obtunded or intubated patients, the evaluation will be based on secondary signs of injury (e.g., bruising, swelling, or deformity) to detect significant fractures, and the use of x-ray can be liberal. These patients require thorough re-evaluation once they are extubated or their mental status clears.

### Radiographs

Although the majority of orthopedic injuries were described prior to advent of x-ray technology (hence the numerous eponyms for fractures), today the mainstay of definitive orthopedic diagnosis is plain radiography. In ordering radiographs in the trauma

patient, two main principles are followed. First, at least two views (at right angles to each other) of each injured area should be obtained, typically an antero-posterior (AP) and lateral view. This allows detection of any displacement and increases the likelihood of elucidating subtle fractures. Second, the x-rays should cover the entire length of the bone in suspect and ideally the joint space proximal and distal to the bone. A dedicated joint series (e.g., shoulder series) is not necessarily required unless injury to that joint is suspected. It is important to consider that radiography is not 100% sensitive, meaning that small fractures may not be apparent. Therefore, if the clinical suspicion is high, a fracture should be assumed and treated as such. For most fractures this means splinting and follow-up in 5 to 7 days for repeat exam or radiography, which is more likely to reveal a fracture that was initially occult. In certain potentially unstable fractures that require an operation (e.g., femoral neck fracture or tibial plateau fracture), a CT scan is often warranted in the setting of normal radiographs if the clinical suspicion is high.

## MANAGEMENT

### Fracture Reduction

Emergent fracture reduction is required if the fracture is causing neurovascular compromise. A classic example of this is an ankle fracture/dislocation that results in absent pedal pulses. This is a procedure that must be done immediately in the ED to restore blood flow to the foot. Another example is a displaced femur fracture with impaired distal pulses or neurologic function. In this case, the management is to place the femur in traction (called Buck's traction) in order to promote straightening and restore function. A displaced humerus fracture with neurovascular compromise can be placed in traction with a coaptation splint.

Otherwise, if distal neurovascular function is intact, fracture reduction is not emergent and is based on the degree of angulation or displacement. In this case, reduction does not necessarily need to occur in the ED. There are countless criteria, beyond the scope of this text, for degree of angulation and displacement for specific fractures that require reduction to optimize long-term function. A guiding principle, however, is that displaced or angulated fractures should be placed in traction until definitive management occurs, whether inpatient or outpatient. This can occur by either mechanical means, as with a Buck's traction device, or with a plaster splint.

Most displaced long-bone fractures will require admission for operative repair (e.g., fractures of the femur, tibia/fibula, humerus, and midshaft radius/ulna), as do open fractures (Box 16-2). In addition, any patient whose fracture is still unstable after splinting should be discussed with an orthopedic surgeon and considered for admission. Box 16-3 lists certain fractures that have high risk for potential complications or need urgent operative repair, thus requiring orthopedic evaluation and likely admission. Many other fractures can be discharged home with orthopedic follow-up (e.g., proximal humerus, distal radius/ulna, distal fibula, or foot and hand fractures), provided intact distal neurovascular func-

tion. Certain fractures can be reduced in the ED and splinted before patient discharge, the classic example being a dorsally displaced distal radius fracture (Colles' fracture). Phalanx fractures can also be reduced and splinted.

### Dislocation Reduction

Joint dislocations require reduction as soon as possible, with the majority being done in the ED. Classic examples of traumatic dislocations that require reduction include shoulder, elbow, hip, and ankle dislocations. Knee dislocations are also possible yet less common. They should typically be reduced in the OR because of the risk of vascular injury with blind reduction and the fact they are universally associated with significant fracture (Box 16-4). Traumatic hip dislocations require prompt reduction in the ED because of the long-term complication of avascular necrosis of the head of the femur. The incidence of this complication increases with the duration of dislocation time, especially after 4 hours. Therefore, reduction is a priority even in the setting of normal distal neurovascular function. Ankle dislocations are associated with fractures, often both distal tibia and fibula (bimaleolar fracture), and ankle ligament disruption. Because of this degree of instability, reduction of an ankle dislocation is generally easy, and a posterior splint is required to maintain this reduction. These patients usually require admission for definitive operative repair and stabilization. Patients with an isolated shoulder dislocation can be reduced in the ED and discharged home with a simple sling. If associated with a proximal humerus fracture, an orthopedist should be consulted for operative reduction, unless of course neurovascular impairment

---

**BOX 16-2  Open fractures require an operation**

Open fractures, with the exception of distal tuft fractures of the phalanx, are generally treated with surgical debridement and wash-out. Additionally, patients with open fractures should receive antibiotics and tetanus promptly. The wound should be covered with a sterile dressing while awaiting operative treatment. Although there have been no specific trials focusing on time to antibiotics, a recent *Cochrane Database System Review* summarized all randomized trials assessing the effectiveness of antibiotics in open fractures, showing that antibiotics clearly reduce the risk of infection. Although the studies did not specify time to antibiotic administration, it is intuitive that they should be administered without delay. It should be noted that even in treated patients, 5% to 6% developed subsequent infection.

The antibiotic regimen should provide good coverage for skin flora (e.g., *Staphalococcus* and *Streptococcus*), with an intravenous

first-generation cephalosporin such as cephalozin (Ancef) being a reasonable choice in nonallergic patients. Gram-negative coverage such as gentamycin should be given for grossly contaminated wounds.

There is sometimes a question of whether a deep laceration in proximity to a joint actually violates the joint capsule. In this instance, the joint can be injected with methylene blue dye through intact skin as if performing an arthrocentesis. The skin is prepped and anesthetized, and an 18-gauge needle is used to enter the joint. Several milliliters of diluted methylene blue (1:9 solution with sterile saline) is injected. If blue fluid is seen extravasating from the wound, then it is an open joint. If not, the diluted methylene blue can be aspirated back into the syringe, although this is not always possible.

---

**BOX 16-3  Specific fractures that should not be sent home without orthopedic evaluation**

**Tibial plateau fracture** involves the articular surface and results in loss of joint congruity. They have a higher likelihood of neurovascular complications, given the close proximity of the popliteal artery (immobile at the level of the tibial plateau) and the peroneal nerve (often injured when the lateral aspect of the tibial plateau is involved). Compartment syndrome is a concern with this fracture. While some are treated nonoperatively, the patient may require admission for observation.

**Midshaft tibial fracture** generally involves a high mechanism injury. Similarly, compartment syndrome is a concern, especially within the anterior compartment (extensor muscles, anterior tibial artery, deep peroneal nerve) and deep posterior compartment (deep flexor muscles, posterior tibial artery, peroneal artery, or tibial nerve).

**Malleolar fracture** that involves two or three of the elements of the ankle ring (either bone or ligament) and tends to be unstable.

**Pilon fracture** is a fracture of the distal tibial metaphysis that disrupts the articular surface. These injuries are generally accompanied by significant soft tissue injury, and swelling should be anticipated. If splinted, it should be padded appropriately. These fractures are often repaired in stages beginning with external fixation to reconstitute alignment and allow time for soft tissue injury to heal. This is followed by ORIF at a later date. These fractures are typically admitted.

**Displaced talus fracture** is significant because the amount of weight bearing per unit area of bone is greatest for the talus compared to any other bone in the body. If splinted, these patients should be strictly nonweight bearing.

**Combined midshaft radius/ulna fracture** is typically displaced given the multiple muscle attachments. These are at high risk for compartment syndrome. Admission for observation and ORIF is the norm.

**Monteggia fracture** is a fracture of the ulna with anterior dislocation of the radial head. These fractures require operative repair. Risk of malunion or nonunion increases if these are not repaired acutely.

**Galeazzi's fracture** is a fracture at the junction of the middle and distal third of the radius and a dislocation at the distal radial-ulnar joint. These fractures tend to be unstable. Yet discharge from the ED with urgent orthopedic follow-up for ORIF is reasonable.

---

necessitates immediate reduction. Elbow dislocations can often be reduced in the ED also, unless they are associated with a fracture, in which case an orthopedist should be consulted for possible operative reduction and repair.

Conscious sedation is required for all joint reductions, not only for the purpose of analgesia but for muscle relaxation as well. Muscles and tendons act to create compressive forces between two articulating bones through the joint space. Therefore, when dislocation and disarticulation occur, the bone ends tend to overlap due to muscle contraction. It often takes a great degree of force to overcome this contractile force, especially in larger joints such as the hip. This is only possible by conscious sedation, which involves the administration of a sedative and relaxing agent, typically midazolam (Versed), and an analgesic agent, typically fentanyl. This should occur while the patient is administered oxygen and placed on a cardiac monitor, and equipment at the bedside is available for intubation if necessary. Typical doses start with midazolam 2 mg IV and fentanyl 100 μg IV. Every 2 to 5 minutes an additional dose can be administered of midazolam 1 mg and fentanyl 100 μg IV. The goal is light sedation, not unconsciousness, and adequate analgesia. Under these conditions, most reductions are successful while providing slow, steady traction and avoiding quick maneuvers that precipitate muscle spasm. Maximum doses of medication should be midazolam 4 to 6 mg and fentanyl 400 to 600 μg IV. If reduction is still unsuccessful with these doses, then reduction must be performed under general anesthesia in the OR.

## Immobilization

All fractures require a splint, especially those that have been reduced or are potentially unstable. External traction devices, such as Buck's traction, are adequate in place of a splint when the patient is being admitted

---

**BOX 16-4  Posterior knee dislocations and popliteal artery injury**

Knee dislocation and popliteal artery injury should always be thought of together, the former so often results in the latter. The popliteal artery has limited mobility at the level of the posterior knee and, given the lack of collaterals distally, the complications because of missed injury are high. Therefore, patients with a knee dislocation or those with multiligamentous instability (assumed to have "spontaneously" reduced) should be worked-up for popliteal artery injury. Patients with signs of distal ischemia require emergent exploration of the politeal fossa. In patients with abnormal pulses but no other evidence of ischemia, an angiogram can be performed to assess the popliteal artery. Whether or not asymptomatic patients require arteriography is debatable. There is conflicting literature addressing this question and, therefore, practice varies.

---

**BOX 16-5 Five general principles of splinting**

1. Immobilize joint above and below the fracture (for midbone fractures)
2. Splint in a "position of function"
3. Avoid compression of peroneal and ulnar nerves
4. Consider postsplint swelling and allow some space for this
5. Check neurovascular status both before and after splinting

---

for surgery. There are five main guiding principles of splinting that are generally followed (Box 16-5). Regardless of these principles, it is important to keep in mind the purpose of splinting: Do not allow the fracture site to move. Therefore, one should not get caught up in the details of making a particular splint but instead make sure in the end that the fracture site is not subject to motion. The wrist is particularly important to immobilize in both hand fractures and forearm fractures, whether distal or proximal. The wrist is unique in that it allows not only motion in flexion and extension, but it also allows rotation with pronation and supination. This latter function creates rotation between the radius and ulna from the wrist up to the elbow. There are exceptions to the first principle of splinting, such as in distal radius or ulna fractures or distal tibia or fibula fractures for which only a single joint is typically immobilized.

It is important to splint an extremity in a "position of function," which incidentally is usually not the neutral position. A splint over time will cause some degree of stiffness, especially in older patients. Therefore, it is crucial to splint the extremity in a position that is functionally useful. For example, most uses of the hand require some degree of extension at the wrist and flexion of the fingers. By splinting the hand in a flexible position (as if holding a beer can), the hand will still be functional even if some stiffness occurs when the splint is removed. This concept can be applied to other parts of the body as well. For example, when applying a long leg cast, the knee should be flexed slightly, allowing the patient to walk with crutches.

It is important to avoid nerve compression when placing a splint. This is especially true for the peroneal nerve, which course takes it in proximity to the head of the fibula laterally below the knee. Prolonged compression of this nerve will result in foot drop. Similarly, the ulnar nerve is subject to compression at the medial aspect of the elbow. Also consider that fractures will cause limb swelling. As a result, a splint should be snug, but not tight, to allow for further swelling. This is the argument for initial splinting followed by casting in several days if needed. A cast is circumferential and does not allow room for swelling. Patients should be

---

**BOX 16-6  Avoid NSAIDs in acute fracture**

There have been multiple reports in the literature linking NSAID use with nonunion of fractures. While a randomized control trial is lacking, the evidence pointing to this association is relatively robust. The theory is that inhibition of the inflammatory pathway interferes with the natural healing process. For this reason, it is recommended that patients be treated with some form of oral narcotics (e.g., oxycodone) for an adequate time period given the severity of fracture (e.g., usually 7 to 10 days for long-bone fractures).

---

instructed to return immediately for increasing pain, numbness, tingling, dusky skin, or weakness distal to a splint or cast, as these are indicators of neurovascular compromise. As a corollary to this, neurovascular status should be assessed both before and after placement of a splint. After splint placement, check distal capillary refill and light touch sensation.

### Follow-up

Many patients with orthopedic injuries can be safely discharged home in the absence of other significant injuries. Follow-up must be ensured for fractures or other significant injuries. Most fractures can be splinted and followed up in 7 to 10 days, provided that further fracture reduction is not required—which should be done within 1 to 2 days. Patients should be given adequate analgesia and instructed to keep the extremity elevated and cool in order to prevent - significant swelling. Of note, orthopedists are now recommending in larger numbers that nonsteroidal anti-inflammatory drugs (NSAIDs) be avoided in the weeks following an acute fracture (Box 16-6). Written instructions should be given for signs and symptoms of compartment syndrome and neurovascular compromise.

---

**BOX 16-7  Fat embolism syndrome**

Fat embolism syndrome (FES) is a clinical entity characterized by respiratory distress, mental status changes, and petechial rash. The suspected pathophysiology is the presence of fat globules in the systemic circulation. While it is not uncommon to have fat droplets present in the circulation after major trauma, the incidence of FES is relatively low. FES is seen most commonly after long-bone fractures (tibia, femur, or fibula) and usually presents 1 to 2 days after the initial injury. Other symptoms and signs, such as renal insufficiency, thrombocytopenia, retinal changes, jaundice, fever, and tachycardia may be present as well. Treatment is supportive in an ICU setting, and the prognosis is typically good.

## KEY POINTS

- Focus first on ABCs, despite despite obvious ortho-
  pedic injuries
- Secondary survey includes vascular, motor, and
  sensory exam distal to injury
- Fractures with distal neurovascular compromise
  require emergent reduction in ED
  - Postreduction splint required and repeat neu-
    rovascular exam
  - Buck's traction or pin traction required for femur
    fractures
- If neurovascular intact, fractures are reduced based
  on displacement and angulation
  - Differing criteria exist, depending on fracture site
  - Does not necessarily need to occur in ED
  - Splint should be placed with fracture fragments in
    traction
- Most long-bone fractures will require admission
  and operative repair because of risk of
  displacement
- Joint dislocations should be reduced as soon as
  possible, most in the ED
  - Generally more difficult to reduce the longer a
    joint is out
  - Reduction of knee dislocation should be done in
    OR if neurovascular intact
    - High risk for popliteal artery injury
  - Traumatic dislocation of hip needs to be emer-
    gently reduced
    - High risk of avascular necrosis of femoral head
      with prolonged dislocation
- It is important to know the five principles of
  splinting
- Avoid NSAIDs in fractures because of potential
  nonunion

# CHAPTER 17

# Burn Injury

## CASE SCENARIO

A 64-year-old male is brought to the ED after he was found at his nearby home in a house fire. By the time rescuers arrived, the fire had been burning for about 15 minutes. At the scene he was found to be awake and alert but confused and anxious. En route to the hospital, two large-bore IVs were placed in his unburned right upper extremity and Ringer's lactate administered wide open. In the ED, his vital signs include a heart rate of 108, blood pressure of 146/82, respiratory rate of 24, and oxygen saturation 100% on a non-rebreather mask. His only complaint is pain in his left lower extremity, which is significantly burned. As he is being undressed, you notice that all of his extremities and chest wall have significant injury. He has two small burns on his left cheek, and you notice that his eyebrows and nasal hairs are singed. You examine his oropharynx and see a small amount of soot by his uvula without edema. You hear faint expiratory wheezes on his lung examination.

1. What is your next step?
   a. Send an ABG and intubate him if his $PaO_2$ is less than 100 mm Hg
   b. Obtain a portable CXR, and intubate if there is evidence of pulmonary edema
   c. Observe him closely, and intubate if further signs of airway compromise develop
   d. Intubate him immediately before he develops significant airway edema

Burn injury to the airway can cause progressive airway edema that makes endotracheal intubation difficult or impossible. Therefore, patients should be intubated early if there are signs of developing airway edema, such as expiratory wheezes. Signs of airway involvement include singeing of nasal hairs, carbonaceous sputum, hoarseness, and soot in the mouth or nose.

You intubate the patient with etomidate 20 mg IV and succinylcholine 120 mg IV without complication and confirm placement of the endotracheal tube with end-tidal $CO_2$ capnometry. You perform a thorough examination of his burns and determine that approximately 54% of his body surface area (BSA) has sustained second-degree and third-degree burns. The nurse asks you how much fluid you want the patient to receive.

2. What do you tell her?
   a. Run normal saline wide open until the patient manifests signs of pulmonary edema
   b. Administer 4 × body weight (kg) × percentage of BSA in mL of NS over 12 hours
   c. Administer 8 × body weight (kg) × percentage of BSA in mL of NS over 24 hours
   d. Administer 2 L bolus of NS and then titrate to urine output of about 0.5 mL/kg/hr

Fluid resuscitation is the mainstay of medical management for the burn patient. The Parkland formula is a commonly quoted tool for calculating the volume of fluid that should be provided over a 24-hour period.

Crystalloid in mL = 4 × body weight (kg) × percentage of BSA.

It is recommended that the first half be administered over 8 hours and the rest over the remaining 24 hours. BSA is determined based on second-degree and third-degree burns. Another method is to start crystalloid at a rate of milliliters per hour determined by body weight (kg) × percentage of BSA burned divided by 8 per hour. Regardless of the method used, crystalloid administration should be titrated to adequate urine output, about 0.5 mL/kg/hr in adults (30 to 40 mL per hr in most adults).

The patient's wife arrives and tells you that the patient was unresponsive for a brief time and subsequently disoriented.

**3.** What is your next step?
   **a.** Observe him since he was responsive on arrival to your facility
   **b.** Obtain a head CT scan to rule out intracranial injury
   **c.** Obtain a carboxyhemoglobin level, and arrange hyperbaric oxygen therapy for syncope.
   **d.** Obtain neurology consultation for altered mental status

Syncope and neurologic deficits (including altered mental status) in the setting of closed-space smoke inhalation are indications to initiate hyperbaric oxygen therapy. A definitive airway and hemodynamic stability should be established before the patient is transferred to the hyperbaric chamber.

Four hours later the patient is transferred from the hyperbaric chamber to the SICU. Now his right forearm is swollen and feels tense. The entire circumference of his arm is burned. His hand is somewhat discolored, yet his radial pulse is still obtainable by Doppler.

**4.** What is the next most appropriate step?
   **a.** Consult orthopedics for possible compartment syndrome
   **b.** Perform fasciotomy for compartment syndrome
   **c.** Perform an emergent escharotomy
   **d.** Decrease the rate of fluid being infused to prevent further edema

Full-thickness circumferential burns of the extremities result in underlying microvascular damage with endothelial leak, resulting in tissue edema and an increase in forearm compartment pressures. This will lead to compartment syndrome that requires emergent escharotomy. This involves several longitudinal incisions only through the dermis into subcutaneous fat with a Bovey to allow underlying tissues to expand. This is different than a fasciotomy, which involves an incision into the muscle compartment itself. It is important to keep in mind that in a burn patient, even in the setting of circumferential burns, pulses are most commonly lost because of hypotension as opposed to compartment syndrome.                    Answers: 1-d; 2-d; 3-c; 4-c

## BACKGROUND

Each year over 50,000 people in the United States are hospitalized with thermal burn injuries. The past two decades have brought major advances in burn care, which have resulted in decreased morbidity and mortality for these patients. The risk of burns is greatest in young adults 18 to 30 years of age. There is a male to female ratio of 2:1 for both injury and death. Neonates, the elderly, and those with comorbid illnesses have poorer outcomes.

The burn wound itself on a histologic level is described as having three zones in concentric order. The innermost zone that is subject to direct burn injury is referred to as the *zone of coagulation*, a necrotic area of irreversible tissue damage because of thrombosis of blood vessels. The middle zone, or *zone of stasis*, is an area of moderate tissue injury where vasoconstriction occurs, resulting in stagnation of the microcirculation. This is an area that can either progress to coagulative necrosis or heal, depending on conditions that are present during treatment and healing. The goal of therapy is to maximize perfusion to this zone, which is partially accomplished through intravascular fluid resuscitation. Lastly, the outer *zone of hyperemia* is an area surrounding the injured tissue where inflammation and

vasodilation occur in response to the injury. This zone is the nidus for healing of tissue in the inner zones.

Skin functions as a semipermeable barrier to evaporative water loss. Thermal injury can disrupt this function, resulting in insensate losses and a free water deficit. A significant burn (greater than 20% BSA with second-degree or third-degree burns) results in systemic activation of an inflammatory cascade, akin to sepsis, with release of multiple mediators such as histamine, prostaglandins, leukotrienes, bradykinins, catecholamines, activated complement, serotonin, thromboxane A, and others. These mediators induce capillary leak and vasoconstriction, both in the tissue surrounding the burn and in remote organs as well. On a systemic level this leads to loss of intravascular volume, increased peripheral resistance, and decreased cardiac output. This may result in tissue hypoperfusion, metabolic acidosis, and multiorgan failure.

## DEFINITIONS

### Burn Depth

Estimating burn depth has important implications in regard to prognosis, course, and treatment (Table 17-1). *First-degree burns* involve only the epidermis and

**TABLE 17-1  Significance of burn depth**

| Type of burn | Findings | Implications |
|---|---|---|
| First-degree | Erythema, blanching, tender | No scarring |
| Superficial second-degree | Erythema, blanching, tender, blistering | Re-epithelialize in 7–14 days from epidermal structures in rete ridges, hair follicles, and sweat glands; minimal discoloration |
| Deep second-degree | Pale erythema, no blanching, pinprick sensation intact | Re-epithelialize in 14–28 days from hair follicles and sweat glands; severe scarring; may require skin graft |
| Third-degree | Hard leathery eschar (black, white, or cherry red), painless | No epidermal appendages remain; requires skin graft |
| Fourth-degree | Involves subcutaneous tissue such as muscle and bone | May require fasciotomy |

are erythematous, blanching, nonblistering, painful, and tender to touch. The classic example is a sunburn. It requires only symptomatic treatment and typically heals within 4 to 7 days with sloughing of the superficial epidermis. *Second-degree burns* (partial thickness burns), which extend into the dermis, are divided into superficial and deep burns. Superficial second-degree burns are erythematous, blanching, blistering, painful, and tender to touch. They involve the superficial dermis and thus spare the rete ridges, hair follicles, sweat glands, and sebaceous glands. This is important because these structures are epidermal in origin and contain keratinocytes that reproduce to form epithelial cells. Also left intact is deep dermal microvasculature, important in promoting wound healing. These burns thus heal spontaneously in 7 to 14 days by re-epithelialization, and they leave minimal residual scars. Deep second-degree burns are more pale than erythematous, and they do not blanch. This is a result of reticular dermis involvement with coagulation of microvasculature. Sensation is markedly decreased, but pinprick sensation remains intact due to deep sensory receptors in the dermis. These wounds can heal spontaneously in 14 to 28 days from residual deep hair follicles and sweat glands in the dermis; however, surgical debridement and skin grafting are often necessary. Scarring is thus extensive. *Third-degree burns* (full-thickness burns) result in charred, leathery eschar (either black, white, or cherry red) that is painless and nonblanching. There is no sensation to pinprick. These burns require skin grafting.

## Burn Size

Burn size is quantified as the percentage of body surface area (% BSA) burned. One method is based on the fact that the area of the back of the hand is approximately 1 percent body surface area. Therefore, BSA can be estimated by the number of "hands" that cover the area of the burn. Another method is the rule of nines. The body is divided into segments that each represent approximately 9%, or multiples thereof, with the remaining 1% dedicated to the perineum (Figure 17–1). The percentages are adjusted for infants and children since their heads are relatively larger in proportion to the rest of the body. A Lund and Browder burn diagram, a chart that accounts for age-based anatomic proportion discrepancies, allows a more accurate assessment of burn size. See Table 17-2 for the American Burn Association classification of major, moderate, and minor burns. It is recommended that patients with moderate to severe burns be transferred to designated burn centers for acute treatment and follow-up.

## Prehospital Care

Prehospital care for the burn patient should begin with extrication of the patient from the burn environment. This includes removing clothing, which still may be smoldering or melted. Early cooling can reduce the depth of burn and reduce pain, although care should be taken to prevent overcooling. Clean sheets should be placed over the patient to protect the wounds. EMS should also establish an airway and administer oxygen, initiate fluid resuscitation, administer analgesics, and transport the patient to an appropriate medical facility. Concern for progressive airway edema should prompt endotracheal intubation. Intravenous fluids should be started using Ringer's lactate solution. Establishing IV access should not delay the patient's transport to a hospital setting.

## PRIMARY SURVEY

### Always Think Inhalation Injury

The primary survey for the burn patient is similar to that of any other trauma victim with the ABCs and

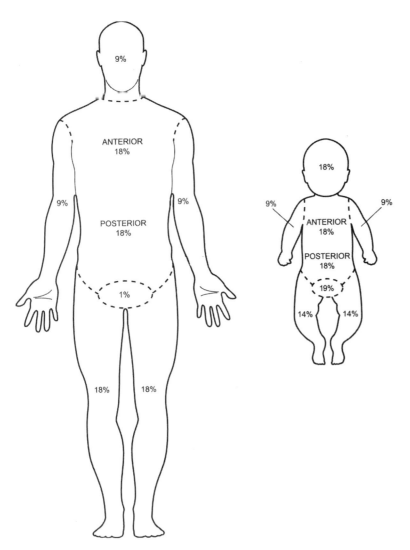

**FIGURE 17-1    Rule of Nines.** (Adapted from Mick NW, Peters JR, Egan D, et al. *Blueprints Emergency Medicine,* 2nd ed. Malden, MA: Blackwell Publishing; 2005)

IV–O₂–monitor, with a special emphasis on the airway. It is important to keep in mind that inhalation injury is the leading cause of mortality in burn patients. Such injuries are more commonly associated with closed-space fires and conditions such as intoxication or head injury that compromise LOC. Direct thermal injury is limited to the upper airway. Inhalation injury damages endothelial cells, causing mucosal edema of the small airways and decreasing alveolar surfactant activity. These result in bronchospasm and airway obstruction. Though airway edema may occur for up to 24 hours after the insult, upper airway edema can be immediate and rapidly progressive. This is especially true for patients with any evidence of facial burns, inhalation injury, hypoxia, or altered mental status on presentation. The symptoms and signs can initially be subtle; but, if action is not taken early, progressive airway edema can lead to a situation in which intubation

is impossible. As a result, endotracheal intubation should be initiated early if there is a suspicion of developing airway edema. Diagnosis of smoke inhalation is based in part on the history and primarily on physical signs that include facial burns, singed nasal hairs, soot in the mouth or nose, hoarseness, carbonaceous sputum, expiratory wheezing, stridor, or uvular edema. In patients with significant respiratory distress, one should be prepared to perform a cricothyrotomy in the event that orotracheal intubation with RSI is unsuccessful.

### Moving Past the Airway

Patients with significant burns will have significant fluid requirements over the first 24 to 48 hours because of large insensate losses, systemic fluid shifts, and intravascular volume depletion. However, during the

**TABLE 17-2 American Burn Association classification of burn severity**

| | |
|---|---|
| Major | Second-degree burns greater than 25% BSA; ages 10–50 years |
| | Second-degree burns greater than 20% BSA; under age 10 or over age 50 |
| | Third-degree burns greater than 10% BSA in any age group |
| | Burns involving the hands, face, feet, or perineum |
| | Burns crossing over major joints |
| | Circumferential burns of an extremity |
| | Burns complicated by inhalational injury |
| | Electrical burns |
| | Burns complicated by fractures or other trauma |
| | Burns in infants or the elderly |
| | Burns in patients with major comorbidities |
| Moderate | Second-degree burns of 15%–25% BSA; ages 10–50 years |
| | Second-degree burns of 10%–20% BSA; under age 10 or over age 50 |
| | Third-degree burns of less than 10% BSA in any age group |
| Minor | Second-degree burns less than 15% BSA; ages 10–50 years |
| | Second-degree burns less than 10% BSA; under age 10 or over age 50 |

**BOX 17-1 Think toxicology in burn victims**

It is a misconception that death from fire is primarily the result of burning. The reality is that the majority of deaths are a result of inhalation injury and respiratory failure. Toxic inhalation must also be a consideration as well, with carbon monoxide (CO) toxicity being the most common. This should be considered for patients involved in a closed-space fire (e.g., house fire) and in those with altered mental status. Of note, CO has an affinity for hemoglobin that is 240 times that of oxygen; and, despite a normal oxygen saturation (i.e., measurement of free oxygen dissolved in blood), little oxygen may be bound to hemoglobin, which carried more than 95% of the total oxygen content of blood. Carbon monoxide levels should be checked in all patients with suspected inhalation injury. Patients should be empirically treated with 100% oxygen until their CO levels return at less than 10%. There is no threshold level that dictates the need for hyperbaric oxygen. However, patients who were unresponsive for a time or have altered mental status in the ED should receive hyperbaric oxygen. In addition, pregnant women with a CO level greater than 25 should also receive hyperbaric oxygen.

Another rarely considered, yet lethal, toxin is hydrogen cyanide, which is formed when nitrogen-containing polymers (e.g., wool, silk, vinyl) are burned. Cyanide causes tissue hypoxia by uncoupling mitochondrial oxidative phosphorylation at the cellular level. So oxygen is effectively being transported to the peripheral tissues, but aerobic metabolism is poisoned. The only alternative is anaerobic metabolism and the result is lactic acidosis. Cyanide toxicity should be suspected in patients with unexplained severe metabolic acidosis, normal arterial oxygen levels, and a low carboxyhemoglobin level. The treatment is sodium nitrite 300 mg IV and amyl nitrate pearls, both of which produce methemoglobin that binds cyanide to form cyanomethemoglobin. These are followed by sodium thiosulfate 12.5 g IV, which provides a sulfur donor that facilitates the natural enzyme rhodanase to convert free serum cyanide and cyanomethemoglobin to thiocyanate (which is safely cleared by the kidneys). Of note, sodium thiosulfate should be used alone in the setting of CO poisoning because the production of methemoglobin, along with carboxyhemoglobin, will exacerbate the blood's decreased oxygen-carrying capacity.

acute phase of injury, the presence of circulatory shock should raise the suspicion for another etiology, such as associated trauma. Thought must also be given to the toxic effects of smoke as well (Box 17-1). Circulation is addressed briefly during the primary survey by checking peripheral pulses and obtaining vital signs. If there is suspicion for blunt trauma, based on history, physical, or unexplained hypotension or shock, then it is appropriate to continue the trauma evaluation with a FAST exam, trauma series, and aggressive resuscitation with large-bore IVs and crystalloid and blood administration. Of note, IV access should be obtained in areas with unburned skin; however, if this is not possible, IV access should be obtained through burned skin, although keep in mind that subcutaneous veins will likely be thrombosed beneath skin with third-degree burns. In the absence of peripheral IV options, central venous catheterization or a saphenous vein cutdown should be done.

## MANAGEMENT

### Fluid Resuscitation Is the Key for Major Burns

Burns cause microvascular injury that manifests as increased vascular permeability with edema formation, resulting in ongoing plasma volume loss. Maximal edema formation occurs 8 to 12 hours after injury for small burns and 24 hours after injury for large burns. In addition, free water loss (referred to as insensate losses) occurs through damaged epithelium. Fluid resuscitation must be initiated to restore effective plasma volume, avoid microvascular ischemia in the zone of stasis, and maintain overall adequate tissue perfusion. It must also be kept in mind that with progressive edema over the first 24 hours, the airway status must be monitored closely and the patient intubated if there are early signs of airway edema or respiratory distress.

Over the past several decades, there have been multiple studies looking to find the optimal fluid type and administration rate for burn patients. In regard to fluid type, both colloid solutions and hypertonic saline have been studied extensively because of the theoretical benefit of increasing intravascular osmotic pressure and thus decreasing capillary leak and third-spacing. It has been established that there is no benefit of colloid in the first 24 hours after injury but that after 24 hours it effectively increases intravascular volume by the amount infused. This effect is thought to be due to restoration of capillary permeability, which some believe is restored within 8 hours. There is still no evidence, however, to suggest that colloid solution actually improves mortality in burn patients. Hypertonic saline has been shown in a head-to-head study to have no benefit over lactated Ringer's solution, and additionally it has been implicated in precipitating renal failure and seizures.

The most noteworthy formula for estimating fluid requirements in burn patients comes from investigators at Parkland Hospital in Texas. The Parkland formula calls for the quantity of Ringer's lactate to be 4 mL × body weight (kg) × % BSA burned, with half over the first 8 hours and the other half over the remaining 24 hours. The percentage of body surface area used includes only second-degree and third-degree burns. A rapid estimation of the initial rate can be made using body weight (kg) × % BSA burned divided by 8, which gives the initial rate for Ringer's lactate in mL per hour. The Brooke formula is a bit more complicated, and it starts with a lower rate of Ringer's lactate followed later by colloid, and then topped off with free water. Regardless of the strategy used, adequate volume resuscitation is measured by monitoring vital signs as well as urine output. Adequate urine output is 1.0 mL/kg/hr in children less than 2 years of age and 0.5 mL/kg/hr in older children and adults, with 30 to 40 mL per hr adequate for most adults.

### Children Lose More Fluid and Heat

Physiologic differences alter some parameters of burn resuscitation in children. The Parkland formula underestimates evaporative fluid loss and maintenance needs in children. Therefore, for burned

### LITERATURE REFERENCE

## Hypertonic versus isotonic fluid for resuscitation in burn patients

Hypertonic solutions and colloid solutions are considered to have a greater ability to rapidly expand blood volume and elevate blood pressure, and they can be infused in a small volume over a short time period. Several studies have investigated such solutions as a feasible alternative to isotonic fluid resuscitation in burn patients and other critically ill trauma patients. A meta-analysis was done to determine whether or not colloid solutions decrease mortality in patients requiring massive resuscitation. Fifty-three trials were studied and several subanalyses were performed to assess the potential benefit of various colloid solutions with isotonic fluid. There was no evidence that resuscitation with colloids reduces the risk of death, compared with isotonic fluid resuscitation, in patients with traumatic injuries or burns. Given the relative expense of such solutions, their routine use cannot be advocated. **[Roberts et al. *Cochrane Database Syst Rev* 2004;18(4):CD00567].**

children, the Galveston formula is used for fluid resuscitation guidelines. The quantity of 5% dextrose in LR solution is $5000 \text{ mL/m}^2$ BSA burned + $1500/\text{m}^2$ BSA burned), with half over the first 8 hours and the rest over the remaining 24 hours. Dextrose is added because children have smaller glycogen stores than adults and are prone to hypoglycemia when under stress. Children also have a greater evaporative water loss per kilogram body weight and a larger body surface area per kilogram body weight than adults and are more prone to hypothermia. Therefore, warming techniques (e.g., heated IV fluids, warm blankets, or heating lamps) are important in children.

### Escharotomy in Circumferential Burns

Deep second-degree and third-degree burns of the extremity result in significant tissue edema. If these burns are circumferential, the extremity is enveloped in a tough, leathery case. The underlying tissues have nowhere to swell or expand, and thus pressure builds within the tissue compartments. This results effectively in a compartment syndrome manifested by muscle ischemia and pain, distal sensory and motor loss, and evidence of decreased distal perfusion. Keep in mind, however, that the presence of distal pulses does in no way rule out a compartment syndrome. Therefore, patients with circumferential extremity burns should be re-examined frequently for the development of compartment syndrome, and those with deep second-degree and third-degree burns should undergo escharotomy. This procedure involves making incisions along the medial and lateral aspects of the affected extremity, extending the length of the eschar, using a scalpel or high-frequency electrical current. Reperfusion injury with reactive hyperemia and compartment muscle edema may occur, necessitating fasciotomy. Circumferential burns to the chest and neck may cause mechanical restriction to ventilation, also necessitating escharotomy. Chest wall escharotomy involves making incisions at the anterior axillary line from the level of the 2nd rib to the level of the 12th rib and then joining these incisions transversely.

## Wound Care

For major burns, wound care should immediately consist of wrapping the patient in a clean dry sheet. If definitive care is going to be delayed, gentle cleansing of the wounds using sterile saline or commercial products containing poloxamer 188 should be initiated. Debridement of blisters, except on the palms and soles, is indicated. A topical antibacterial agent should be applied after cleansing. Silver sulfadiazine, mafenide acetate, and 0.5% silver nitrate solution are used frequently. The treated wounds should be covered with sterile gauze. The temptation to give prophylactic antibiotics is great, given that antibiotics are often used to treat minor infections, and a burn seems like a major nidus for potential infection. The current teaching is to withhold antibiotics unless there is evidence of infection.

Minor burns should be cleansed. Blisters large enough to interfere with application of a dressing should be aspirated or incised sterilely. Palm and sole blisters should be left intact. Tetanus toxoid should be given if not up to date. Topical antimicrobial agents are not indicated for the outpatient management of minor burns. The reason for this is that patients tend not to fully cleanse the wound on a daily basis because of pain, and they apply a new layer of antimicrobial cream over the old layer. This actually increases the risk of infection. It is more effective to cleanse the wound thoroughly once in the ED, and then apply gauze soaked in sterile saline. This should be wrapped with a fluff gauze dressing. This can be left intact for 5 to 7 days while re-epithelialization takes place. As much as possible, the site of injury should

**LITERATURE REFERENCE**

## Should we give antibiotics to acute burn patients?

Ergun et al. conducted a study to determine whether prophylactic antibiotics decreased rates of infection and whether they affected outcomes if septicemia occurred. Forty-seven patients with moderate to severe burns received prophylactic antibiotics, and 30 did not. Both groups of patients were similar in terms of age, wound depth, day of admission, mechanism of burn injury, and type of local wound care received. Wound infection rates were slightly higher in the prophylaxis group. Septicemia rates and length of hospital stay were higher in the prophylaxis group [Ergun et al. *Eur J Pediatr Surg* **2004;14(6):422–426**].

In a study by Gang et al., staphylococcal septicemia in 1,516 burn patients admitted over a period of 7 years were analyzed in terms of type of *Staphyloccus*, age of patient, percentage of total body surface area affected, type of burn, and outcome. No significant difference was noted in mortality among the septicemic patients, whether or not they received prophylactic antibiotics. Survival was due to early detection of the organism in the blood, appropriate wound care, and appropriate antibiotic therapy after positive blood cultures were obtained [Gang et al. *Burns* **2000;26(4):359–366**].

A follow-up study was performed by Bang et al. to analyze the outcomes and role of fluid resuscitation that was more aggressive than that of Parkland formula parameters, wound care, and prophylactic antibiotics in two groups of burn patients. These patients were comparable in terms of age, percentage of total body surface area burned, and type of burn injury. Septicemia most commonly occurred within 2 weeks after the burn event in both groups. The group that was more aggressively managed in terms of initial resuscitation had a lower incidence of both septicemia and death. Comparing septicemic patients from both groups demonstrated no role of prophylactic antibiotics in decreasing mortality [Bang et al. *Burns* **2002;28(8):746–751**].

be elevated to prevent edema to expedite return to normal function. On follow-up when the dressing is removed, the damaged skin will have sloughed onto the dry dressing, leaving underlying viable epithelium intact.

## KEY POINTS

- Pathophysiology is important in understanding principles of treatment
  - Zones of coagulation, stasis, and hyperemia
  - Massive inflammatory response with release of multiple mediators
  - Attributes to capillary leak, vasoconstriction, tissue ischemia, and multiorgan failure
- Severity is detemined by burn depth and size
  - First-degree, superficial second-degree, deep second-degree, and third degree
  - Rule of nines used to estimate percentage body surface area (BSA) involved
- Inhalational injury is the most common cause of mortality in burn patients
  - Airway edema may be rapid and catastrophic
  - Any signs of airway involvement should prompt intubation
- Initial hypotension should prompt a search for associated trauma
- The Parkland formula is used to determine fluid resuscitation needs for the burn patient.
  - Total fluid $= 4 \times$ body weight (kg) $\times$ % BSA in mL
  - Half of fluid over first 8 hours then the rest over remaining 24 hours
  - BSA takes into account only second-degree and third-degree burns
  - Urine output should be maintained at 0.5 mL/kg/hr (30 to 40 mL per hr)
- Carboxyhemoglobin and cyanide toxicity should be considered in closed-space fires
- Circumferential extremity burns are at risk for compartment syndrome
  - Escharotomy is necessary to allow release of subcutaneous pressure
- The keys to treatment are wound cleansing and sterile dressing
  - Topical antimicrobial agents are also effective
  - Oral or IV antibiotics are not indicated unless evidence of infection develops
- Tetanus toxoid should be given if not up-to-date

# CHAPTER 18

# Trauma in Pregnancy

## CASE SCENARIO

A 32-year-old G3P2 female, at 32 weeks gestation, presents to ED after a moderate-speed MVC. She was the restrained front seat passenger in a vehicle that was hit head-on by another vehicle traveling at 30 to 40 mph. The patient's airbag deployed. She was ambulatory at the scene and remained awake and alert on transport. She was c-spine immobilized and transported on a backboard. On arrival in the trauma bay, she has an obvious laceration on her right scalp that is bleeding through the gauze placed over it. She is crying and demands that you immediately make sure that her baby is all right.

1. What is your first step in the management of this patient?
   a. Consult obstetrics
   b. Obtain a Doppler to listen for a fetal heart beat
   c. Check for vaginal bleeding
   d. Perform primary survey on the mother

It is a common pitfall to concentrate on the pregnancy and fetus when caring for a pregnant trauma patient, especially late in the pregnancy. Caring for the mother should always be the first priority because fetal circulation is contingent on maternal circulation. It is reasonable to gather information about the fetus and the pregnancy early; however, fetal assessment begins after maternal airway, breathing, and circulation are ensured. You explain this to the patient and continue with her evaluation. Her vitals signs are a pulse of 95, blood pressure of 88/54, respiratory rate of 22, and oxygen saturation 98% on oxygen. The patient is alert and following commands appropriately. Her airway and breathing are intact, she has clear breath sounds bilaterally, and she has palpable radial pulses.

2. What is the next step in her management?
   a. Transfuse 2 units of uncrossmatched blood
   b. Perform a diagnostic peritoneal lavage to search for intra-abdominal blood
   c. Turn the backboard to displace the uterus from the inferior vena cava
   d. Perform a FAST exam

Blood pressure declines slightly during the first trimester, levels out in the second trimester, and then returns to prepregnancy levels as the third trimester progresses. Heart rate rises throughout pregnancy but does not increase by more than 10 to 15 beats per minute. This can make interpretation of vital signs difficult when assessing for shock. As pregnancy progresses, compression of the inferior vena cava by the gravid uterus causes decreased venous return to the heart; hypotension can result. All pregnant trauma patients should be placed in a lateral decubitus position, both during transport and in the ED. During transport, the patient should be tilted to the left about 15 degrees on the backboard. After the patient is taken off the backboard, several towels can be placed under the right hip to keep the uterus displaced to the left. After you place the patient into the left lateral decubitus position, her blood pressure is 108/76. She denies any pain or discomfort anywhere except over her laceration.

3. What is the next step?
   a. Perform a secondary survey, including vaginal exam and assessment of fetal heart rate
   b. Order a trauma series consisting of a CXR, c-spine x-ray, and pelvic x-ray
   c. Order an abdominal CT scan to assess the fetus
   d. Send the patient to labor and delivery for observation and fetal assessment

Trauma evaluation is the same in the pregnant patient as in the nonpregnant patient except that a vaginal examination must be performed. Additionally, the secondary survey includes determination of fetal heart rate and movement. The secondary survey reveals a 5 cm laceration over the right forehead with extension to the galea. The pelvic exam reveals blood in the vaginal vault and bleeding from the os. The patient denies vaginal bleeding prior to her accident. A bedside ultrasound shows a viable fetus with heart rate of 140; a formal ultrasound shows no evidence of placental abruption.

**4.** What do you do next?
   **a.** Observe the patient for 2 hours in the ED, and discharge home if her vitals remain normal
   **b.** Discharge her since her vital signs, hematocrit, and ultrasound are normal
   **c.** Repeat an ultrasound in 4 hours, and discharge her if it is normal
   **d.** Admit her to the obstetrics service for continuous fetal heart monitoring

Ultrasound can be falsely negative in placental abruption, especially if the placenta lies posteriorly, which can hide hematoma. Hematoma may also be absent because of active bleeding from the os. The most sensitive indicator of abruption is fetal distress reflected by a decrease in the fetal heart rate. Therefore, this patient must be admitted for continuous fetal monitoring. Depending on level of distress, immediate c-section may be warranted. You repair your patient's scalp laceration, administer tetanus toxoid, which is safe for the fetus, and admit her to the obstetrics service. An hour later her vaginal bleeding increases, and the fetal heart rate drops to 114. She is immediately taken for c-section where she is found to have placental abruption. The newborn is delivered with a normal Apgar score at 5 minutes. Both mother and baby have a good recovery.      Answers: 1-d; 2-c; 3-a; 4-d

## BACKGROUND

Trauma is the leading cause of nonobstetrical death in pregnant women. The most common mechanism is motor vehicle collisions, followed by assaults and falls. Though the basic principles of running trauma prevail in the pregnant patient, there are a number of special conditions that must be considered. Pregnancy causes altered physiology and anatomic changes involving all organ systems. This can alter the signs and symptoms of injury, the responses to resuscitation, the evaluation of the extent of injury, and the interpretation of diagnostic tests. Though there are two lives involved, preservation of maternal life takes priority. Indirectly, this is also in the best interest of the fetus.

## ANATOMIC CHANGES IN PREGNANCY

Until the 12th week of gestation, the uterus remains an intrapelvic organ. By 20 weeks, it reaches the umbilicus; and by 34 to 36 weeks, it reaches the costal margin. As the uterus enlarges, the bowel is pushed upward, resting mainly in the upper abdomen and becoming somewhat protected in blunt trauma. Conversely, the uterus and fetus become more vulnerable to injury. Pain location patterns may also be altered because of the upward displacement of abdominal contents. Furthermore, because of the stretching of the abdominal wall, signs of peritoneal irritation may be masked.

As the uterus emerges from the pelvis during pregnancy, the uterine wall stretches and thins out. During the third trimester, the fetus is in the vertex position (head down), and maternal pelvic injuries may cause fetal skull fractures or intracranial injuries. Because the placenta has little elasticity, it is susceptible to shear forces at the uteroplacental interface, resulting in abruptio placentae. Though the placental vasculature is maximally dilated, it is extremely sensitive to catecholamine release. Thus, abrupt decreases in maternal intravascular volume may result in uterine vascular constriction, reducing fetal oxygenation despite relatively normal maternal vital signs. The bladder also becomes displaced out of the pelvis during late pregnancy, making it a target for injury.

Other differences in pregnancy include an elevated diaphragm with compensatory flaring of the ribs. Tension pneumothorax may develop more quickly as a result. Thoracostomy tubes should be placed 1 to 2 interspaces higher than usual to account for diaphragmatic elevation. Also, the ligaments of the symphysis pubis and sacroiliac joints are loose during pregnancy, which can cause baseline diastasis of the pubic symphysis, mimicking pelvic disruption on x-ray. Lastly, compression of the ureters by the gravid uterus can cause some degree of baseline hydronephrosis during pregnancy.

| TABLE 18-1   Summary of physiologic changes in pregnancy | |
|---|---|
| Blood volume | Increased plasma volume by 30%–40% |
| | Anemia with hematocrit 31%–35% |
| | Increased total RBC mass |
| | Increased WBC count 15,000–20,000 |
| Cardiovascular | Increased heart rate by 10–15 bpm (mean of 90) |
| | Blood pressure reaches low in second trimester (mean of 100/60) |
| | Blood pressure returns to normal in third trimester (mean of 110/70) |
| | Increased cardiac output by about 20% |
| | Decreased peripheral vascular resistance |
| Respiratory | Decreased total lung volume |
| | Decreased functional residual capacity |
| | Increased tidal volume |
| | Increased minute ventilation |
| | Chronic respiratory alkalosis |
| Gastrointestinal | Decreased GI motility |
| | Decreased GE sphincter tone |
| | Increased acid production |
| | (All these result in increased aspiration risk.) |

# PHYSIOLOGIC CHANGES OF PREGNANCY

## Blood Volume and Composition

A physiologic anemia occurs during pregnancy as a result of an increase in plasma volume out of proportion to the increased red blood cell count. Because of this increased plasma volume, a hematocrit of 31% to 35% is normal in late pregnancy. Despite the lower hemotocrit, which represents the concentration of RBCs per unit volume of blood, there is actually an overall increase in oxygen-carrying capacity because of an increased total RBC mass. The white blood cell count increases during pregnancy, peaking in late pregnancy at 15,000 to 20,000/mm$^3$. Prothrombin (PT) and partial thromboplastin (PTT) levels may be shortened, but bleeding and clotting times remain unchanged. There are, however, increased amounts of clotting factors and fibrinogen, resulting in a hypercoagulable state.

## Cardiovascular Changes

Depending on the trimester of pregnancy, normal hemodynamic changes of pregnancy can either mimic or hide shock. Cardiac output is increased from about 5.0 L to 6.0 L per minute, or by about 20%, after the 10th week of pregnancy. During the second half of pregnancy, vena cava compression in the supine position can decrease cardiac output by up to 30% due to decreased blood return to the heart. Heart rate increases gradually throughout pregnancy, with a maximal increase of 10 to 15 beats per minute (mean of about 90 bpm). Tachycardia is therefore more prevalent in pregnancy. Blood pressure falls during the second trimester, with expected drops of 2 to 5 mm Hg in systolic pressure and 5 to 15 mm Hg drops in diastolic pressure. By the end of the third trimester, blood pressure returns to prepregnancy norms. At its nadir in the second trimester, the mean blood pressure is about 100/60, and it returns in the third trimester to a mean of about 110/70.

## Respiratory and Gastrointestinal Changes

Because of a decrease in functional residual capacity from diaphragmatic elevation and a high oxygen requirement of the fetus and placenta, the pregnant woman has a markedly reduced oxygen reserve. Minute ventilation increases, resulting in hypocapnea. An otherwise normal PaCO$_2$ of 35 to 40 mm Hg may indicate impending respiratory failure in pregnancy. Gastrointestinal motility and gastroesophageal sphincter tone are both reduced during pregnancy. The stomach's acid production is increased. The combination of these alterations increases the likelihood of aspiration of particularly noxious material. Therefore, early gastric decompression should be considered in appropriate situations.

# MECHANISMS OF INJURY

The leading cause of blunt trauma during pregnancy is motor vehicle collisions. A major factor affecting outcome in pregnant women is proper seatbelt use. One fear of many pregnant women regarding seatbelt use is the potential for causing fetal injury. However, unbelted women are two times more likely to have premature birth within 48 hours of an accident and four times more likely to have fetal demise. Correct positioning of the seatbelt involves placing the lap belt underneath the abdomen and the shoulder belt to the side of the abdomen, between the breasts. Incorrect placement over the abdomen can cause increased force transmission through the uterus, resulting in abruptio placenta or uterine rupture. Physical abuse is a significant cause of blunt trauma during pregnancy. The abdomen is the most common target of abuse in pregnant women. Falls occur more frequently after the 20th week of pregnancy due to the protuberant abdomen, lower back strain, and fatigue. Repeated falls may

### Are we educating pregnant women enough about proper seatbelt use?

Seatbelt use reduces the incidence of fatal injury after motor vehicle collision, and this holds true in pregnancy for both the mother and fetus. There are many misconceptions about the use of seatbelts during pregnancy, which raises the question of whether we are educating pregnant women about the proper use of restraints. A large survey reported that 37% to 57% of women reported being counseled by their obstetrician or primary care provider during pregnancy. Younger, non-Hispanic, black, and less educated women were more likely to have been counseled **[Beck et al. *Am J Obstet Gynecol* 2005;192(2):580–585]**. A recent study showed that offering informational materials to prenatal care clinic patients, along with verbal education, led to an increase in the correct placement and use of seatbelts from 70% to 83%. Only 25% of women in the pre-education group received instruction on the proper use of seatbelts compared with 77% of posteducation group patients **[McGwin et al. *J Trauma* 2004;56(5): 1016–1021]**.

cause premature contractions, but immediate labor is unlikely.

In penetrating abdominal trauma, the gravid uterus alters the injury patterns. Upper abdominal penetration is more likely to injure the bowel, spleen, or liver. In the third trimester, the uterus shields abdominal organs. The uterine musculature can absorb a significant amount of energy from penetrating objects, such as a gunshot wound. Furthermore, amniotic fluid and the placenta also contribute to absorbing the impact of missiles, thereby sparing other viscera. Uterine injury is assumed with gunshot wounds below the umbilicus.

## PRIMARY SURVEY

The rule for trauma in pregnancy is that the mother comes first. Airway, breathing, and circulation are assessed in the standard fashion. It is important to keep in mind the decreased pulmonary reserve in pregnant women because of decreased lung volumes, which is exacerbated in the supine position. Therefore, any

signs of respiratory difficulty or hypoxia should be addressed with immediate endotracheal intubation, as maternal hypoxia rapidly leads to fetal hypoxia and demise. There are no contraindications to rapid sequence intubation in the pregnant patient.

In regard to assessing circulation, several factors must be kept in mind, which increase the risk of end-organ hypoperfusion. The first is compression of the inferior vena cava by the gravid uterus, which results in decreased venous return to the heart (preload) and in turn decreases cardiac output. Foremost in the assessment of circulation is to place the mother in a left lateral decubitus position. Second, the uterus requires a significant proportion of the total body oxygen demand; therefore, oxygen is taken away from overall maternal perfusion to vital organs. As stated above, this is in part compensated for by increased maternal plasma volume and RBC mass, thus providing more oxygen-carrying capacity. However, in the setting of trauma and maternal blood loss, there is little reserve. Signs of maternal shock (e.g., tachycardia, hypotension, altered mental status, decreased pulses, or poor peripheral perfusion) should be treated aggressively with crystalloid and blood replacement. Keep in mind these signs will be delayed due to physiologic hypervolemia; therefore, resuscitation should be started early. Vasopressors should be avoided because they cause vasoconstriction of uterine vessels and decreased uterine blood flow. Titrating fluid resuscitation to central venous pressure (CVP) via an internal jugular or subclavian central line can be helpful. Normal CVP during pregnancy is about 12 mm Hg.

## SECONDARY SURVEY

The unique aspect of the secondary survey for the pregnant patient is the pelvic exam; and, when possible, an obstetrician should be present. During the third trimester, this should be performed with sterile gloves. The exam should assess for vaginal discharge or blood, cervical dilation or effacement, and the presence of uterine tenderness or contractions. Clear fluid in the vagina suggests ruptured chorioamniotic membranes. Nitrazine paper can be used to confirm this with a change in color from green to deep blue. Ruptured membranes increase the risk for uterine infection and uterine cord prolapse, the latter of which will result in fetal demise. Blood-tinged amniotic fluid or frank bleeding suggests placental abruption or uterine rupture.

### Fetal Evaluation

After the primary and secondary surveys are completed and the mother has been stabilized, the focus can be turned to the fetus. The first task is to determine gestational age, which can be as simple as taking a history in the alert patient. If the patient is unconscious, gestational age can be estimated by the height of the fundus. A rule of thumb is the distance from the symphysis pubis to the fundus in centimeters is equivalent to gestational age in weeks. The importance of gestational age is to determine fetal viability, considered to be greater than 24 weeks. In general, a fundus above the umbilicus should be considered a viable pregnancy. The next step is to determine fetal heart rate, the best indicator of fetal well-being. Fetal heart rate can be determined with a handheld Doppler after 10 weeks of gestation and with a stethoscope beyond 20 weeks gestation. A normal fetal heart rate ranges from 120 to 160 bpm. If the fetus is nonviable (less than 24 weeks gestation), intermittent monitoring of fetal heart rate is appropriate. After 24 weeks gestation, continuous external monitoring should be performed and maintained throughout all diagnostic and therapeutic maneuvers. Signs of fetal distress include any decrease in heart rate. Other more subtle signs include decreased heart rate variability and fetal decelerations with uterine contractions.

### Bedside Ultrasound for FAST and Fetal Evaluation

The FAST exam is equally effective in pregnancy for evaluation of free intraperitoneal fluid in the hepatorenal and splenorenal spaces. It is important as part of the routine FAST exam in females to look for retrovesicular free fluid in the pelvis. It is not unheard of to discover a pregnancy in a young woman who is severely injured or did not otherwise know she was pregnant. Additionally, the ultrasound is a good tool for assessing fetal well-being. The heart can be directly visualized after about 12 weeks gestation, and a fetal heart rate determined. After 18 weeks gestation, spontaneous fetal movement should be visualized.

### Concerned about Radiation Exposure?

The fetus is extremely sensitive to radiation. However, the risk of exposure to 1 rad (1,000 mrads) is about a 1,000-fold smaller than the baseline risk of malformations, miscarriage, and genetic diseases. Studies have demonstrated that exposure to less than 5 to 10 rads (5,000 to 10,000 mrads) causes a small increase in the risk of childhood cancer, but it does not increase the risk of malformations or growth retardation. If indicated, radiologic studies should be performed in pregnant patients as in any other trauma patient. The risk of missed injury to the mother far outweighs the risk of radiation exposure to the fetus. Plain films often obtained for trauma evaluation have low fetal radiation exposure—with the exception of pelvic or lumbar x-rays, which impart about 0.2 rads (200 mrads). C-spine, thoracic spine, chest, and extremity x-rays each cause less than 0.001 rads (1 mrad) of exposure to the fetus. Despite the low radi-

---

**LITERATURE REFERENCE**

 ## Utility of the FAST exam for blunt abdominal trauma in pregnancy

Bedside ultrasound is becoming standard in the initial evaluation of trauma victims. Several studies have been conducted to evaluate the accuracy of the focused abdominal sonography in trauma (FAST) exam for the detection of clinically significant blunt abdominal injury in pregnant patients. Brown et al. prospectively compared 101 pregnant patients who sustained blunt abdominal trauma. The results of the FAST exam were compared with surgical findings, CT results, cystography, clinical course, and repeat ultrasound. Of the patients found to have intra-abdominal injury upon exploratory laparotomy, 80% had abnormal FAST exams. The specificity of the FAST exam was 100%, meaning that an abnormal FAST exam assured intra-abdominal injury upon exploratory laparotomy **[Brown et al. *J Ultrasound Med* 2005;24(2):175–181; quiz 183–184].**

Richards et al. conducted a retrospective review of emergency ultrasounds in pregnant trauma patients presenting to a Level I trauma center from 1995 to 2002. The goal was to determine the accuracy of ultrasonography for the detection of clinically significant blunt abdominal injury and to compare differences in accuracy between pregnant and nonpregnant patients. For pregnant women, the sensitivity of ultrasonography was 61%, compared with 71% in nonpregnant patients. The specificity was 94% and accuracy 92% in pregnant patients. This shows that the FAST exam is positive in only 61% of pregnant trauma patients with intra-abdominal injury; therefore, further workup is required if the suspicion for injury is high **[Richards et al. *Radiology* 2004;233(2): 263–270].**

**TABLE 18-2 Estimated radiation dose to the fetus with various imaging modalities**

| Type of Exam | Dose (mrad) |
|---|---|
| C-spine x-ray | <1 |
| Thoracic spine x-ray | <1 |
| CXR | <1 |
| Extremity x-rays | <1 |
| Lumbar spine x-ray | >200 |
| Pelvic x-ray | >190 |
| Hip x-ray | >125 |
| KUB | >200 |
| Head CT | <50 |
| Chest CT | <1,000 |
| Upper abdominal CT | <3,000 |
| Lower abdominal CT | 3,000–9,000 |

ation exposure, efforts should be made to shield the uterus with lead when possible. See Table 18-2 for a summary of fetal exposure to various radiographic studies.

CT is becoming an oft-used diagnostic tool in trauma. It has largely taken the place of observation and serial abdominal exams in the setting of blunt abdominal trauma. The indications for CT should be the same in the pregnant patient, but consideration should be given to fetal radiation exposure for abdominal and pelvic CT. Head and c-spine CTs impart less than 0.05 rads (50 mrads) to the fetus with proper shielding; CT of the chest can impart up to 1 rad (1,000 mrads). CT of the abdomen and pelvis can impart between 3 and 9 rads (3,000 and 9,000 mrads) to the fetus, which is not insignificant. CT scan of the abdomen and pelvis should not be withheld if the suspicion for significant injury is high; although observation and fetal monitoring should be used more liberally in patients with a lower mechanism of injury, benign abdominal exam, and normal vital signs.

## MANAGEMENT

### Stable Mother

In general, specific management of trauma in pregnancy depends on the stability of the mother and fetus. The algorithm for trauma in pregnancy, assuming a fetus greater than 24 to 26 weeks gestation, first considers maternal stability (see the algorithm at the end of this chapter). Once maternal stability is established by the primary survey, then the focus turns to the fetus (e.g., Doppler FHTs, or bedside ultrasound) and the continued trauma workup for the mother (e.g., FAST exam, trauma series, or CT scans). If fetal heart tones are absent or the heart is not beating on ultrasound, then full attention is turned to the mother's trauma workup. In this scenario, there is no utility to performing a c-section in order to evacuate the fetus. Most fetal demises will pass spontaneously within a week. However, a c-section may be required if there is evidence of placental or uterine rupture with significant intraperitoneal or vaginal bleeding.

In the case where the mother is stable but there is evidence of fetal distress (fetal heart rate < 120 bpm), then an emergency c-section is indicated. This should be performed by an obstetrician in the OR. Infant survival rate is about 75% for an emergency c-section if a fetal heart rate is detectable. For the simplest case where both mother and fetus are stable, fetal monitoring is recommended for at least 4 hours even for minor trauma. In the absence of other maternal injuries, admission is recommended for extended fetal monitoring if there is any evidence of placental or uterine injury, fetal distress, or preterm labor during that first 4 hours (e.g., uterine tenderness, vaginal blood, transient abnormality in fetal monitor strip, ruptured membranes, or greater than 3 contractions per hour).

### Unstable Mother

If the mother is unstable during the primary survey, then the initial focus is on stabilization done in the standard fashion for trauma (e.g., intubation, chest tubes, large-bore IVs, crystalloid bolus, type O blood transfusion, FAST exam, trauma series, and wrapping pelvis). If the mother is stabilized, then attention can be focused on the fetus as discussed above. If an indication for operative care is found (e.g., massive hemothorax, intra-abdominal blood, or peritonitis) during the primary survey, then the patient should go directly to the OR. In this case, after the initial lifesaving operation is performed, a c-section can then be considered if there are fetal heart tones present and the mother is deemed fit to tolerate the additional procedure, anticipating an extra 1,000 cc blood loss from the c-section.

If there is no clear indication for operative management but the mother remains unstable, then the presence of fetal heart tones should prompt consideration for emergency c-section in the OR. In these cases, however, the priority should remain saving the mother's life, even at the expense of fetal demise if necessary. The reasoning for this is that in the face of maternal shock, the infant is likely to do poorly anyway, and the odds of salvaging the mother are potentially greater. Alternatively, emergency c-section may actually help the mother in some cases where shock is because of placental abruption or uterine rupture. If fetal heart tones are absent, then there is no specific indication for emergency c-section unless placental abruption or uterine rupture is the etiology of maternal instability.

## Perimortem Cesarean Section

If the mother is severely injured and death is certain (e.g., gunshot wound to the head), then fetal viability should be rapidly assessed. Perimortem emergency c-sections are rarely indicated but can sometimes spare one life where otherwise both mother and baby would die. If the fundus is below the umbilicus or fetal heart activity is absent, either by Doppler or bedside ultrasound, then perimortem cesarean section is not indicated. The most critical factor in determining fetal outcome is the time elapsed since the mother's demise. C-sections performed within 5 minutes of maternal death can result in up to a 70% fetal survival rate, provided that maternal circulatory collapse was rapid (no prolonged shock) and no traumatic injury has occurred to the fetus. As stated above, in some instances, delivery of the fetus will increase maternal blood return to the heart and facilitate maternal resuscitation.

## SPECIFIC INJURIES

### Fetomaternal Hemorrhage and the Betke-Kleihauer Test

Introduction of fetal blood into the maternal circulation via transplacental bleeding is a potential complication of abdominal trauma during pregnancy. Though this can occur as early as 4 weeks gestation, it is more likely after 12 weeks as the uterus emerges from the pelvis, making it more susceptible to injury. Fetomaternal hemorrhage is more commonly associated with motor vehicle collisions, anteriorly located placentas, and uterine tenderness on exam. The Betke-Kleihauer test detects fetal cells in maternal blood. The ratio of fetal cells to maternal cells can be extrapolated to determine the volume of fetal blood introduced into maternal circulation. All Rh-negative mothers with abdominal trauma should receive Rho (D) immune globulin (RhIG) 300 µg IM. This will prevent the mother from developing antibodies to the fetal Rh factor, if the fetus is Rh-positive, which can result in fetal demise in a future Rh-positive fetus. The Betke-Kleihauer test can detect fetomaternal hemorrhage of 5 ml or more, but Rh-negative women can be sensitized by less than 5 ml of fetal blood. The main use of the Betke-

**LITERATURE REFERENCE**

## Can the Betke-Kleihauer test predict increased risk for preterm labor?

Fetal heart monitoring and bedside ultrasound are used in the acute trauma setting to determine fetal well-being and the need for emergency c-section. However, it is difficult to predict which mothers are at higher risk for preterm labor after the acute trauma resuscitation. The Betke-Kleihauer test has been postulated as a predictor of preterm labor. Meunch et al. studied pregnant trauma patients who underwent the Betke-Kleihauer test over a 6-year period. All patients were assigned a trauma score based on injury severity, underwent fetal heart monitoring, were assessed for uterine contractions, and were followed for preterm labor and serious perinatal complications. Of 46 women who were Betke-Kleihauer positive (defined as great than 0.01 mL of fetal blood in the maternal circulation), 95% had documented contractions, and 45% had preterm labor. Of the 25 women with a negative Betke-Kleihauer test, none had uterine contractions or preterm labor. Of note, the trauma scoring systems did not predict preterm labor. These data suggest that a negative Betke-Kleihauer test is reliable to exclude preterm labor; however, it is still standard to use fetal monitoring to observe patients who have sustained significant trauma **[Meunch et al.** *J Trauma* **2004;57(5):1094–1098].**

Kleihauer test is in determining which women require more than the standard RhIG dose of 300 µg, although it has recently been suggested that the test can be useful for predicting preterm labor after traumatic injury.

### Placental Abruption

Abruptio placentae, a condition that may occur even after relatively minor trauma, is the leading cause of fetal death after blunt trauma. Signs and symptoms include vaginal bleeding, abdominal pain and tenderness, amniotic fluid leakage, uterine rigidity, and maternal shock. Up to one-third of abruptions do not produce vaginal bleeding. The most sensitive sign of placental abruption is fetal distress, thus emphasizing the importance of fetal monitoring. Ultrasonography is not accurate in diagnosing abruption, especially if blood is exiting through the os or the placenta is implanted posteriorly. There is a close correlation between uterine activity and placental abruption, with a frequency greater than four contractions per hour as an indication for prolonged observation. Intervention is based on fetal well-being. Emergency c-section is indicated for fetal bradycardia in the stable mother. It is also important to keep in mind that the gravid uterus can contain up to 2 L of blood and cause hypovolemic shock in the mother.

## CONCLUSION

It is important to reiterate that stabilization and treatment of the mother takes priority over the well-being of the fetus because maternal instability uniformly leads to fetal demise. Minor trauma to the mother does not definitively exclude the fetus from serious injury, and fetal monitoring looking for signs of uterine injury, placental abruption, or fetal distress for at least 4 hours is mandatory. Once the mother is stable, attention can be focused on the fetus, assessing gestational age and fetal heart tones. If the mother is stable, emergency c-section should be considered in the setting of fetal distress, provided a gestation greater than 24 weeks and a mother who can tolerate the procedure. Alternatively, if the mother is unstable in the setting of fetal distress or demise, continued resuscitation and treatment should focus on the mother. In this case, emergency c-section may be indicated if placental abruption or uterine rupture is the etiology of maternal instability. A perimortem c-section should be done with an unsalvageable mother and a viable fetus (fundal height above umbilicus) with fetal heart tones.

## KEY POINTS

- There are important physiologic changes during pregnancy
  - Increased plasma volume and relative anemia
  - Increased heart rate, decreased blood pressure, and increased cardiac output
  - Decreased GI motility and GE sphincter tone
- Seatbelt use is clearly beneficial to mother and fetus
- Guiding principle is that maternal resuscitation takes first priority
  - Left lateral decubitus positioning of mother is part of ABCs
  - Adequate airway management important to provide blood oxygen for fetus
  - Aggressively manage signs of early shock with crystalloid and blood administration
  - Inadequate maternal resuscitation will lead to fetal demise

- Secondary survey includes pelvic exam
  - Look for blood, fluid, cervical dilation or effacement, and uterine tenderness
- Fetal evaluation comes after stabilization of mother
  - Determine gestational age either based on history or fundal height
  - Viable is generally considered 24 weeks or older
  - Doppler to determine fetal heart rate; normal is 120 to 160 bpm
  - FAST exam should include assessment of fetal heart motion
- Radiation exposure should not be major concern
- In stable mother, emergency c-section indicated for fetal distress (FHT <120 bpm)
  - No c-section indicated if no fetal heart movement (fetal demise)
- If mother unstable and operative cause found, go to OR to treat mother (e.g., ex-lap)
  - After initial procedure, c-section can be considered if mother stable
- If mother unstable and no obvious source, aggressively resuscitate and consider c-section
  - Especially if signs of placental abruption or uterine rupture
- Perimortem c-section should be performed if maternal death is certain
  - FHT must be detectable, otherwise futile
  - Must be completed within 5 minutes of maternal death for any chance of good outcome

## TRAUMA IN THE PREGNANT PATIENT
### (for gestational age >24 weeks)

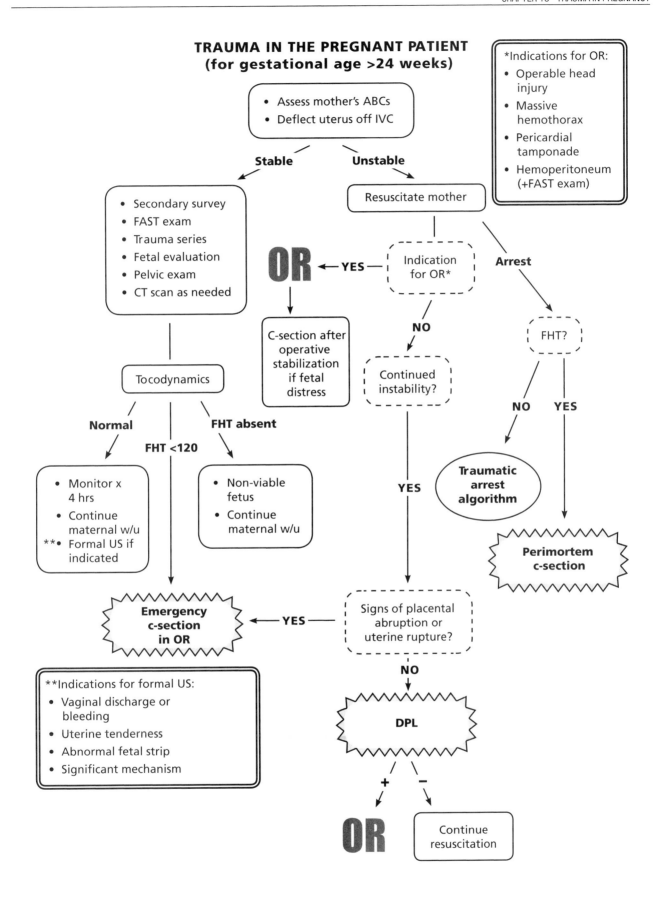

**\*Indications for OR:**
- Operable head injury
- Massive hemothorax
- Pericardial tamponade
- Hemoperitoneum (+FAST exam)

- Assess mother's ABCs
- Deflect uterus off IVC

**Stable**

- Secondary survey
- FAST exam
- Trauma series
- Fetal evaluation
- Pelvic exam
- CT scan as needed

**Unstable**

Resuscitate mother

**OR**   ← **YES** ← Indication for OR*

**Arrest**

**NO**

C-section after operative stabilization if fetal distress

Continued instability?

FHT?

**NO**   **YES**

Tocodynamics

**Normal**   **FHT <120**   **FHT absent**

**YES**

**Traumatic arrest algorithm**

- Monitor x 4 hrs
- Continue maternal w/u
\*\*• Formal US if indicated

- Non-viable fetus
- Continue maternal w/u

**Perimortem c-section**

**Emergency c-section in OR**   ← **YES** ← Signs of placental abruption or uterine rupture?

**\*\*Indications for formal US:**
- Vaginal discharge or bleeding
- Uterine tenderness
- Abnormal fetal strip
- Significant mechanism

**NO**

**DPL**

**+**   **−**

**OR**   Continue resuscitation

# CHAPTER 19

# Pediatric Trauma

## CASE SCENARIO

A 2-year-old male weighing approximately 13 kg is brought into the ED after a motor vehicle crash. The child was a rear seat passenger restrained in a car seat. The car was T-boned by a small truck, which impacted the side on which he was sitting. He is brought in on a pedi-backboard with a c-collar in place. His last set of vital signs recorded by EMS were a pulse of 168, blood pressure 100/68, respiratory rate of 24, and oxygen saturation 100% on a nonrebreather mask. He has a 22-gauge IV in his right arm.

1. What is the first priority in assessment?
   **a.** Check pupils for reactivity
   **b.** Order a STAT head CT to check for intracranial injury
   **c.** Check for a patent airway and the presence of breath sounds
   **d.** Repeat his vital signs

As in adult patients, pediatric trauma evaluation starts with the ABCs while the IV–$O_2$–monitor is attended to. On primary survey, he is crying but is alert and responds to your voice. His airway is intact, anterior neck unremarkable, and breath sounds equal bilaterally. He is well-perfused with a bounding femoral pulse, and he moves all four extremities. On secondary survey, he has a 4 cm boggy hematoma over his left parietotemporal area. His pupils are equal and reactive, and there is no evidence of facial trauma. His chest is nontender without ecchymoses. He cries out when you press on the left side of his abdomen. He has ecchymosis on his left flank. His pelvis is stable, and his extremities are nontender with good peripheral pulses. A FAST exam shows no obvious intraperitoneal blood. The nurse asks you if you want to start IV fluids.

2. What is your answer?
   **a.** No fluids for now as his blood pressure is normal for his age
   **b.** $D_5$ 1/2 normal saline infusion at 5 cc/kg/hr
   **c.** Normal saline bolus of 20 cc per kg
   **d.** PRBC transfusion 10 cc per kg

The most appropriate initial fluid in this situation is a NS bolus given the child's tachycardia. Blood pressure will be maintained in the setting of significant hypovolemic shock and should not be used to gauge the need for fluids in a tachycardic pediatric trauma. While the child may need red blood cells as well, the response to a rapid crystalloid bolus should be assessed.

After the bolus, repeat vitals signs are a pulse of 170, blood pressure 94/68, respiratory rate of 28, and oxygen saturation of 100%. The trauma series shows no obvious c-spine fracture, normal chest and mediastinum, and a normal pelvis. His mother is in the room and is having difficulty consoling him.

3. What other radiologic tests do you want to order?
   **a.** Formal ultrasound and skull films
   **b.** Abdominal CT given the left-sided tenderness
   **c.** Head CT, c-spine CT, and abdominal CT
   **d.** No further imaging at this point

Advanced imaging is indicated in this child because of the significant mechanism and possible significant head and torso injuries. Given the boggy parietal hematoma, he needs a head CT to rule out skull fracture or intracranial injury. Skull films may be helpful in minor head injury, but CT is required given the high probability for significant injury. Splenic and renal injuries are a concern given his left-sided abdominal tenderness and flank ecchymosis. While ultrasound can be done to evaluate for these, the sensitivity of CT scan is much greater, in addition to the advantage of detecting other injuries such as occult pelvic fractures or a retroperitoneal hematoma. A c-spine CT is also required given the mechanism.

The imaging tests show a subdural hematoma without midline shift or herniation, a normal c-spine, and a Grade I splenic laceration without intraperitoneal free blood. After a second 20 cc per kg bolus of NS, his vital signs now are now a pulse of 160, blood pressure 96/64, respiratory rate of 12, and oxygen saturation 98% on a nonrebreather mask. He is more lethargic and less responsive. You decide the child needs to be intubated.

**4.** What medications should you give to facilitate this?
   **a.** Etomidate 0.3 mg/kg and succinylcholine 2 mg/kg
   **b.** Atropine 0.02 mg/kg, ketamine 1 mg/kg, and succinylcholine 2 mg/kg
   **c.** Atropine 0.02 mg/kg, etomidate 0.3 mg/kg, and succinylcholine 2 mg/kg
   **d.** Midazolam 0.3 mg/kg and rocuronium 1 mg/kg

Clearly you are making the right call intubating this child, who now has an inadequate respiratory effort (RR is too low for age and situation) and who has decreasing mental status, but you must know the right drugs to use. While either rocuronium or succinylcholine are acceptable paralytics, given that he is less then 10 years old, he has a high risk for reflex bradycardia with airway manipulation. Therefore, you must pretreat him with atropine, even though he is currently tachycardic. In this situation, either etomidate or midazolam are acceptable induction agents (although etomidate might be a better choice since it is far less likely to cause hypotension). Ketamine would be unacceptable given the child's intracranial injury, since it has been shown to increase ICP.

Answers: 1-c; 2-c; 3-c; 4-c

## BACKGROUND

Injury is one of the leading causes of death among children from infancy to adolescence, with motor vehicle crashes accounting for approximately 50% of accident-related mortality. While many basic principles of adult trauma management (e.g., the ABCs, IV–O$_2$–monitor) can be applied to the pediatric patient, there are other aspects of approach and management that must be tailored specifically to the care of a child. In particular, it is important to remember that the child's body is pliable and thus can absorb a large amount of kinetic energy without showing obvious external signs of trauma. The size of the patient and the stage of development (infancy, childhood, or early adolescence/prepubertal) are the two major factors driving the need to alter the approach to the pediatric trauma patient. This chapter will highlight the main differences in the approach to the pediatric trauma patient, as well as review some injuries and injury patterns unique to childhood.

## PRIMARY SURVEY

The primary survey is essentially the same as in an adult, with the caveat that the astute clinician will rec-ognize that the awake child will have special psychological needs that must be met early on in order to make the resuscitation run smoothly. Most younger children will be scared and confused by the many new faces and experiences in the trauma bay. Thus, the physician should work to console the child and explain in simple terms what the team will be doing. Below, the crucial points of the ABCs as applied to children are highlighted.

### Airway and Breathing

Older children and adolescents can be managed essentially with the same airway techniques used in adults; however, there are importance differences in the approach to younger children and infants. The first major difference is in the location of the glottic opening, which is highest (C1 level) in infancy and gradually "descends" to its adult position at the C4–C5 level. Additionally, the angle between the epiglottis and the opening of the trachea is much more acute, increasing the difficulty of visualizing the airway adequately and making blind nasotracheal intubation all but impossible. Furthermore, the child's airway is prone to obstruction by the relatively large tongue, thus proper

> **BOX 19-1 Pediatric airway considerations**
>
> *Intubation:*
> - ETT size: 4 + (age in years/4)
> - ETT depth: 3 × ETT size
> - Uncuffed ETT should be used if the child is less than 8 years old
>
> *Surgical airway in the rare occation of failure to intubate and failure to ventilate:*
> - Needle cricothyrotomy (temporizing measure) if younger then 10 years
> - Surgical cricothyrotomy if older than 10 years

bag technique and oral airways are crucial in pediatric airway management. Finally, the adenoids and tonsils are more likely to bleed in the child than in the adult, obscuring visualization of the airway. To further complicate airway management, the child's rate of oxygen consumption is far greater and the functional residual capacity much smaller than the adult, leading to more rapid desaturation after apnea is induced. The time to desaturation is slightly greater than 4 minutes even with maximum oxygenation. Despite these concerns, rapid sequence intubation is generally the method of choice for pediatric trauma patients. It is important to remember that, in children younger than 10 years, bradycardia is common with airway manipulation and especially with administration of succinylcholine. Therefore, 0.02 mg/kg of atropine is administered as a pretreatment medication prior to rapid sequence intubation. See Box 19-1 for other considerations for airway management in children.

### Circulation

Circulation is assessed in the small child largely based on appearance, vital signs, and central pulses (e.g., carotid and femoral). Hypovolemic shock can be insidious in the child as he or she will compensate until the end, at which point he or she can die rapidly. It is therefore important to assess adequate circulation early. Hypotension is an ominous sign and carries a mortality of at least 25%. Peripheral IV access may be difficult to obtain in a small child, especially if hypovolemic. If peripheral access is unsuccessful, intraosseous (IO) access should be attempted in children younger than 10 years of age. The preferred site for IO access is just inferior to the tibial tuberosity, except in cases where a tibial fracture is suspected, in which case the distal femur or uninjured leg should be used. If an IO line is contraindicated, a femoral venous catheter is the next best option for access in young children. Of note, infants often have large forehead veins that usually allow easy access. For the purposes of

trauma, the blood volume of a child can be estimated at 80 mL/kg. When a child presents in shock, the standard initial crystalloid bolus should be 20 mL/kg, which can be repeated up to three times if the patient remains hypotensive. However, once the second bolus is being given, it is important to prepare PRBCs for transfusion. Blood is administered in 10 mL/kg boluses. The use of these guidelines obviously requires a determination of the child's weight. This is best accomplished with the Broselow Pediatric Resuscitation Measuring Tape, which estimates the child's weight based on height and also provides drug doses and other useful information.

### Deformity

Assessing neurologic status in the child presents some unique challenges. The approach must be modified based on the patient's age. Table 19-1 contains a version of the modified Glascow Coma Scale (GCS) for used in infants. For older children and adolescents, the adult GCS scale can be used. For younger children, it may be necessary to estimate the score based on a combination of the standard score and the infant scale.

### Exposure

The ratio of body surface area to body mass is greatest in the neonatal period and decreases as a child ages. This means rapid heat loss for infants and young children if they are left exposed. In order to prevent

**Table 19-1 Pediatric Glascow Coma Scale**

| Category | Response | Score |
|---|---|---|
| Eye opening | Spontaeous | 4 |
| | To voice | 3 |
| | To Pain | 2 |
| | None | 1 |
| Verbal response | Coos, babbles | 5 |
| | Irritable cry, consolable | 4 |
| | Cries to pain | 3 |
| | Moans to pain | 2 |
| | None | 1 |
| Motor response | Normal movements | 6 |
| | Withdraws to touch | 5 |
| | Withdraws to pain | 4 |
| | Flexion posturing | 3 |
| | Extension posturing | 2 |
| | Flaccid | 1 |

complications of hypothermia (e.g., prolonged coagulation times, CNS depression, refractory shock, or increased oxygen consumption), it important to prevent excessive heat loss. This can be accomplished by using warmed IV fluids, minimizing exposure time, completely removing wet clothing, warming the room with heat lamps, and covering the patient with warmed blankets.

### Foley

More seriously injured children may require strict calculations of their urine output and thus require placement of a Foley catheter. Normal urine output decreases with age from 2 mL/kg/hr in infancy to 1 mL/kg/hr in older children and adolescents. For comparison, normal adult urine output is 0.5 mL/kg/hr. These guidelines will need to be altered in special circumstances, such as burns and rhabdomyolysis to favor more brisk urine output.

## SECONDARY SURVEY AND BEYOND

### Physical Exam

In the pediatric trauma patient, as in the adult, the secondary survey is a head-to-toe examination aimed at identifying remaining injuries not discovered in the primary survey. As in the adult, it is important to frequently reassess vital signs and return to the ABCs if the patient's condition changes. There is also data to indicate that a tertiary survey is helpful to diagnose injuries (generally musculoskeletal) missed in the primary and secondary surveys. This can either be done after the patient returns from radiologic studies or before the patient is admitted or discharged.

### Laboratory Studies

Reliance on ancillary studies is notoriously determined by institutional policy, which is unfortunately often based more on tradition than science. In general, "screening labs" (e.g., liver function tests, general chemistries, amylase, lipase, toxicology screen, or cardiac enzymes) sent from the ED are of no value. The sensitivity and specificity of these tests are too low to be helpful in reliably identifying or excluding injuries. In the setting of significant injury, where the patient may need an operation, it is reasonable to send a CBC, basic chemistries, coagulation studies, urinalysis, and a blood bank specimen. Base deficit is defined as the amount of base needed to titrate a liter of fully saturated arterial blood at 37°C to a pH of 7.40. This test has been shown to correlate with mortality, with a base

deficit of −11 mEq/L corresponding to a mortality of 25%. Base deficit can be useful to monitor the effectiveness of resuscitation in the critically ill child.

### Imaging Studies

As with adults, the ATLS guidelines recommend a trauma series (c-spine, chest, and pelvic plain films) in pediatric trauma patients. In practice, these may or may not be useful, depending on the clinical scenario. For hemodynamically unstable children, a portable chest and pelvic x-ray can be helpful to identify a source of hypotension. If the suspicion is high, a lateral c-spine x-ray can be helpful in identifying significant fractures before the child is manipulated any further or transported to radiology. In the stable child who requires a CT scan based on physical exam (e.g., abdominal tenderness or head contusion), parts of the trauma series can be bypassed. The focused abdominal ultrasound in trauma (FAST) exam is also an important aspect of the initial workup of pediatric trauma.

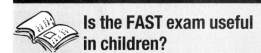

**LITERATURE REFERENCE**

## Is the FAST exam useful in children?

Theoretically, the focused abdominal ultrasound in trauma (FAST) exam should be useful in pediatric trauma patients. Several studies have been done to determine whether this is true. Soudack et al. studied 393 pediatric trauma patients and found that the FAST exam missed no injuries requiring surgical intervention. Additionally, it was used as the primary radiologic screening test in 60% of patients who did not undergo CT scanning. None of the children who only received a FAST exam required delayed surgical intervention **[Soudack et al.** *J Clin Ultrasound* **2004;32(3):53–61].** Suthers et al. demonstrated that the FAST exam, when used in conjunction with physical exam, had a much lower false-positive rate than when used alone **[Suthers et al.** *Am Surg* **2004;70(2):164–167; discussion 167–168].** When using the FAST exam in children, remember that solid organ injuries are less likely to lead to hemoperitoneum than are similar injuries in adults. While these injuries are often handled nonoperatively, they may have importance in determining need to refrain from certain activities until healing is complete.

## INJURIES AND INJURY PATTERNS PARTICULAR TO CHILDHOOD

### Head Trauma

Head trauma is common in the pediatric population and accounts for a significant percentage of the mortality in pediatric trauma. There are three fundamental anatomical concepts to remember regarding pediatric head trauma. First, the ratio of head size to body size is greater in the child than in the adult. Thus, the brain is subject to higher forces during rapid deceleration or falls. Second, the sutures and fontanels are open in younger children. While this does permit more cerebral swelling or bleeding within the cranial vault, the child is subject to precipitous decompensation once the room for expansion is filled. Furthermore, hypotension in an infant can be caused solely by blood loss into the epidural or subgaleal space. Lastly, the pediatric brain is not as well myelinated as the adult brain and thus is more subject to shear injury.

A frequent question in pediatric head trauma is whether or not the child needs head imaging; and, if so, whether a CT scan or skull films should be performed. The answer to this depends on the age of the child and whether or not the head injury can be classified as minor (Box 19-2). Severe head injury is treated as in the adult. Patients who have a GCS of 8 or less should be intubated for airway protection and proper ventilation. A quick neurologic exam should be attempted before intubation to get a baseline level of function. Similar to adult head injury, the bed should be inclined so that the body is at a 30 degree angle with the head up. In conjunction with neurosurgical consultation, mannitol, hypertonic saline, mild hyperventilation ($PaCO_2 = 35$), and barbiturate coma are all treatments to consider. There is also some data that children given prophylactic anticonvulsants, most commonly phenytoin or phenobarbital, have both decreased incidence of seizures and improved mortality.

---

**BOX 19-2  Definition of minor head injury in children older than 2 years**

No history of bleeding diathesis or neurologic problems

Normal mental status on presentation (GCS 15)

Normal neurologic exam

No palpable skull depression

Absence of Battle's sign, raccoon eyes, hemotympanum, and CSF rhinorrhea

No evidence of other major trauma

No concern for abuse or neglect

These children *may* give a history of brief (<1 minute) loss of consciousness, a brief seizure immediately after the incident with rapid return to normal mental status (impact seizure), and temporary lethargy or vomiting after the injury.

---

### Spinal Cord Injury

Small children have heads that are larger when compared to the size of the rest of their bodies. Therefore, greater forces are imparted on the c-spine during rapid deceleration injuries. At the same time, the bones and connecting ligaments of the c-spine are not as well developed as they are in the older child or adult, giving it greater flexibility and resulting in a lower incidence of cervical fracture or ligament disruption. If a fracture does occur, greater than 70% occur at C3 or above. However, up to 50% of spinal cord injuries associated with neurologic deficits have no accompanying radiographic abnormalities and are referred to as spinal cord injury without radiographic abnormality (SCIWORA). This emphasizes the importance of a thorough neurologic exam in pediatric trauma and that a normal radiograph should not necessarily be reassuring. Of note, children can have subluxation apparent on x-ray that is normal, referred to as physiologic pseudosubluxation. This is most common at the level of C2 and C3. Radiographs and cervical injury patterns approach that of adults after the age of 10 years.

### Chest Trauma

Since the child's chest wall is so pliable, significant pulmonary contusions can occur in the absence of rib or sternal fractures. Thus, information such as mechanism of injury, respiratory rate, oxygen saturation, and CXR will help determine the initial management of pediatric patients with chest trauma. Smaller chest tubes are used in children, their length estimated by the distance between the lateral chest wall and superior, aspect of the hemithorax. Although cardiogenic shock secondary to cardiac contusion is much less common in children than in adults, it must be considered in the presence of chest trauma and circulatory shock.

### Pediatric Abdominal Trauma

Since the child's abdominal wall generally contains less muscle and adipose than that of the adult, there is an increased likelihood of significant injury in penetrating trauma and of solid organ laceration and hollow organ perforation with blunt abdominal trauma. Furthermore, diagnosis of perforation is commonly delayed because these children may not present with obvious free air or peritonitis. The absence of free air can be attributed to the lack of air in the small bowel, which perforates more commonly than the stomach. There are several specific abdominal injuries and injury patterns to consider (Box 19-3). As in adults, nonoperative management of splenic and liver lacerations is the standard of care in children, given hemodynamic stability. Transfusion requirements of

---

**BOX 19-3  Handlebars and seatbelts**

A classic pediatric abdominal injury is the bicycle "handlebar injury." This injury pattern, while initially appearing innocuous, can result in serious injury. It results from a child falling forward on a bike and the end of the handlebar being driven into the epigastrium. More common injuries as a result of this mechanism are duodenal hematoma, pancreatic contusion or laceration, and splenic laceration. These should be considered given the right mechanism, abdominal tenderness, epigastric ecchymosis, or vomiting. In motor vehicle crashes the lap belt, especially when used without a shoulder harness, may cause a hyperflexion injury. This may result in a Chance fracture of the thoracolumbar spine, or bowel hematoma or rupture. This emphasizes the importance of a thorough back exam in the setting of abdominal tenderness.

---

40 mL/kg (about 50% of blood volume) to maintain stability is an indication for operative repair.

## Musculoskeletal Trauma

The musculoskeletal system of children is more pliable because of open growth plates, relative plasticity of children's bones, and loose ligamentous connections. As a result, there are a number of fractures and fracture patterns unique to childhood, such as greenstick and torus fractures. Joint dislocations and sprains are unusual before the closure of associated growth plates. Several fractures specific to children are highlighted. See Box 19-4 for the Salter-Harris classification for physeal injuries, significant for fractures in the vicinity of open growth plates. This classification is significant in predicting long-term prognosis and outcome, with subsequent growth disturbance much more likely in type IV and type V epiphyseal fractures.

---

**BOX 19-4  Salter-Harris Classification of Physeal Injuries (SALTR)**

**I  S**lipped—Epiphyseal separation, injury isolated to growth plate, and x-ray may look normal
**II  A**bove—Fracture of metaphyseal bone above and into growth plate
**III  L**ow—Fracture of epiphyseal bone below and into growth plate
**IV  T**hrough—Fracture extends across the epiphysis, growth plate, and metaphysis
**V  R**uined—Growth plate crushed with vascular disruption, loss of epiphyseal space on x-ray

---

## Supracondylar Fractures

Supracondylar fractures generally occur in children between 3 and 10 years of age who fall on an outstretched arm, a result of hyperextension at the elbow because of immature ligamentous integrity at the joint. This fracture is at risk for compartment syndrome and injury to the median nerve and brachial artery that course anterior to the distal humerus. In cases of minimal displacement with intact neurovascular structure, the child can be placed in a long arm posterior splint with the elbow at 90 degrees. Displaced fractures, or those with associated neurologic deficits, require orthopedic intervention to prevent long-term disability.

## Radial Head Subluxation (Nursemaid's Elbow)

This is the most common pediatric orthopedic injury and occurs in children from a few months to 5 years of age. It occurs when there is axial traction applied to an extended and pronated arm, usually when a parent lifts the child off the ground by the wrist. This causes the annular ligament to partially detach from the radial head and become trapped in the radiohumeral groove. After the injury, the child refuses to use the arm, and it is held in pronation and slight flexion. This subluxation can be reduced by placing pressure over the radial head with a thumb while supinating and flexing the arm simultaneously.

## Toddler's Fracture

This oblique, nondisplaced fracture of the distal tibia commonly occurs in children 9 to 36 months of age and often presents as a new limp. The injury is the result of torsional forces, typically from a fall from trivial height or while running or walking. In general, spiral fractures should raise the suspicion of child abuse, which would be more of a concern with a midshaft tibial fracture in this age group or a Toddler's fracture in a child who is not yet ambulatory (younger than 9 months of age).

## KEY POINTS

- There are crucial anatomic differences in the airway of infants and small children
  - Anterior location of glottis making laryngoscopy potentially challenging
  - Large tongue that can cause airway obstruction when trying to bag ventilate
  - Narrow subglottic trachea
  - Use only uncuffed ETT in children younger than 8 years

- – Cricothyrotomy impossible in children younger than 10 years
  – Atropine is required as pretreatment in RSI because a child less than 10 years old has a high risk of reflex bradycardia with airway manipulation
- Hypotension is a late sign of circulatory shock in children and is ominous
- Volume resuscitation starts with NS 20 cc per kg bolus that can be repeated several times
  – If persistent shock, administer PRBCs 10 cc/kg
- Beware of inducing hypothermia in small child
- Trauma series useful in some situations as in adult, especially in setting of instability
- FAST exam shown to be useful in conjunction with physical exam
- CT scan indicated if patient is stable and there is potential for serious injury

# Case Scenarios

## CASE SCENARIO #1

You are told that a 32-year old male is being brought to your ED from a local nightclub where he was stabbed in the left chest. On arrival to the scene, the paramedics found the patient to be anxious and slightly combative. His vital signs were a heart rate of 122 bpm, blood pressure 101/56, and oxygen saturation 99% on high-flow oxygen via a nonrebreather facemask. The EMTs call en route and inform you they have placed a 16-gauge IV and are preparing to intubate. You are preparing the resuscitation bay when the paramedics call back. The patient is now unresponsive, and they are having difficulty intubating him because of his large body habitus. The patient is now pulseless, and CPR is initiated in the ambulance.

1. Which is the most important to this patient's survival?
   a. Successful intubation and ventilation by EMS
   b. Rapid administration of normal saline by EMS
   c. Rapid transport to trauma center and continued CPR
   d. Needle decompression to relieve possible tension pneumothorax

Although resuscitation should be initiated in the field, rapid transport to a trauma center is crucial to survival. Because hypovolemia is the most common cause of traumatic arrest, establishing intravenous access and initiating crystalloid administration is important. Needle thoracotomy is also reasonable, given the possibility of tension pneumothorax. Rapid transport to the ED is of utmost importance in critical trauma. Of note, prehospital intubation has never been shown to increase survival. Although it is sometimes necessary, it should not be done at the expense of delayed transport, especially when bag-valve-mask (BVM) ventilation is possible.

On arrival to the ED the patient is unresponsive and pulseless. You notice two stab wounds to his left chest, one in the midclavicular line and the other just lateral to the sternal border.

2. What is your first action?
   a. Intubate the patient
   b. Start CPR, and obtain portable CXR
   c. Start CPR, obtain central access, and administer high-volume blood transfusion
   d. Perform an ED thoracotomy

CPR is ongoing, and it is obvious that the patient will likely need several procedures. However, the first priority is airway, and intubation should be performed immediately. This is done without difficulty. The patient remains pale and pulseless.

3. What is the next step?
   a. Place left chest tube
   b. Start blood transfusion
   c. Perform ED thoracotomy
   d. Perform FAST exam to assess for pericardial fluid

This scenario requires rapid action if the patient is to survive. Patients with penetrating chest trauma who become pulseless en route or on arrival to the ED require an ED thoracotomy. This should begin simultaneously with intubation. Bilateral needle thoracostomy should be done initially to check for a tension pneumothorax. Given the call that the patient became pulseless en route, you have a thoracotomy tray prepared with a scalpel ready to open the chest when the patient arrives.

4. Which procedure should be performed simultaneously by a second physician?
   a. Right tube thoracostomy
   b. Diagnostic peritoneal lavage
   c. Right subclavian central venous line placement
   d. Pericardiocentesis

The right side of the chest should be decompressed simultaneously in case a stab wound crossed the midline, causing right-sided pneumothorax or hemothorax. Simultaneous central venous access is also reasonable, yet a femoral line is more accessible during a thoracotomy. Trauma to the left chest should also raise concern for great vessel injury, and a subclavian should be avoided on the side of injury. A pericardiocentesis is not necessary when doing a thoracotomy. Of note, an orogastric tube should be placed to differentiate between the aorta and esophagus if aortic clamping is necessary.

You make an incision through skin and subcutaneous tissue from the sternum to past the midaxillary line at the level of the fifth interspace, or just below the left nipple. You make a deeper incision down to intercostal muscle. Being careful not to injure the lung, you then use the Metzenbaum scissors to cut the intercostal muscles so that lung is visible. You place the rib spreaders and ratchet the chest apart, exposing the heart and lung. There is some blood pooling around the lung.

5. What is the next step in the procedure?
   a. Dissect the soft tissues of the mediastinum to clamp the aorta
   b. Inspect the entire lung for lacerations, and apply direct pressure as needed
   c. Perform pericardiotomy
   d. Start internal cardiac compressions

In unstable penetrating chest trauma, there can only be a few explanations for decreased cardiac output. These include tension pneumothorax, injury to great vessel or lung causing massive hemothorax, or cardiac injury resulting in pericardial tamponade. The first two of these have essentially been ruled out, despite there being some blood in the chest cavity. The first step once the chest is open is to open the pericardial sac to relieve a potential tamponade.

You identify the phrenic nerve and make a small nick anterior to this structure. Blood squirts out of your incision, and you continue with the Metzenbaum scissors to open the pericardium. While the heart is contracting weakly, you identify a laceration in the left ventricle, place a Foley catheter in the hole, and inflate the balloon to stop the bleeding. As uncrossmatched blood is administered rapidly, the heart begins to beat more vigorously, and a carotid pulse becomes palpable. You transport the patient immediately to the OR.

Answers: 1-c; 2-a; 3-c; 4-a; 5-c

## CASE SCENARIO #2

A 7-year-old male presents approximately 3 hours after falling from his bicycle. He had been riding down a hill and lost control of the bike. Mom was inside the house at the time but saw the whole accident through a window. She states that the wheel seemed to turn to the left, and he fell forward onto the handlebars. When she got to him, he was a bit confused, and his helmet was cracked on the left side. After an hour she brought him to the ED because he became more lethargic and vomited several times. His vital signs are a pulse of 104, blood pressure 90/56, respiratory rate of 22, and oxygen saturation of 100% on room air.

His primary survey reveals a somnolent child with an intact airway, bilateral breath sounds, and strong symmetric radial pulses. A c-collar is placed. He opens his eyes to painful stimulus, moans incomprehensible words, and withdraws his extremities only to pain. Mom says this is different from how he was 5 minutes ago. The nurse places a 20-gauge IV in his left arm and places him on oxygen and a monitor.

6. What is your next move?
   a. Intubate the patient
   b. Perform the secondary survey
   c. Transfuse 10 cc of PRBCs for hypotension
   d. Send the patient for a head CT

This patient has a GCS of 8, and your suspicion is traumatic brain injury. He requires intubation to optimize oxygenation and ventilation, in addition to protecting his airway and preventing aspiration. While the nurse is retrieving intubation medications, you perform a secondary survey. He has a 2 cm hematoma over his left temporal bone, and he has no facial trauma. His anterior neck and chest appear normal. You notice a circular ecchymosis on the right side of the epigastrum, and he has epigastric guarding to palpation. His extremities are well perfused with no evidence of fracture. A FAST exam is normal.

He receives a 20 cc/kg bolus of NS, and you prepare to intubate him.

7. What is the correct tube size, type, position, and laryngoscope blade for this patient?
   a. 6-0 cuffed tube inserted to 15 cm at the lip, #1 straight blade
   b. 5-0 uncuffed tube, inserted to 15 cm at the lip, #2 curved blade
   c. 4-0 uncuffed tube inserted to 12 cm at the lip, #2 straight blade
   d. 6-0 uncuffed tube, inserted to 12 cm at the lip, #3 curved blade

The formula for determining tube size is $4 + $ (age in years/4). The formula for insertion is three times the tube size. In general, children younger than 8 years require an uncuffed tube to prevent pressure necrosis of the narrow trachea. Either a #2 straight or curved blade can be used in this age group.

8. The nurse asks you what drugs you want to administer. What is your reply?
   a. Lidocaine, pentothal, and rocuronium
   b. Lidocaine, fentanyl, ketamine, and succinylcholine
   c. Fentanyl, pentothal, and succinylcholine
   d. Lidocaine, atropine, etomidate, and succinylcholine

As in adults, there is controversy as to the effectiveness of pretreatment agents in mitigating increases in ICP with laryngoscopy. Lidocaine is likely the most beneficial of pretreatment agents, having been shown to help mitigate the sympathetic response to laryngeal stimulation. Fentanyl has also been suggested as a cerebroprotective agent, although there is conflicting data as to its effectiveness. Ketamine is an induction agent that results in a sympathetic response, increasing blood pressure and ICP. It should be avoided in head injury patients. Pentothal is an induction agent that is cerebroprotective; however, it can cause hypotension. Etomidate is an ideal sedative agent for head injury as it tends not to induce hypotension. Succinylcholine is the paralytic of choice for children.

Intubation is successful, and good color change is seen on the $CO_2$ detector; breath sounds are clear bilaterally. You rapidly obtain a lateral c-spine and CXR in the bay. His vital signs are essentially unchanged. You take the child immediately to CT, which shows a left subdural hematoma with 1 to 2 cm of midline shift. You consult neurosurgery and alert the OR. While still in radiology, you review the trauma series and notice good tube position and normal mediastinum and lungs. You also notice two large bubbles of gas within the abdomen.

9. Given this finding and the mechanism of injury, what does this likely represent?
   a. Liver laceration
   b. Gastric perforation
   c. Traumatic pancreatitis
   d. Duodenal hematoma

The "double bubble sign" with epigastric pain, nausea, and vomiting in the setting of a handlebar injury points toward a duodenal hematoma. Liver laceration and traumatic pancreatitis have been documented with handlebar injuries but do not cause a double bubble sign. Gastric perforation is also possible but quite uncommon.

The patient is brought back to the trauma bay, the head of his bed elevated to 30 degrees, and mannitol started. The nurse places a Foley catheter and a second IV line. He is taken to the OR by neurosurgery 10 minutes later. Upon review of the labs, you notice the patient has 50 to 100 RBCs per high powered field in his urine.

10. What test will he likely need after he has his subdural hematoma drained?
   a. Renal ultrasound
   b. Serial KUB
   c. Abdominal/pelvic CT scan with IV contrast
   d. Retrograde cystogram

Following decompression of his subdural hemorrhage, he should have a CT scan of the neck and abdomen. The traditional cutoff for working up microscopic hematuria in kids is 50 RBCs per hpf, and this practice is coming into question in the absence of hypotension. Given his epigastric tenderness and ecchymosis, a CT scan is obtained that confirms your diagnosis of duodenal hematoma. He is observed in the ICU and is extubated the next day. He made a good neurologic recovery.

Answers: 6-a; 7-b; 8-d; 9-d; 10-c

# CASE SCENARIO #3

A 26-year-old woman is a restrained passenger in a high-speed MVC in which the car ran off the road and rolled over several times. On EMS arrival, she is still in the car, screaming about her unborn baby because she is 8 months pregnant. Extrication takes 15 minutes. Her pulse is 126 and blood pressure 96/56. EMS places her in a c-collar and in a lateral decubitus position on a backboard. She complains of abdominal, left chest, and back pain. En route to the hospital, 2 large-bore IVs are established and normal saline started. In the ED, she looks pale but is oriented; her airway is intact; her breathing is mildly tachypneic; neck is without ecchymosis or contusions; and breath sounds are decreased on the left. She has ecchymosis of her left chest and left upper abdomen, as well as over her lower abdomen. She has a small amount of vaginal blood. Her vital signs are a pulse of 136, blood pressure 86/46, and oxygen saturation of 88% on oxygen.

11. What is the most appropriate first step in her management?
   a. Orotracheal intubation with etomidate and succinylcholine
   b. Place left-sided chest tube using lidocaine for local anesthesia
   c. Obtain fetal monitor to assess fetal heart rate
   d. Perform bedside ultrasound to assess viability of fetus

The first priority in assessing a pregnant trauma victim with a potentially viable fetus (age >24 weeks) is to stabilize the mother. This woman appears to be in shock with hypotension and evidence of a left-sided hemothorax or pneumothorax. Intubation should be a strong consideration at this point as she will likely require an operative procedure; however, she is oriented and does not appear to have immediate airway issues. B of the ABCs is to assure adequate ventilation, and part of this is relieving a hemothorax or pneumothorax. She likely has intra-abdominal or pelvic injuries as well, but these are addressed after the primary survey.

A left-sided chest tube is placed with return of air and about 300 cc of blood. The tube is attached to a suction device and reservoir. Her pulse is now 126 with a blood pressure of 96/48. The second liter of normal saline is just finishing. On secondary survey, she has tenderness and crepitus over her left lower chest wall, as well as tenderness and guarding in the LUQ of the abdomen.

She is also tender with palpation of the pelvis. There is blood at the vaginal introitus, and the cervix is palpated with a sterile glove. The cervix is dilated to one finger breadth and is not effaced. There is a good amount of blood on the glove.

**12.** What is the next priority?
   **a.** Notify the obstetrician
   **b.** Test for ruptured amniotic sac with use of nitrazine paper
   **c.** Perform a FAST exam
   **d.** Place an external fetal heart monitor to assess fetal heart rate

At this point the mother is somewhat stable, although a search for serious and operable injuries must still be carried out. Quick attention must be turned to the fetus as fetal distress would be an indication for immediate transport to the OR for a c-section. An obstetrician should be notified as early as possible, ideally before the patient even arrives in the ED. Determining whether the amniotic sac ruptured is important in the case where the fetus is stable in order to predict potential infection or prolapsed umbilical cord. At this point, determining the fetal heart rate (FHR) is the priority. A normal fetal heart rate is 120 to 160 bpm. Fetal bradycardia of less than 120 bpm is a sign of fetal hypoxia and distress and should prompt immediate action. A FAST exam is also important given her significant abdominal tenderness; but, even in the setting of free intraperitoneal blood, the patient is currently hemodynamically stable.

The fetal heart monitor is placed on the mother's abdomen, and an FHR of 130 bpm is detected. Uncrossmatched type O blood is started, and the mother's repeat blood pressure is 104/68. She appears better but still has significant abdominal pain. A FAST exam shows a small amount of fluid in the splenorenal space, and fetal movement is observed along with fetal heart activity. A Foley catheter is placed with return of pink urine.

**13.** What should be done next?
   **a.** Trauma series in the bay
   **b.** Retrograde urethrogram (RUG)
   **c.** Operative ex-lap for c-section and identification of abdominal injuries
   **d.** CT scan of the chest and abdomen with IV contrast

The extent of this woman's injuries is still unclear. She had a period of hypotension that is now resolved, but the concern for significant life-threatening injury still exists, especially given the small amount of intraperitoneal fluid seen on the FAST exam. Given the stability of the mother and fetus, the evaluation in the ED can proceed, with the next step being a trauma series to evaluate for significant injury before sending the patient to the CT scanner. The CXR will be valuable specifically to assess the mediastinum, as the potential for aortic injury still exists. A significant pelvic fracture is also possible given her pelvic tenderness and hematuria. Radiation exposure should not be a concern at this point given the age of the fetus and the need to identify life-threatening injuries.

The CXR shows the left-sided chest tube in good position with a left lower lobe opacity consistent with pulmonary contusion. The mediastinum looks normal. The pelvic x-ray shows bilateral pubic symphisis fractures with 6 mm diastasis of the pubic symphysis. At this point, the trauma surgeon and the obstetrician are fully aware of the case, and the OR has been alerted for a potential operation. As the patient is being packaged to go to CT scan, she becomes pale, sweaty, and confused. Her repeat blood pressure is 76/palp, and she has a thready carotid pulse. The fetal heart monitor is reading 105 bpm. There is a pool of blood on the bed under her pelvis.

**14.** What step should be taken next?
   **a.** Immediate c-section in the bay
   **b.** Diagnostic peritoneal lavage
   **c.** Immediate intubation and administration of PRBCs
   **d.** ED thoracotomy

If at any time during trauma workup the patient's condititon changes, the ABCs are readdressed. Starting from the top, this is a minimally responsive trauma patient in shock who needs to be intubated immediately and administered large volumes of blood. In any case, an ED c-section or thoracotomy would not be possible in an awake patient who is not intubated.

The intubation is uncomplicated, with the administration of etomidate 10 mg IV and succinylcholine 120 mg IV. Blood transfusion is continued with pressure bags assisting. Her pulse is now 134 bpm and blood pressure 86/58. The FHR is 110 bpm.

15. What is the next action?
    a. Continue immediately to CT scan and then to the OR
    b. Go directly to the OR for emergency c-section and ex-lap
    c. Perform emergency c-section in the ED with obstetrics present
    d. Perform DPL in trauma bay, and go to OR if grossly positive

This woman now has a clear indication for immediate operative intervention with repeat hypotension, profuse vaginal bleeding, and fetal distress, as well as intraperitoneal fluid on a FAST exam. An ED c-section would be considered if maternal death was assured or impending in the setting of a viable fetus. This procedure should be done in the OR whenever feasible. She is taken immediately and found to have a ruptured uterus; a baby boy is delivered and resuscitated; his Apgar score is 9 after 5 minutes. The mother was found to have about 1 L of free intraperitoneal blood, an intraperitoneal bladder rupture, and a grade III splenic laceration. Her spleen was removed and her bladder repaired. Both the mother and baby eventually had full recoveries.

Answers: 11-b; 12-d; 13-a; 14-c; 15-b

## CASE SCENARIO #4

You receive a call from EMS saying that they are 15 minutes from the hospital with a 29-year-old male who was involved in a head-on collision with a tractor-trailer truck. The patient was driving a large, modern SUV and had a lap belt and shoulder harness on. His airbags did deploy. The extrication was prolonged and took about 25 minutes. The patient was initially unconscious, but he awoke while the firemen were cutting the doors off the SUV. He has since been slightly confused, repeatedly asking what happened. He also complains of abdominal pain and is tender bilaterally in the upper quadrants. His vital signs are a pulse of 102, blood pressure 144/58, and oxygen saturation 100% on high-flow oxygen via nonrebreather facemask. He is becoming lethargic and is breathing at about 10 per minute. EMS asks to give midazolam 5 mg to facilitate intubation.

16. What is your response?
    a. Continue with high-flow oxygen by facemask, and closely monitor respiratory status
    b. Go ahead with the Versed, but give him succinylcholine 160 mg as well
    c. Go ahead with the Versed, and call back if need a second dose
    d. Go ahead with the Versed, but start first with a pretreatment dose of lidocaine 100 mg IV

While this patient will likely require intubation on arrival in the ED, he will not benefit at this point from intubation in the field, given the less-than-ideal conditions and the complications that go along with a sedation-only intubation (e.g., inadequate relaxation, gagging, vomiting, hypoxia). Given the patient is still breathing, he would benefit from high-flow oxygen to maximize tissue oxygen saturation and then intubation under more controlled conditions with the availability of RSI medications in the ED. A series of trials, the San Diego Paramedic RSI Trials, cast doubt over the safety of field intubation of head injury patients. Although it is not entirely clear why, it appears that intubating these patients in the field increases mortality and the rate of poor outcomes. It is postulated that this may be because of a period of hypoxia incurred during paralysis and attempted intubation in the absence of assistance to rapidly administer BVM ventilation when necessary. Versed alone has been shown in multiple studies to be a poor choice to facilitate intubation, and repeat dosing has not been shown to help. Lidocaine is a pretreatment agent commonly used in the setting of head injury because of its effect of blunting the sympathetic response to laryngoscopy. The indication to intubate this patient in the field would be absent or agonal respiratory effort and inability to BVM ventilate.

The medics arrive, and the patient appears somewhat more awake, although he repeatedly asks, "How'd we do today?" His vital signs are a pulse of 122, blood pressure 121/50, and oxygen saturation 100% on high-flow oxygen. He has bilateral breath sounds and palpable radial pulses. He moves all extremities purposefully to command. On secondary survey he has a large, boggy contusion on his right parietal scalp, ecchymosis over his anterior chest, and bilateral upper quadrant abdominal tenderness. He again becomes somnolent during the secondary survey and by the end is no longer consistently following commands.

17. What is your next priority?
    a. Intubate the patient using RSI techniques
    b. Take patient immediately to radiology for head CT
    c. Continue high-flow oxygen, and continue with FAST and trauma series
    d. Notify neurosurgery and OR regarding likely operative intracranial hemorrhage

Whereas in the field the conservative approach to airway management is often the right choice, in the ED a patient with likely head injury who is becoming unresponsive requires immediate intubation using RSI techniques. This will allow optimal oxygenation and ventilation to maximize oxygen delivery to the injured brain, allow for adequate sedation for CT scan, and prevent vomiting and aspiration. Alcohol is often a confounding factor in patients with head injury, as it contributes to altered mental status. Patients with potential head injury should be treated as if they were sober, never assuming a decline in consciousness is the result of intoxication.

You are preparing for intubation, and the nurse asks you what meds you want to give. His repeat vital signs are a pulse of 110, blood pressure 136/56, and oxygen saturation 99% on high-flow oxygen.

18. What is the best combination of medications for this average-sized adult?
    a. Lidocaine 100 mg IV (pretreatment), etomidate 20 mg IV, succinylcholine 120 mg IV
    b. Fentanyl 200 mg IV and etomidate 20 mg IV
    c. Lidocaine 100 mg IV (pretreatment), propofol 180 mg IV, and succinylcholine 120 mg
    d. Pentothal 250 mg IV and vecuronium 10 mg IV

There are various acceptable pharmacologic agents used for intubating head injury patients. The goals of RSI are to rapidly render the patient unconscious and fully relaxed, minimize ICP increases, and avoid hypotension and hypoxia. A suggested pretreatment regimen includes lidocaine, fentanyl, and a "defasciculating" dose of a nondepolarizing neuromuscular blocker. Fentanyl, however, must be used with caution in trauma patients because it has the effect of removing physiological sympathetic drive and can result in hypotension. Lidocaine has been shown in human studies to have a protective effect on ICP in the setting of laryngoscopy. On the other hand, the defasciculations because of succinylcholine have not been proven to significantly increase ICP; therefore, the utility of a defasciculating dose of a nondepolarizing agent (e.g., vecuronium or pancuronium) is of questionable benefit. It has been demonstrated that laryngoscopy without paralysis significantly increases ICP and should not be done unless there is concern that intubation or BVM ventilation may be difficult. Pentothal was commonly used for induction because of its cerebroprotective properties; however, its disadvantage is causing hypotension. The same is true for propofol as an induction agent. Etomidate is a commonly used induction agent today, because it is cerebroprotective and does not result in significant hypotension. Vecuronium is a nondepolarizing paralytic agent that is not ideal for RSI because it has a slow onset (2 to 3 minutes) and it renders the patient paralyzed for 30 to 40 minutes.

The patient is intubated without difficulty with good color change on the $CO_2$ detector and good breath sounds bilaterally. The nurse is preparing the patient for CT when the neurosurgeon comes into the bay. A repeat exam shows a slightly sluggish right pupil. He withdraws to pain in all extremities. You rush the patient to the CT scanner, while the neurosurgeon calls the OR to make sure the room is ready. As the patient is placed on the CT scanner, you notice that his heart rate is trending down (now about 70 bpm), and his blood pressure is 162/88. The head CT reveals a large right-sided epidural hematoma with some evidence of herniation; the neurosurgeon tells you the OR is ready. The CT tech goes to reposition the patient for the chest and abdominal CT.

19. What should you do now?
    a. Rapidly scan the c-spine, chest, and abdomen
    b. Repeat the exam to look for signs of herniation

    **c.** Take the patient directly to the OR

    **d.** Return to trauma bay, hyperventilate, and administer mannitol

This patient requires immediate decompression in the OR, and every second counts. The patient is demonstrating Cushing's reflex (hypertension and bradycardia), seen in patients with herniation and compression of the brainstem. C-spine, thorax, and abdominal injuries are of secondary importance, and the workup can be delayed until the epidural hematoma is evacuated. As a bridge to decompression, hyperventilation and mannitol may have some effect; however, there should be no delay in transferring the patient directly from CT scan to the OR.

The patient is transported to the operating room and prepared for evacuation of his cerebral clot by neurosurgery.

**20.** How are his potential abdominal injuries best assessed?

    **a.** Perform ex-lap after evacuation of epidural hematoma

    **b.** Perform a DPL while the epidural hematoma is being evacuated

    **c.** After evacuation, obtain CT scan of c-spine, chest, and abdomen if stable

    **d.** Follow serial abdominal exams in the ICU if stable

A DPL should be done in the OR simultaneously with the neurosurgical procedure. This is a relatively noninvasive procedure that is a sensitive indicator of intra-abdominal injury. Aspiration of gross blood would indicate a significant injury requiring ex-lap. The lavage fluid cut-off for injury is 100,000 RBCs per hpf in the setting of blunt abdominal trauma; however, given a normal FAST exam, the absence of gross blood, and hemodynamic stability, many surgeons might choose to observe in the setting of positive lavage. Serial abdominal exam is not reliable in patients who are intubated and sedated. If the DPL is negative, the patient can wait to go for CT scans of the c-spine, chest, and abdomen at a later time. In addition, a portable CXR can be done in the OR to look for evidence of significant thoracic trauma and to check for ETT position.    Answers: 16-a; 17-a; 18-a; 19-c; 20-b

---

## CASE SCENARIO #5

A 22-year-old man is an unrestrained driver in a head-on collision on the freeway. When EMS arrived, the passenger of the car was found dead 30 feet away in a ditch, and the driver of the other car was dead as well. The patient was unresponsive in the driver's compartment of the car. He was moved immediately onto a backboard and intubated. A faint carotid pulse was obtained, and a c-collar was placed. En route, two large-bore IVs were placed, and normal saline initiated. In the ED, the patient is opening his eyes and is noted to move all extremities. He has a large abrasion over his left face with a depressed zygomatic arch. His neck is abraded but without swelling or tracheal shift. His lungs are clear bilaterally with a large contusion over the anterior chest. His vital signs include a pulse of 120, blood pressure 108/66, and oxygen saturation of 96% intubated.

**21.** What should be done next?

    **a.** Extubation, given he is awake and moving all extremities

    **b.** Trauma series in the bay

    **c.** Paralyze and sedate the patient with vecuronium and midazolam

    **d.** Perform a detailed secondary survey

The ABCs have been stabilized with a definitive airway, clear breath sounds with effective ventilation, and a reasonable blood pressure. The patient is waking up, and his neurologic status should be rapidly assessed as part of the secondary survey before he is paralyzed and sedated. The secondary survey reveals reactive pupils bilaterally, no hemotympanum, and a clear oropharynx. As he is looking around, his left eye does not seem to track to the left of the midline. He has crepitus over his left cheek bone, with an obvious depressed zygomatic fracture. He has significant sternal tenderness; but, his heart sounds are normal, and he has no chest wall crepitus. His abdomen is soft and nontender, and his pelvis is stable. He is log rolled and found to have tenderness over his thoracic spine, but no ecchymosis or obvious step-off. His rectal exam reveals normal tone and no blood. He has deformity of his right humerus with intact radial pulses bilaterally. He is able to squeeze your fingers bilaterally to command and can wiggle his toes.

You then decide to sedate him with a propofol drip, given its short duration of action, so that you can turn it off and reassess his neurologic status if needed. A trauma series is done, which shows an intact c-spine, bilateral patchy opacities in both lungs, a narrow mediastinum but indistinct aortic knob on the left. The pelvic x-ray is normal. The FAST exam shows a possible fluid stripe in the hepatorenal space (Morrison's pouch). His blood pressure remains stable.

**22.** What is the most concerning potential injury at this point in the patient's workup?
   **a.** Tripod fracture of the face with lateral rectus entrapment
   **b.** Intra-abdominal injury requiring exploratory laparotomy
   **c.** Aortic rupture
   **d.** Diffuse bilateral pulmonary contusions

At this point, the most concerning features of the patient's workup are the indistinct aortic knob and the fluid stripe on the FAST exam. A small fluid stripe in the setting of hemodynamic stability is not an indication for ex-lap. In contrast, traumatic aortic rupture with a contained hematoma is an indication for immediate operative repair even in the setting of hemodynamic stability.

**23.** What is the best way at this point to approach a potential aortic injury?
   **a.** Angiography given the patient's stability and its superior test characteristics
   **b.** CT scan of the head, c-spine, chest, and abdomen with contrast
   **c.** Transesophageal echocardiography (TEE), given the patient is already intubated
   **d.** Transthoracic echocardiography (TTE)

A CT scan of the head, c-spine, chest, and abdomen with IV contrast is ideal for this patient, whose likely has multiple injuries include a zygomatic fracture, pulmonary contusions, and probably intra-abdominal injuries. Also concerning are potential intracranial injury and c-spine fracture. CT scan will answer all these questions, in addition to providing information about the aorta. The sensitivity and specificity of aortography versus CT scan for aortic injuries is similar. The disadvantage of aortography is that it only gives information about the aorta and nothing else, and it requires the patient to go to the angiography suite—which is not ideal if hemodynamic instability occurs.

As the patient is being wheeled to CT scan, he begins to look more pale. His radial pulse is no longer palpable, and his carotid pulse is faint. The nurse turns around and brings the patient back into the trauma bay. Uncrossmatched type O+ blood is started with pressure bags. His pulse is 134, blood pressure 80/palp, and oxygen saturation 94% on an $FiO_2$ of 1.0. A repeat FAST exam is done to reconfirm no pericardial effusion. The small fluid stripe in Morrison's pouch is unchanged.

**24.** What should be done next?
   **a.** Start norepinephrine for possible cardiac contusion with heart failure
   **b.** Diagnostic peritoneal lavage and transesophageal echocardiography (TEE)
   **c.** Take the patient directly to the OR for exploratory thoracotomy
   **d.** Consult neurosurgery to place an ICP bolt

This patient has become unstable, and the ABCs are readdressed. The question now is: Where is the blood? Another consideration is decreased cardiac output either from a pericardial tamponade (ruled out by repeat FAST exam) or severe cardiac contusion with myocardial stunning. The first consideration, however, should be a bleeding source that can be repaired. At this point, the suspect body cavities that can hide blood have been investigated, including the thorax, abdomen, pelvis, and extremities. It is reasonable to do a DPL to rule out the possibility of gross blood that would prompt immediate ex-lap. The only potential space that has not been evaluated for significant bleeding is the mediastinum and retroperitoneal space. An exploratory thoracotomy is not ideal without a known aortic injury, and a diagnosis should be secured. TEE is the best way to make this diagnosis in a patient who is too unstable to go to CT scan. Ideally, the TEE should be done in the OR so that preparations can be made for the open thoracotomy. Cardiac contusion is also a consideration given the mechanism, and dobutamine or dopamine can be started if the patient is in circulatory shock despite administration of large-volume blood transfusion.

The DPL is done without return of gross blood upon aspiration. The lavage aspirate is sent to the lab for evaluation. The patient is transported to the OR where a TEE is done. An aortic intimal disruption is seen at the distal aortic arch after the take-off of the left subclavian artery, with a large hematoma in the surrounding mediastinum. There is no dissection proximally or distally.

**25.** What is true regarding surgical management of this injury?
   **a.** Open thoracotomy, aortic clamping, removal of injured segment, and reconstruction is standard
   **b.** Open thoracotomy and primary repair of aortic lesion is common
   **c.** Intravascular stenting is well established and considered standard in BAI
   **d.** Open thoracotomy and graft repair is only considered for aortic arch injuries

Surgical repair of a traumatic aortic injury is complicated because of difficult exposure, the need to isolate the injury to control bleeding, and the frequent need for pump-assisted cardiopulmonary bypass. The latter requires the use of heparin, which can be tricky in the setting of multiple traumatic injuries, especially intracerebral bleeding. The basis for repair is open thoracotomy with clamping and direct reconstruction for all injury types, whether ascending, arch, or descending. Once proximal and distal control of the injured aorta is achieved, the injured portion of the aorta is entirely resected. If the injury is small, end-to-end anastomosis can be used to close the defect. Most injuries require replacing the injured segment with a Dacron graft. For patients who make it to the OR alive, which is a minority, the mortality ranges from 50% for ascending injuries to 5% to 25% for descending injuries.

Answers: 21-d; 22-c; 23-b; 24-b; 25-a

## CASE SCENARIO #6

A 20-year-old man is at a fraternity party, drinking heavily, when he decides to jump from a second story balcony into a swimming pool. He jumps into the shallow end and strikes his forehead on the bottom. After a few seconds, he does not resurface, and his friends jump in after him and roll him over onto the concrete poolside. When EMS arrives he is unconscious but breathing, and he has a strong carotid pulse. A c-collar is placed, and he is transferred onto a backboard. En route to the ED, two large-bore IVs are placed. He is also placed on oxygen. In the ED, he is minimally arousable to voice, with incomprehensible mumbling. His pupils are equal and reactive; his oropharynx is clear. He has no anterior neck hematomas, and his breath sounds are equal bilaterally. He does not withdraw his extremities to pain. His vital signs include a pulse of 86, blood pressure 168/96, respiratory rate of 10, and oxygen saturation of 98% on oxygen.

**26.** What is the best method for managing his airway?
   **a.** Maintain the patient on high-flow oxygen by facemask, and obtain CT head and c-spine
   **b.** Orotracheal intubation without medication, given decreased level of consciousness
   **c.** Orotracheal intubation with lidocaine, etomidate, and succinylcholine
   **d.** Orotracheal bronchoscopic intubation with topical anesthetic and a sedative agent

This patient requires intubation based on his GCS of less than 8, given the likelihood for significant head injury and risk for vomiting and aspiration. It also seems evident that he has a high c-spine injury given that he does not withdraw his extremities to pain. Therefore, bronchoscopic intubation is the ideal method. This should be performed by an experienced operator under controlled conditions, with administration of topical anesthetic to the oropharynx (e.g., atomized lidocaine 4% solution or benzocaine spray 20% solution). Once the upper airway is sufficiently anesthetized, a bite block is inserted between the teeth, and a bronchoscope loaded with an ETT is inserted into the oropharynx. A sedative agent should also be administered to minimize gagging and the potential for vomiting. Once the bronchoscope is inserting into the trachea, the ETT is advanced forward. Direct laryngoscopy with in-line stabilization of the c-spine is also a reasonable method if fiberoptics are not available or practical. Pretreatment (e.g., lidocaine), induction (e.g., etomidate), and paralytic (e.g., succinylcholine) agents should be administered as well in order to optimize conditions for intubation.

The patient is intubated over a bronchoscope without complication. Good purple-to-yellow color change is observed with the $CO_2$ capnometer, and his breath sounds are clear bilaterally. On secondary survey, he has no evidence of trauma below the clavicles. Of note he has absent rectal tone on exam and the absence of a bulbocavernosus reflex (contraction of the anus) when his Foley catheter is pulled.

27. What should be the next step in his management?
    a. Hyperventilate to a $PCO_2$ of 25 mm Hg
    b. Obtain trauma series in the bay
    c. Administer solumedrol 30 mg per kg bolus then 5.4 mg per kg drip
    d. Take the patient directly for CT of head and c-spine

In some centers a trauma series would be obtained at this point in the workup. However, it is clear that there may be significant head and c-spine injuries, and manipulation of the patient should be kept to a minimum. The added benefit of a portable chest and pelvic x-ray is minimal at this point. If there is a question of thoracic, abdominal, or pelvic trauma, a CT scan through the chest and abdomen should be obtained, given the patient is hemodynamically stable.

The patient is transported to radiology for a CT scan of his head, c-spine, chest, and abdomen. His head CT shows bilateral frontal contusions with a small amount of subarachnoid blood. The c-spine CT shows a burst fracture of the body of C3 with retropulsion of bone fragments into the spinal canal, with canal narrowing greater than 50%. Neurosurgery is contacted for management of both the head and c-spine injuries.

28. What is true regarding the administration of high-dose steroids in the setting of acute spinal cord injury?
    a. Administration of steroids has a clear benefit in spinal cord injury
    b. High-dose steroids have no documented adverse effects
    c. Two large studies have shown marginal neurological improvement with steroids
    d. High-dose steroids are clearly contraindicated for acute spinal cord injury

The administration of high-dose steroids for acute spinal cord injury has been extremely controversial for the past two decades. An initial randomized controlled trial involving 330 patients in NASCIS I **Bracken et al.** *JAMA* **1984;251:45–52** concluded that there is no improvement in neurologic outcome with administration of high-dose steroids, and there was a trend toward higher mortality, in addition to increased incidence of infection. Two subsequent trials (NASCIS II and III **[Bracken et al.** *N Engl J Med* **1990;332:1405–1411; Bracken et al.** *JAMA* **1997;277:1597–1604]**) concluded that there was a statistically significant improvement in neurologic function at 6 weeks and 6 months if methylprednisolone is administered within 8 hours of injury, with no difference in mortality. The debate remains as to whether the neurologic improvement is clinically significant, or whether it is a statistical phenomenon without clinical relevance. The potential adverse effects of high-dose steroids are increased incidence of infection and sepsis. The current guideline calls for methylprednisolone 30 mg/kg over the first hour followed by 5.4 mg/kg/hr over the next 23 hours if started within 3 hours of injury. If started between 3 and 8 hours after injury, the guideline calls for continuing the steroid drip for 48 hours.

The patient is brought back to the trauma bay, the bed tilted slightly head-up to keep ICP to a minimum. Phenytoin 1000 mg IV over 1 hour is started at the request of the neurosurgeon.

29. Which of the following is true regarding stabilization of this c-spine fracture?
    a. Immediate surgery is clearly indicated to remove fragments from the spinal canal
    b. This particular burst fracture is considered unstable but requires only halo traction
    c. A reasonable treatment plan is halo traction with delayed surgery within 72 hours
    d. Surgery is unnecessary given a complete spinal cord level on exam

The indications for surgery in c-spine injury are variable and controversial, but the majority of injuries are treated without surgery. Absolute indications for immediate surgery are progressive neurological deterioration and facet dislocations with incomplete or no neurologic deficits. Complete neurologic compromise below a certain cord level is not necessarily an indication for immediate surgery given that cord injury is complete. It is a reasonable practice to apply a traction device in an attempt to realign the fragments and decompress the cord. Surgery is indicated at a later time for structurally unstable fractures. Determining stability is in itself complicated and controversial, and it varies for each type of fracture. For burst fractures, instability is considered greater than 50% loss of vertebral body height, greater than 25 degrees angulation, greater than 50% canal compromise, or the presence of neurologic deficits.

Answers: 26-d; 27-d; 28-c; 29-c

## CASE SCENARIO #7

An 18-year-old man is involved in a high-speed motorcycle accident. EMS finds him approximately 50 feet from his motorcycle, with his helmet still intact. He lost consciousness initially but opens his eyes to command and is moving his upper extremities. His helmet is halfway off his head, so EMS removes it and places him in a c-collar and onto a backboard. En route, two large-bore IVs are established, and normal saline started. He has no recollection of the events and denies alcohol or drugs. On arrival to the ED, he is arousable but confused. His airway is intact, anterior neck normal, and he has clear breath sounds bilaterally. His vital signs include a pulse of 138, blood pressure 88/palp, respiratory rate of 24, and oxygen saturation of 94% on high-flow oxygen. Secondary survey reveals a mildly distended and tender abdomen and pelvic instability to rocking. His right thigh is externally rotated. His extremities appear mottled with decreased pulses throughout.

**30.** What is your first priority at this point?
  **a.** Intubate the patient
  **b.** Perform a DPL
  **c.** Perform a FAST exam
  **d.** Call for type O+ blood

Calling for type O+ blood could be considered C of the ABCs. This patient has evidence of circulatory shock that seems likely because of blood loss either into the abdomen or the pelvis. This will likely require a large-volume blood transfusion, and it is wise to call for blood early. His airway is stable for the time being, although that could change as well, especially given that his oxygen saturation is only 94% on high-flow oxygen.

He remains hypotensive after 2 L of normal saline and type O+ blood is transfused. A FAST exam reveals a normal pericardium and no obvious intraperitoneal fluid. The trauma series is completed, which shows a normal lateral c-spine, diffuse haziness of the left lung, a normal mediastinum, and an open book pelvic fracture with 12 mm diastasis, bilateral pubic rami fractures, and right-sided sacroiliac joint disruption. He also has a right hip dislocation. His repeat vital signs include a pulse of 142, blood pressure 84/42, respiratory rate of 28, and oxygen saturation 90% on high-flow oxygen.

**31.** What is the next immediate step?
  **a.** Intubate the patient using lidocaine, etomidate, and succinylcholine
  **b.** Place a left-sided chest tube
  **c.** Wrap the pelvis tightly with a bed sheet
  **d.** Relocate right hip

This is a loaded question because all of these actions need to be done with exception of relocating the hip. Typically a traumatic hip dislocation should be relocated as quickly as possible in order to minimize the risk of avascular necrosis; however, in this case, traction on the femur may displace the pelvic fracture even more and result in further hemorrhage. In this scenario, it is best to go back to the ABCs. Now his respiratory status is deteriorating and he is becoming hypoxic, likely because of hemorrhagic shock.

Intubation will not only allow administration of 100% oxygen directly into the lungs, but it will eliminate the work of breathing and will allow sedation for the painful procedures that are about to ensue.

The patient is intubated without complication with half-dose etomidate 10 mg IV and succinylcholine 120 mg. Simultaneously, the left chest is prepped for a chest tube, which is placed shortly after intubation while the etomidate still has its sedative effect. The chest tube initially drains 400 cc of blood from the left chest, which is collected in an autotransfuser. Now the patient becomes pale and loses his peripheral pulses while maintaining a faint carotid pulse. He is receiving his fourth unit of PRBCs.

**32.** What is the next most important step?
   **a.** Place a left subclavian single-lumen catheter for large-volume blood transfusion
   **b.** Take the patient to the OR for ex-lap and pelvic packing
   **c.** Wrap the pelvis tightly with a bedsheet
   **d.** Insert a Foley catheter

This patient's workup has not yet gotten past the C of the ABCs. Now that A and B have been adequately addressed, this patient needs maximum circulatory resuscitation. Now it is important to wrap the pelvis tightly with a bedsheet to bring together fracture fragments and tamponade bleeding. This, in fact, should be done initially when pelvic instability was detected on exam in the setting of hypotension. As in many trauma cases, things always seem clear in hindsight when the diagnosis is known. Yet there are several tasks to be accomplished in the unstable trauma patient initially; they are all important and must all be prioritized based on the ABCs. In the absence of intraperitoneal blood, there is no indication for an ex-lap.

The pelvis is wrapped tightly with a bedsheet, tied off, and taped down. A left subclavian single-lumen catheter is placed and blood rapidly transfused under pressure. Within 10 minutes, he develops more color in his face, and his carotid pulse is stronger. His blood pressure is now 90/58. A Foley catheter is placed with the return of gross blood.

**33.** What is the next most approporiate step?
   **a.** Perform a DPL to help decide whether to go to OR or to angiography
   **b.** Perform a retrograde cystogram
   **c.** Go directly to angiography for pelvic arterial embolization
   **d.** Obtain CT scans of head, c-spine, chest, and abdomen, including CT cystogram

An ideal study for this patient would be a CT scan of the head, c-spine, chest, abdomen, and pelvis, including CT cystogram. Given that he nearly died in front of you minutes earlier and that he is still hypotensive, it is clear that he is too unstable to spend the next 45 minutes at the CT scanner. It seems apparent that the bleeding is secondary to his pelvic injury. However, gross intraperitoneal blood would persuade you to take the patient to the OR for an ex-lap, despite the fact that the FAST exam was negative.

A DPL is performed without aspiration of gross blood. The patient is then taken to angiography where he is found to have extravasation from a branch of the right internal iliac artery, which is embolized. He is then taken to the OR for placement of an external fixator followed by closed reduction of the right hip dislocation. Retrograde cystography is also performed in the OR and shows extravasation of contrast through the extraperitoneal portion of the bladder.

**34.** Which of the following is appropriate management for his bladder injury?
   **a.** Suprapubic tube for 4 weeks
   **b.** Foley catheter for 14 days, repeat cystography to confirm healing
   **c.** Cystoscopy and embolization of bladder tear
   **d.** Exploratory laparotomy and direct repair

Genitourinary injuries are rarely life threatening and should be a low priority in unstable polytrauma victims. However, if the patient is going to the OR for another reason and gross hematuria exists, a workup must be done in case operative intervention is required. The primary concern is to identify intraperitoneal bladder rupture, where urine extravasates directly into the intraperitoneal space. This is an indication for exploratory laparotomy and direct repair. The more common injury is extraperitoneal bladder rupture with extravasation into pelvic soft tissues. This does not require operative repair and is treated conservatively with a Foley catheter for 14 days and a repeat cystogram to confirm healing.          Answers: 30-d; 31-a; 32-c; 33-a; 34-b

## CASE SCENARIO #8

A 48-year-old female with no past medical history is brought in via EMS after being trapped in a house fire. Per the paramedics, she was in the basement when something exploded, and a fire broke out. She was initially unable to get out and was trapped inside for more than 15 minutes before the firefighters could get to her. She was unconscious when they found her, but she awoke once she was out of the house and was placed on oxygen. Her vital signs initially were a pulse of 122, blood pressure 162/76, and oxygen saturation 99% on high-flow oxygen. The paramedics established two 14-gauge IVs and started normal saline wide open. There was no apparent sign of trauma, but she had erythema and blistering over her face, anterior chest, and arms. She began to have seizure activity en route, and the paramedic administered lorazepam 2 mg IV with resolution. She is screaming in pain on arrival.

On exam, her repeat vital signs are essentially unchanged. She has second-degree burns to her face with singed nose hairs. She is groggy and somewhat confused but able to phonate relatively normally. She has soot in her oropharynx, but there is no obvious airway swelling. Her breath sounds are clear bilaterally with mild expiratory wheezing. On secondary survey she has second-degree burns to the anterior chest and second-degree burns to the anterior arms. She has a circumferential third-degree burn to her right forearm. She has equal and strong radial pulses and can move her fingers and toes on both sides.

**35.** What is the next priority of management in this patient?
   **a.** Rule out intracranial injury with head CT, given LOC and seizure
   **b.** Intubation with RSI technique
   **c.** Perform immediate escharotomy on right forearm
   **d.** Transfer to a hyperbaric oxygen chamber

This patient has evidence of significant inhalation injury with second-degree burns to the face, singed nose hairs, soot in the oropharynx, and wheezing on exam. Airway edema is progressive in the setting of burn injury, and expectant airway management can lead to a situation later in which intubation is impossible. Therefore, intubation should always be performed early if there is potential for inhalation injury, regardless of normal oxygen saturation.

The patient is intubated using RSI technique. Blood is drawn from the IV in the left antecubital space, and the nurse shows you the blood which looks arterial. A blood gas analysis is done that returns with a pH of 7.16, $PaO_2$ 680 mm Hg, $PaCO_2$ 37 mm Hg on 100% $FiO_2$. Her chemistries show a sodium of 139, potassium 3.8, chloride 101, $HCO_3$ 14, BUN 14, Cr 0.8, and glucose 100.

**36.** What do you want to do next?
   **a.** Send an HbCO level
   **b.** Send an HbCO level, serum lactate, and treat empirically with sodium thiosulfate
   **c.** Immediately transfer to hyperbaric oxygen chamber
   **d.** Get a STAT head CT

While it is not unreasonable to get a head CT given the question of the explosion, the patient has no signs of trauma and has a potential reason for seizure given her acidosis and high venous oxygen tension. This is consistent with cyanide poisoning, because cyanide inhibits mitochondrial oxidative phosphorylation, thus preventing tissue extraction of oxygen. Oxygen saturation will be 100%. This also results in anaerobic metabolism and a profound metabolic acidosis. The patient should be treated empirically with sodium thiosulfate without waiting for a cyanide level, which could take days. Sodium nitrite, which induces methemoglobinemia, is also standard treatment for cyanide poisoning but is contraindicated in the setting of potential CO poisoning because methemoglobinemia further limits the oxygen-carrying capacity of hemoglobin that is already present with carboxyhemoglobin. Hyperbaric oxygen should also be considered given the likelihood of coexisting CO poisoning.

You estimate that she weights 70 kg and has a 25% total body surface area with second- and third-degree burns (9% are third degree).

**37.** Which of the following describes the proper management of this patient's burns?
  **a.** 7 L NS over 24 hours, debridement, and sterile dressing of burns
  **b.** 7 L NS or LR over 8 hours, debridement, and prophylactic broad-spectrum antibiotics
  **c.** 14 L NS over 24 hours, prophylactic antibiotics, and leave blisters intact
  **d.** 14 L NS over 16 hours, debridement, and early skin grafting in OR the next morning

The Parkland formula calls for 4 mL × body weight (kg) × % BSA of IV fluid (either LR or NS) over 24 hours, with the first half given in the first 8 hours and the remainder given over the next 16 hours. In practice, fluids are generally titrated to urine output, with the goal of 0.5 to 1.0 cc/kg/hr for an adult burn patient. Additionally, her burns should be debrided and dressed with sterile gauze. Typically, topical antibacterial agents are applied to the skin. Most centers use silver sulfadiazine (Silvadene) to areas with average blood flow (e.g., arms, chest, back, and legs) and mafenide (Sulfamylon) to areas of low blood flow (e.g., ears, distal extremities), and triple antibiotic ointment to areas of high blood flow (e.g., face). Oral or intravenous antibiotics are not indicated in acute burns. Skin grafting will eventually be necessary in the area of the third-degree burn, but this is not done in the acute phase of injury.

Re-examination of the right arm reveals a mildly diminished radial pulse and discoloration. She appears to wince when you passively flex and extend her hand. The circumferential burn extends from her wrist to her elbow, with noncircumferential burns extending all the way to her shoulder.

**38.** What should you do now?
  **a.** Check compartment pressures in her forearm
  **b.** Elevate her arm and reassess in 2 to 3 hours
  **c.** Perform an escharotomy of the forearm
  **d.** Reduce crystalloid administration as she is developing capillary leak edema

This patient has signs of compartment syndrome and needs emergent escharotomy. This entails making longitudinal incisions, usually with a Bovey, along the medial and lateral aspects of the forearm from the wrist up to the elbow. The incisions should only go as deep as the subcutaneous adipose tissue and not into the muscle beds. This will allow the hard, charred dermis to expand, thus releasing the pressure from subcutaneous edema. Hand elevation decreases arterial perfusion pressure and may actually be counterproductive. There is no need to check compartment pressures in the setting of a circumferential third-degree burn, and escharotomy is indicated even without evidence of distal ischemia because of the high incidence of compartment syndrome. Continued crystalloid resuscitation is important to provide adequate intravascular volume and prevent tissue ischemia in the salvageable zone of stasis.

Her labs reveal an HbCO level of 15% and methemoglobin level less than 5%. The lactate level is 11 mmol/L. Her repeat vital signs are a pulse of 102, blood pressure 122/56, and oxygen saturation 99% on an $FiO_2$ of 1.0.

**39.** What is the next step?
  **a.** Arrange for hyperbaric oxygen treatment if available
  **b.** Continue mechanical ventilation, and admit to the burn unit
  **c.** Transfuse PRBCs 2 units, admit to burn unit, and arrange for delayed hyperbaric treatment
  **d.** Administer bicarbonate 2 amps IV for lactic acidosis

It has been shown that acute hyperbaric oxygen treatment can be effective in reducing long-term neuropsychiatric sequelae of CO poisoning. The decision of whether to undergo treatment is more based on clinical signs rather than a specific carboxyhemoglobin level. Typically, a level of 15% would cause only a slight headache, nausea, and possibly some difficulty breathing. The serum level however is not always indicative of tissue levels. Patients with neurologic symptoms (e.g., altered mental status, syncope, or seizure) should undergo hyperbaric oxygen therapy if available. Otherwise, continued mechanical ventilation with $FiO_2$ of 100% and admission to a burn unit is reasonable.

Answers: 35-b; 36-b; 37-a; 38-c; 39-a

## CASE SCENARIO #9

EMS calls ahead to the ED to inform that they are bringing in a 20-year-old male with a single gunshot wound (GSW) to the abdomen. The entrance wound is just inferior and lateral to the umbilicus on the right side. The initial vital signs on EMS arrival are a pulse of 138, blood pressure 90/46, and oxygen saturation of 99% on high-flow oxygen via a nonrebreather facemask. You notify the OR of a potential emergent case. On arrival, EMS personnel inform you that his abdomen is significantly more tense than it was 15 minutes ago when they arrived at the scene. The patient had already received 1,500 cc NS via a 14-gauge antecubital IV.

Repeat vitals on arrival in the bay are a pulse of 140, blood pressure 84/32, respiratory rate of 6, and oxygen saturation of 98% on high-flow oxygen. He does not respond to voice but groans occasionally. His airway and breathing are intact, and you notice a single gunshot wound to the right abdomen. He has palpable femoral pulses, and you notice spontaneous movement in both legs. The trauma cooler is in the ED with 4 units of type O+ blood.

**40.** What is your first priority?
  **a.** Start type O+ blood, and transfer the patient directly to the OR for ex-lap
  **b.** Administer naloxone (Narcan) 2 mg IV for suspected concurrent heroin use
  **c.** Perform FAST exam
  **d.** Intubate the patient while starting type O+ blood

This patient has obvious signs of severe hypovolemic shock that cannot be explained by heroin use alone (e.g., tachycardia, hypotension despite 1,500 cc NS). Furthermore, his GCS is 7 (E1, V2, M4), and his respiratory effort is poor. Rather than administering Narcan and potentially escalating the situation, it is better at this point to simply intubate the patient and start blood transfusion. Based on instability, he needs to go directly to the OR after an airway is secured. The FAST exam does not change the management for a patient with penetrating abdominal trauma and unstable vital signs or peritonitis.

You intubate him on the first pass using half-dose etomidate 10 mg IV and succinylcholine 160 mg. There is good color change on the $CO_2$ detector. He remains hypotensive after intubation. You roll the patient to check for an exit wound or other injury, but none is found. The remainder of his exam is normal except for a firm abdomen and decreased femoral pulse on the right. He has been in the bay for 5 minutes and is now ready to go to the OR; however, now his blood pressure is unobtainable, and his carotid pulse is absent despite a continued sinus tachycardia on the monitor.

**41.** What should you do next?
  **a.** Place a single-lumen central venous catheter
  **b.** Perform an ED thoracotomy
  **c.** Perform CPR, and go directly to the OR
  **d.** Stop resuscitation

The patient has lost his vital signs and pulses with a rhythm on the monitor, known as pulseless electrical activity, or PEA arrest. Given the location of his GSW and decreased femoral pulse, he likely has an arterial injury, either aortic or common iliac artery. While the CPR should be initiated and a rapid infuser should be used to administer blood, the patient is now "newly dead" and may not survive the time it takes to get to the OR. His best chance for neurologically intact survival is to perform an ED thoracotomy. The literature is quite clear that patients with a GSW to the abdomen who lose vital signs have a reasonable survival rate (10% to 20%) if ED thoracotomy is promptly performed.

**42.** What is the first action on gaining access to the chest?
  **a.** Pericardiotomy
  **b.** Cross-clamp the descending aorta
  **c.** Place a central line directly in the right atrium
  **d.** Extend the incision in a "clamshell" fashion since the wound is on the right

In this case, the problem leading to the arrest is most likely rapid arterial blood loss. Therefore, the goal of thoracotomy is to halt blood flow below the diaphragm until surgical control of the damaged vessel can be obtained. This can be accomplished by cross-clamping the aorta. Pericardiotomy is not necessary in this case unless pericardial blood was noted on direct inspection. CPR should be started while the chest is prepped, which should take less than 5 seconds. It should take less than 30 seconds to get into the chest, at which time direct cardiac massage should be initiated. A clamshell thoracotomy is generally only needed for right-sided chest wounds.

While you are performing the thoracotomy, a third physician arrives and asks what else needs to be done.

**43.** What do you say?
   **a.** Place a single-lumen right subclavian central line
   **b.** Place a single-lumen femoral central line since it will be easier to access the groin
   **c.** Place a right-sided chest tube
   **d.** Place an arterial line for blood pressure monitoring

The next thing this patient needs is large-bore central venous access above the diaphragm, which can be accomplished with a single-lumen right subclavian catheter. In a code situation, subclavian or internal jugular access is always better than femoral access because of proximity to the heart. It is especially true in this case, given the potential vascular injury and the risk of administering crystalloid and blood through a venous tear directly into the retroperitoneal space. A right-sided chest tube can be placed, especially if there is concern that the bullet may have tracked into the right chest and caused a hemothorax or pneumothorax; however, that is unlikely in this case, and no time should be wasted to get this patient to the OR.

A thoracotomy is performed and the aorta cross-clamped. A right subclavian central venous catheter is placed concurrently, through which he rapidly receives 2 more liters of type O+ blood. His heart begins to pump more vigorously, and a carotid pulse is palpable. His blood pressure is now 84/40 with a heart rate of 144.

**44.** What should you do now?
   **a.** Take the patient directly to the OR for ex-lap
   **b.** Obtain a pelvic and abdominal x-ray to look for the location of the bullet
   **c.** Get a CXR for confirmation of ETT and central line position
   **d.** Administer vasopressors for continued hypotension

Now that you have revived the patient, he needs to go directly to the OR for an ex-lap and repair of his injuries. The only goal is to identify the source of abdominal or pelvic bleeding and gain proximal control so that the aortic cross-clamp can be released to avoid further ischemia below the diaphragm. The location of the bullet is immaterial at this point and will not alter operative management. Vasopressors are of no utility in hemorrhagic shock.

The patient is taken to the OR and found to have a right common iliac artery disruption, which is repaired with a graft. The iliac vein was partially damaged as well and required repair. There was approximately 3 L of blood in his abdomen. Additionally, a piece of small bowel was perforated and had to be resected. The patient remained intubated and was transferred to the SICU postoperatively.

Answers: 40-d; 41-b; 42-b; 43-a; 44-a

## CASE SCENARIO #10

You receive a radio call from EMS that they are bringing in a pedestrian who was struck by a car traveling approximately 25 mph. You are in a Level IV trauma center, and the nearest Level I center is an hour by helicopter flight. As the ED physician, you are the only doctor in house, as it is a Saturday afternoon and the general surgeon on call lives approximately 45 minutes away. There is no orthopedist on call. The basic EMTs report that the patient is a 44-year-old female with no significant medical problems. Her vital signs are a pulse of 122, blood pressure 96/54, and oxygen saturation 94% on high-flow oxygen via a nonrebreather facemask. She initially lost consciousness but now is awake and alert. She complains of abdominal pain, and she has an obvious deformity of her left lower leg with a palpable DP. Her right thigh is swollen and painful to touch, and her right DP pulse is absent. They report an ETA of 5 minutes.

**45.** What do you want to do with the 5 minute lead time?
   **a.** Alert air medical services, the general surgeon, and blood bank; prepare the trauma bay
   **b.** Call a "trauma consult" to discuss the case with the trauma surgeon at the Level I center
   **c.** Finish caring for the patient with an ankle sprain as you will likely be tied up for a while
   **d.** "Divert" the EMTs to a Level III center that is 40 minutes by ambulance

From the report, the patient likely has multisystem trauma and the potential for instability. In a situation like this, where you are caring for a sick patient who clearly will exceed your center's resources, it is important to alert necessary help early. It will take the helicopter service a while to get to your center, and thus alerting them sooner rather than later is crucial. Alerting the surgeon is also important in case the patient needs operative stabilization before transport. Preparing the trauma bay for intubation and chest tubes is important as rapid action may be required. Since you are the only available physician, you will be doing all procedures and should have the equipment ready so no time is wasted once she arrives. It is not safe to have EMS bypass your center and transport an unstable patient to another center.

The patient arrives in the bay with a pulse of 124, blood pressure 90/42, respiratory rate of 28, and oxygen saturation of 90% on high-flow oxygen. She is alert but in clear respiratory distress and is unable to speak more than a few words at a time. She has no obvious airway trauma or blood in her mouth. Her trachea is midline. She has subcutaneous air over the right chest and has decreased breath sounds on the right as well. Her femoral pulses are palpable bilaterally. She was transported by BLS ambulance and thus has no IV. You have two nurses working with you.

**46.** In what order do you wish to proceed?
   **a.** Ask a nurse to place a 14-gauge IV while you simultaneously place a chest tube
   **b.** Ask a nurse to place a 14-gauge IV, and then you intubate the patient
   **c.** Proceed with the secondary survey while a nurse places a 14-gauge IV
   **d.** Place a right subclavian central line for rapid administration of PRBCs

Now, more then ever, knowing the ABCs is crucial. This patient does not have an airway issue, so A is fine, and you can proceed to B. She does have a breathing issue, with evidence of a pneumothorax causing respiratory distress. She needs a chest tube immediately, and this should not be delayed even for intubation. The nurse should concurrently gain IV access and administer a normal saline bolus.

Within 30 seconds, you create an opening in the pleura and get a rush of air in return. Her breathing becomes less labored, and her oxygen saturation drifts slowly up to 95%. The nurse has established an IV, has started normal saline wide open, and is working on getting a second IV placed. Repeat vital signs include a pulse of 110, blood pressure 98/42, respiratory rate of 20, and oxygen saturation of 98% on a nonrebreather facemask. She is alert and complains mostly of leg pain. You proceed with the secondary survey that reveals a small hematoma over her frontal bone, a tender left upper quadrant with guarding, a tense right thigh with deformity at the level of the midfemur, absent right DP pulse, and a left lower leg deformity with a diminished left DP pulse. Her pelvis is stable and nontender. She also has a large laceration over her right palm with lacerated underlying tendons. She is able to move all extremities to command.

**47.** What is your next task?
   **a.** Obtain trauma series, and prepare patient for CT scan
   **b.** Intubate the patient to sedate for painful procedures
   **c.** Place right leg in traction after administering fentanyl 100 µg
   **d.** Call the receiving trauma center to give pass off

This patient is now stable, at least temporarily, from the point of airway, breathing, and circulation. Now attention can be turned to limb-threatening orthopedic injuries. Given the thigh deformity and significant swelling, it is likely that a midshaft femur fracture with resulting hemorrhage may be the cause of her hypovolemic shock, as the thigh can hold up to 1.5 L of blood. This fracture should be reduced without delay because of distal neurovascular compromise. Manipulation of the leg will be painful, and fentanyl is an ideal analgesic because of its hemodynamic stability, although deleterious blunting of physiologic sympathetic tone must be considered in the setting of hemorrhagic shock.

You place her in traction after administering fentanyl 100 μg, and she has significant relief of her pain. Repeat vital signs are a pulse of 118, blood pressure 96/50, respiratory rate of 22, and oxygen saturation of 96%. You call the receiving trauma center, and air medical transport is still 30 minutes away. You obtain CT scans of her head, c-spine, chest, abdomen, and pelvis. The images are downloaded onto a CD for transport with the patient. The CT scans show subcutaneous air in the chest wall, right-sided rib fractures, a well-placed chest tube, fully expanded right lung, a large right pulmonary contusion, a small (< 10%) left pneumothorax with left-sided contusions, and a grade III splenic laceration with about 200 cc of free fluid in the left paracolic gutter. Plain films show a midshaft tibia and fibula fracture on the left and a now reduced midshaft femur fracture on the right.

The patient's vital signs are now a pulse of 122, blood pressure 108/54, respiratory rate of 28, and oxygen saturation 94% on high-flow oxygen. She is receiving her second unit of PRBCs. On exam, you note she has pain with passive motion of her ankle and toes on the left. Her left calf is getting progressively more swollen.

**48.** What injury is most likely to result in instability during the helicopter trip?
   **a.** Splenic laceration
   **b.** Pulmonary contusions
   **c.** Left-sided pneumothorax
   **d.** Left lower extremity fracture

This patient is again becoming more tachypneic and hypoxic, likely a result of the large pulmonary contusions. While the small pneumothorax and splenic laceration are also potential sources of instability, the likelihood of her respiratory status worsening as a result of pulmonary contusions is almost assured. She needs to be intubated prior to transport and, in addition, receive a left-sided chest tube to prevent development of a tension pneumothorax with mechanical ventilation. Both of these procedures before transport will minimize the risk of decompensation during flight.

You intubate her with good color change on $CO_2$ detector and breath sounds bilaterally. You place an NG tube and a left-sided chest tube. The helicopter has not arrived yet.

**49.** What else should be done prior to transport?
   **a.** Transport the patient with no further intervention
   **b.** Ask the general surgeon to travel with the patient in the helicopter
   **c.** Check compartment pressures in left leg prior to transport
   **d.** Take the patient to the OR for a splenectomy

This patient has signs of developing compartment syndrome in the left lower extremity, and re-evaluation will not be for at least another 1 to 2 hours. By checking compartment pressures, you can relay critical information to the Level I center. She does not have an indication for emergent splenectomy, as the CT did not show a large amount of intra-abdominal blood, and she has only received 2 units of PRBCs so far. Air ambulance crews are usually quite comfortable with critical patients, so sending a physician with this patient will not provide additional benefit.

The anterior compartment pressure is 52 mm Hg; the general surgeon quickly performs a fasciotomy in the trauma bay. The air ambulance crew arrives and transports the patient to the Level I center. When you call for follow up a few days later, the trauma surgeon tells you that she had her femur and tibia-fibula fractures repaired by orthopedics and that her splenic laceration was managed nonoperatively. He congratulates you on your excellent management of such a complicated case.

Answers: 45-a; 46-a 47-c; 48-b; 49-c

# Index

*Note:* Page numbers followed by b indicate boxed material; those followed by f indicate figures; those followed by t indicate tables.